Eating Disorders in Boys and Men

Jason M. Nagata • Tiffany A. Brown
Stuart B. Murray • Jason M. Lavender
Editors

Eating Disorders in Boys and Men

Springer

Editors
Jason M. Nagata
Division of Adolescent and Young Adult Medicine, Department of Pediatrics
University of California, San Francisco
San Francisco, CA
USA

Stuart B. Murray
Department of Psychiatry and Behavioral Sciences
USC Keck School of Medicine, University of Southern California
Los Angeles, CA
USA

Tiffany A. Brown
Department of Psychiatry
University of California, San Diego
San Diego, CA
USA

Jason M. Lavender
Department of Medicine
Military Cardiovascular Outcomes Research (MiCOR) Program, Uniformed Services University of the Health Sciences
The Metis Foundation
Bethesda, MD
USA

ISBN 978-3-030-67126-6 ISBN 978-3-030-67127-3 (eBook)
https://doi.org/10.1007/978-3-030-67127-3

This Springer imprint is published by the registered company Springer Nature Switzerland AG
The registered company address is: Gewerbestrasse 11, 6330 Cham, Switzerland

Foreword

Among the "Nine Truths about Eating Disorders," Truth #5 states, "Eating disorders affect people of all genders, ages, races, ethnicities, body shapes and weights, sexual orientations, and socioeconomic statuses" [1]. Despite this fact, the notion that eating disorders are a "female problem" has created a systemic gap in the recognition, understanding, prevention, and treatment of eating disorders in boys and men. This gap is widened by the decreased likelihood of boys and men seeking treatment for their eating disorders or even volunteering for research on eating disorders. The resulting reliance on information based on female patients and participants contributes to a vicious cycle in which eating disorders have been defined, assessed, and treated based on their clinical presentation in girls and women, and then these same definitions, assessments, and interventions exclude boys and men. *Eating Disorders in Boys and Men* represents a must-read text for every clinician, researcher, and student to break this vicious cycle by offering the most up-to-date clinical information describing clinical presentation, assessment and diagnosis, medical considerations, prevention, treatment, and the intersection of gender with race, ethnicity, culture, sexual orientation, athletics, social media, and age.

My own interest in this topic dates back to a 1998 article I authored titled "Disordered eating in adolescent males from a school-based sample" [2]. In the opening paragraph of this article, I stated:

> Published research of eating disorders in males is sparse compared to the estimated proportions of males with eating disorders. For example, Carlat and Camargo (1991) reported that males comprise 10–15% of all subjects diagnosed with bulimia nervosa (BN); however, far less than 10% of BN studies screened by Carlat and Camargo (1991) included data or hypotheses concerning males. Similarly, a recent report concluded that "lack of familiarity with AN [anorexia nervosa] in males leads to a delay in evaluation, diagnosis, and referral," and increased risk for medical complications (Siegel, Hardoff, Golden, & Shenker, 1995:452). Early estimates indicate that 40% of binge-eating disorder (BED) occurs in males (Spitzer et al., 1992, 1993), but similar tendencies to exclude male subjects from empirical investigations have occurred (e.g., Arnow, Kenardy, & Agras, 1992; deZwaan, Nutzinger, & Schoenbeck, 1993; Berkowitz, Stunkard, & Stallings, 1993). Given these patterns, determining the development of AN, BN, and BED in males may be hindered if findings for females do not generalize to males.

The article proceeded to provide correlational analyses of eating pathology in adolescent boys because that represented a significant contribution to the literature at that time! In the two decades since this paper was published, the field has made significant advances in determining the prevalence of eating disorders in boys and men from representative population-based studies, identifying prospective risk factors for the development and maintenance of eating disorders in boys and men from adolescence to late mid-life in longitudinal studies, and examining interventions that reduce eating pathology in men using randomized controlled trials. However, the value of this information depends entirely upon making it accessible outside academic and medical journals.

The editors of this essential text bring a wealth of expertise based on their ground-breaking contributions to identifying medical complications of eating disorders in adolescent boys (Dr. Nagata), developing and evaluating prevention and treatment of eating disorders in late adolescent and young adult men (Dr. Brown), identifying clinical presentations more prevalent in boys and men (Dr. Murray), and contributing to more refined assessments tailored to these clinical presentations (Dr. Lavender). Prior to *Eating Disorders in Boys and Men*, each editor published scientific findings in leading academic and medical journals and shared their insights at national and international conferences. However, these methods of dissemination reach a small fraction of those who need the information most. Collecting the expertise of the top researchers and clinicians for each chapter provides readers with an accessible resource for all of their questions.

Pamela K. Keel, PhD
Department of Psychology
Florida State University
Tallahassee, FL, USA

References

1. https://www.aedweb.org/resources/online-library/publications/nine-truths
2. Keel PK, Klump KL, Leon GR, Fulkerson JA. Disordered eating in adolescent males from a school-based sample. Int J Eating Disord. 1998;23:125–32.

Preface

The eating disorders field developed primarily through a female-centric lens. Although there has been progress in recognizing the diversity of individuals who are affected by eating disorders, certain stereotypes remain that may perpetuate stigma in particular groups. The goal of this book is to highlight boys and men, a population that has been historically underrecognized and underserved with regard to eating disorders research and clinical care. The first section offers a background and overview of eating disorders and body image in boys and men. The second section focuses on the diagnosis and assessment of eating disorders and related symptoms. The third section addresses medical considerations, nutrition, and appearance/performance-enhancing substance use. The fourth section focuses on prevention and treatment. The final section is devoted to addressing specific populations and sociocultural considerations. We conclude with a brief review of the core points raised within each section, as well as a discussion of future directions in this area.

We wish to acknowledge at the outset that, although this book is focused on boys and men, many of the empirical findings and clinical topics may have some degree of relevance across individuals with other gender identities. We also recognize that the majority of existing knowledge in this area derives from research on samples of predominantly cisgender boys and men. We further note that the opinions and assertions expressed herein are those of the editors or contributing authors, and do not necessarily reflect the official policy or position of any academic or governmental institutions or agencies with which the editors or authors are affiliated.

In sum, our goal for this book is to provide a comprehensive and empirically informed synthesis of the most up-to-date information on important topics relevant to research and clinical care with boys and men with eating disorders.

San Francisco, CA, USA — Jason M. Nagata
San Diego, CA, USA — Tiffany A. Brown
Los Angeles, CA, USA — Stuart B. Murray
Bethesda, MD, USA — Jason M. Lavender

Acknowledgments

We would like to thank each of the chapter authors for their thoughtful contributions. We appreciate the support of the editorial office at Springer, particularly Eugenia Judson and Miranda Finch. We also thank Samuel Benabou for editorial assistance. This book is dedicated to anyone who has experienced an eating disorder.

To my husband, Ryan,
and to my parents, Ronnie and Ada
-Jason M. Nagata

To my family and friends,
for their support and encouragement.
-Tiffany A. Brown

To Emilíana and Lucíana,
my inspiration.
-Stuart B. Murray

To my family and friends,
for their unwavering support.
-Jason M. Lavender

Contents

Part I Overview and Perspectives

1 **A Historical Overview of Eating Disorders in Males** 3
Stuart B. Murray

2 **Models of Body Image for Boys and Men** 7
Tracy L. Tylka

3 **Muscularity-Oriented Disordered Eating in Boys and Men** 21
Mitchell L. Cunningham, Jason M. Nagata, and Stuart B. Murray

4 **Epidemiology of Eating Disorders in Boys and Men** 37
Nora Trompeter, Kay Bussey, and Deborah Mitchison

Part II Assessment and Diagnosis

5 **Assessing and Diagnosing Eating Disorders in Boys and Men: An Overview** 55
Brittany K. Bohrer and Joseph M. Donahue

6 **Avoidant/Restrictive Food Intake Disorder** 67
Jessie E. Menzel and Tana Luo

7 **Using Eating Disorder and Body Image Assessment Questionnaires with Boys/Men** 83
Jason M. Lavender

8 **Muscle Dysmorphia** 103
William Grunewald and Aaron J. Blashill

Part III Medical and Substances

9 **Medical Complications of Eating Disorders in Boys and Men** 119
Jason M. Nagata, Kyle T. Ganson, and Neville H. Golden

10 Medical Management of Eating Disorders in Boys and Men: Current Clinical Guidance and Evidence Gaps 127
Kyle T. Ganson, Neville H. Golden, and Jason M. Nagata

11 Nutritional Considerations for Boys and Men with Eating Disorders 137
Melissa Whitelaw and Jason M. Nagata

12 Appearance- and Performance-Enhancing Substances Including Anabolic-Androgenic Steroids Among Boys and Men 149
Mitchell L. Cunningham and Scott Griffiths

Part IV Prevention and Treatment

13 Prevention of Eating Disorders in Boys and Men 169
Marie Nebel-Schwalm and Tiffany A. Brown

14 Psychotherapy with Men with Eating Disorders: The Influence of Gender Socialization and Masculine Gender Norms on Engagement and Treatment 197
Douglas W. Bunnell

Part V Specific Populations and Social Cultural Considerations

15 Racial and Ethnic Considerations in the United States. 217
Kimberly Yu and Marisol Perez

16 Cross-Cultural Considerations in Latin American Boys and Men . . 229
Emilio J. Compte and Eva Trujillo

17 Eating Disorders and Related Symptomatology in Sexual Minority Men and Boys 253
Alexandra D. Convertino, Christopher A. Albright, and Aaron J. Blashill

18 Eating Disorders Among Transgender and Gender Non-binary People 265
Allegra R. Gordon, L. B. Moore, and Carly Guss

19 Eating Disorders in Boys and Men: Considerations in Sport and Exercise. 283
Eva Pila and Sasha Gorrell

20 Social Media and Eating and Body Image Concerns Among Men and Boys. 307
Alexandra Rhodes Lonergan, Deborah Mitchison, Kay Bussey, and Jasmine Fardouly

21 Eating Disorders and Body Image Across the Lifespan: A Focus on Boys and Men in Midlife and Beyond 317
Tiffany A. Brown and Jason M. Lavender

22 Eating Disorders in Boys and Men: Conclusions and Future Research Directions 335
Jason M. Nagata, Tiffany A. Brown, Stuart B. Murray, and Jason M. Lavender

Index 341

Contributors

Christopher A. Albright San Diego State University/University of California San Diego Joint Doctoral Program in Clinical Psychology, San Diego, CA, USA

Aaron J. Blashill, PhD Department of Psychology, San Diego State University, San Diego, CA, USA

Department of Psychology, San Diego State University/University of California San Diego Joint Doctoral Program in Clinical Psychology, San Diego, CA, USA

Brittany K. Bohrer Department of Psychiatry, UC San Diego Health Eating Disorders Center for Treatment and Research, San Diego, CA, USA

Tiffany A. Brown Department of Psychiatry, University of California, San Diego, San Diego, CA, USA

San Diego State University Research Foundation, San Diego, CA, USA

Douglas W. Bunnell Private Practice, Westport, CT, USA

Kay Bussey Centre for Emotional Health, Department of Psychology, Macquarie University, Sydney, NSW, Australia

Emilio J. Compte Research Department, Comenzar de Nuevo Treatment Center, Monterrey, Nuevo León, Mexico

School of Psychology, Universidad Adolfo Ibáñez, Peñalolén Santiago, Chile

Alexandra D. Convertino San Diego State University/University of California San Diego Joint Doctoral Program in Clinical Psychology, San Diego, CA, USA

Mitchell L. Cunningham School of Psychology, The University of Sydney, Sydney, NSW, Australia

Joseph M. Donahue Department of Psychiatry, UC San Diego Health Eating Disorders Center for Treatment and Research, San Diego, CA, USA

Jasmine Fardouly Centre for Emotional Health, Department of Psychology, Macquarie University, Sydney, NSW, Australia

Kyle T. Ganson Factor-Inwentash Faculty of Social Work, University of Toronto, Toronto, ON, Canada

School of Social Work, Simmons University, Boston, MA, USA

Neville H. Golden Department of Pediatrics, Stanford University School of Medicine, Stanford, CA, USA

Allegra R. Gordon Department of Community Health Sciences, Boston University School of Public Health, Boston, MA, USA

Sasha Gorrell Department of Psychiatry, Weill Institute for Neurosciences, University of California San Francisco, San Francisco, CA, USA

Scott Griffiths School of Psychological Sciences, The University of Melbourne, Melbourne, VIC, Australia

William Grunewald, MA Department of Psychology, San Diego State University, San Diego, CA, USA

Carly Guss Division of Adolescent/Young Adult Medicine, Boston Children's Hospital and Department of Pediatrics, Harvard Medical School, Boston, MA, USA

Jason M. Lavender Department of Medicine, Military Cardiovascular Outcomes Research (MiCOR) Program, Uniformed Services University of the Health Sciences, Bethesda, MD, USA

The Metis Foundation, San Antonio, TX, USA

Alexandra Rhodes Lonergan Centre for Emotional Health, Department of Psychology, Macquarie University, Sydney, NSW, Australia

Tana Luo, PhD Department of Psychiatry, University of California, San Diego, San Diego, CA, USA

Jessie E. Menzel, PhD Department of Psychiatry, University of California, San Diego, San Diego, CA, USA

Deborah Mitchison Centre for Emotional Health, Department of Psychology, Macquarie University, Sydney, NSW, Australia

Translational Health Research Institute, School of Medicine, Western Sydney University, Sydney, NSW, Australia

L. B. Moore Framingham LGBTQ+ Adolescent Social Services (Framingham GLASS), Justice Resource Institute, Health Division, Framingham, MA, USA

Stuart B. Murray Department of Psychiatry and Behavioral Sciences, USC Keck School of Medicine, University of Southern California, Los Angeles, CA, USA

Jason M. Nagata Division of Adolescent and Young Adult Medicine, Department of Pediatrics, University of California, San Francisco, San Francisco, CA, USA

Marie Nebel-Schwalm Illinois Wesleyan University, Department of Psychology, Bloomington, IL, USA

Marisol Perez Department of Psychology, Arizona State University, Tempe, AZ, USA

Eva Pila School of Kinesiology, Western University, London, ON, Canada

Nora Trompeter Centre for Emotional Health, Department of Psychology, Macquarie University, Sydney, NSW, Australia

Eva Trujillo Psychiatry Department, Comenzar de Nuevo Treatment Center, Monterrey, Nuevo León, Mexico

Tracy L. Tylka Department of Psychology, The Ohio State University, Columbus, OH, USA

Melissa Whitelaw Department of Adolescent Medicine, Department of Nutrition and Food Services, The Royal Children's Hospital, Melbourne, VIC, Australia

Kimberly Yu Department of Psychology, Arizona State University, Tempe, AZ, USA

Part I
Overview and Perspectives

Chapter 1
A Historical Overview of Eating Disorders in Males

Stuart B. Murray

Learning Objectives
1. Overview the history of eating disorders in males.
2. Evaluate how males were excluded from eating disorder research.
3. Synthesize how this has impacted the recognition of eating disorders in males.

Key Points
- Males were reported among the first reported cases of eating disorders, although, subsequently, males were excluded from eating disorder research.
- It has been thought that eating disorders in males are rare, although this may have been due to the female-centricity of research examining EDs.
- The increasing recognition of EDs in males suggest physicians will likely see an upsurge in male presentations of EDs.

Eating disorders (EDs) are among the most pernicious of psychiatric disorders, characterized by elevated rates of mortality, suicidality, multi-systemic medical complexities, and an often chronic and relapsing illness course which may extend over several decades [1–4]. Phenomenologically, EDs have historically been considered one of the most gendered of psychiatric disorders, demonstrating a striking sexual dimorphism. Yet, while many associate the term "eating disorder" with stereotypes of affluent, middle-class, young White females, EDs have been reported in male patients for as long as they have been reported in female patients.

In fact, the very first case description of the cluster of symptoms that would later be termed anorexia nervosa included a careful description of one female patient and one adolescent male patient [5]. Similarly, the simultaneous work of Gull [6] and Lasegue [7], which was critical in identifying the phenotype they later termed

S. B. Murray (✉)
Department of Psychiatry & Behavioral Sciences, USC Keck School of Medicine, University of Southern California, Los Angeles, CA, USA
e-mail: stuartmu@usc.edu

J. M. Nagata et al. (eds.), *Eating Disorders in Boys and Men*,
https://doi.org/10.1007/978-3-030-67127-3_1

anorexia nervosa, described the characteristics and sequelae of this disorder in male patients. Further reflecting the centrality of males in this seminal literature relating to EDs, even the term anorexia *nervosa* itself was coined to underscore the presence of male patients with this syndrome. An alternatively considered moniker at the time, anorexia *hysterica*, was ruled out due to the commonly held belief at the time that males could not be hysterical [8].

Beyond these seminal works, however, the history of EDs is characterized by a striking absence of male patients, and it wasn't until almost 300 years after the work of Morton [5] and 100 years after the simultaneous work of Gull [6] and Lasegue [7] that the presence of EDs in males was systematically studied by leading authorities in the field [9, 10]. Crucially, the misnomer that EDs did not afflict males prevailed for large parts of the twentieth century, during a period of rapid evolution for the field of EDs in which the first (i) diagnostic framework, (ii) treatment modalities, and (iii) measures of symptom profiles were developed [11]. As such, all critically important developments relating to diagnostic criteria were predicated on clinical trials exclusively comprising female patients, which inherently excluded male patients. The lack of utility of these diagnostic criteria in accounting for male presentations was broadly misconstrued as evidence that males cannot be afflicted by EDs.

This is perhaps best exemplified by the argument that, owing to the absence of a direct endocrine equivalent of the amenorrhea criterion of anorexia nervosa, which for many decades was a key diagnostic feature of this disorder, males could not meet diagnostic criteria for anorexia nervosa [12]. Indeed, despite weight loss being occasionally documented in clinical reports of male patients, it was thought that any dietary restriction or disordered eating was not a primary concern and was secondary to a more general psychiatric illness such as depression [13, 14]. This was exacerbated by the active exclusion of male patients from clinical trials on the basis of their proposed atypicality or rarity [15]. Consequently, the marginalization of male ED patients is apparent today, with less than 1% of all contemporary eating disorder-related scientific manuscripts relating specifically to male patients [16].

Where Are We Now?

It wasn't until the 1980s that clinical data began to illustrate a limited number of male patients in specialist ED clinics [17–20], which forced the field to reconsider the premise that EDs don't afflict males. More systematic research in the 1990s examined the prevalence and correlates of male presentations in specialist ED clinics, noting that males accounted for 5–10% of cases [12, 21–23], although this was likely an underrepresentation, since males have faced unique stigma in seeking treatment for EDs. Notwithstanding, this emerging evidence was critical in dispelling the long-held misnomer that EDs did not afflict males [12].

However, evidence from specialist ED clinics now suggest that males represent more than one in four EDs among young adolescents in Australia [24] and up to

Table 1.1 An overview of the earliest accounts of eating disorders and their findings relating to male patients

Year	Author	Findings
1689	Richard Morton	Reported "nervous consumption caused by sadness and anxious cares" in a 16-year-old boy
1874	Sir William Gull	Noted that anorexia nervosa occurs in males
1874	Ernest-Charles Lasegue	Described the family dynamics of male patients with anorexia nervosa

33% in the UK [25]. Moreover, ED diagnoses in non-ED settings (i.e., gastroenterology settings) may be *more* prevalent among males than females, where up to 67% of avoidant/restrictive food intake disorder (ARFID) diagnoses, for instance, are accounted for by males [26]. Even in specialist ED settings, male presentations of "selective eating" may account for up to 50% of all cases [27].

More broadly, epidemiological surveillance has recently illustrated shifting trends around the prevalence of anorexia nervosa and bulimia nervosa in males. In the USA, evidence now suggests that males may account for one in four cases of AN and BN [28]. Similarly, in Australia, epidemiological data suggest that one third of those reporting ED behaviors in community settings are male [29]. In light of these findings, it no longer appears tenable to assume that EDs are uncommon among males nor that males account for only a negligible proportion of the public health burden of EDs and disordered eating [16]. As such, efforts to advance research around clinical practice relating to the treatment of males with EDs are now critical (Table 1.1).

References

1. Berkman ND, Lohr KL, Bulik CM. Outcomes of eating disorders: a systematic review of the literature. Int J Eat Disord. 2007;40:293–309.
2. Fichter MM, Quadflieg N, Crosby RD, Koch S. Long-term outcome of anorexia nervosa: results from a large clinical longitudinal study. Int J Eat Disord. 2017;50:1018–30.
3. Mitchell JE, Crow S. Medical complications of anorexia nervosa and bulimia nervosa. Curr Opin Psychiatry. 2006;19:438–43.
4. Smink FRE, van Hoeken D, Hoek HW. Epidemiology of eating disorders: incidence, prevalence and mortality rates. Curr Psychiatry Rep. 2012;14:406–14.
5. Morton R. A treatise of consumptions. London: Princess Arms Press; 1694.
6. Gull W. Anorexia nervosa (Apepsia Hysterica, Anorexia Hysterica). Cfin Sot Trans London. 1874;7:22.
7. Lasegue CH. de I'anorexie hystbrique. ArchsgPn. M&d. XXI, 1873: 385–403.
8. Wooldridge T. Understanding anorexia nervosa in males: an integrative approach. New York: Routledge; 2016.
9. Beumont PJV, Beardwood CJ, Russell GFM. The occurrence of the syndrome of anorexia nervosa in male subjects. Psychol Med. 1972;2:216–31.
10. Bruch H. Anorexia nervosa in the male. Psychosom Med. 1971;33:31–47.
11. Murray SB, Nagata JM, Griffiths S, Calzo JP, Brown TA, Mitchison D, Blashill AJ, Mond JM. The enigma of male eating disorders: a critical review and synthesis. Clin Psychol Rev. 2017,57:10–1.

12. Andersen AE. Males with eating disorders. New York & London: Routledge; 1990.
13. Dally PJ. Anorexia nervosa. New York: Grune and Stratton; 1969.
14. Selvini-Palazzoli M. Interpretation of mental anorexia. In anorexia nervosa. Stuttgart: Thieme Verlag; 1965.
15. Goldberg SC, Halmi KA, Eckert ED, Casper RC, Davis JM. Cyproheptadine in anorexia nervosa. Br J Psychiatry. 1979;134:67–70.
16. Murray SB, Griffiths S, Mond JM. Evolving eating disorder psychopathology: conceptualizing muscularity-oriented disordered eating. Br J Psychiatry. 2016;208:414–5.
17. Andersen AE, Mickalide AD. Anorexia nervosa in the male: an underdiagnosed disorder. Psychosomatics. 24:1066–75.
18. Crisp AH, Hsu LKG, Chen CN, Wheeler M. Reproductive hormone profiles in male anorexia nervosa before, during and after restoration of body weight to normal. A study of twelve patients. Int J Eating Disord. 1982;1:3–9.
19. Hall A, Delahunt JW, Ellis PM. Anorexia nervosa in the male: clinical features and follow-up of nine patients. J Psychiatr Res. 1985;19:2–3.
20. Vandereycken W, Van den Broucke S. Anorexia nervosa in males: a comparative study of 107 cases reported in the literature (1970–1980). Acta Psychiatr Scand. 1984;70:447–54.
21. Carlat DJ, Camargo CA, Herzog DB. Eating disorders in males: a report on 135 patients. Am J Psychiatr. 1997;154:1127–32.
22. Fairburn CG, Beglin SJ. Studies of the epidemiology of bulimia nervosa. Am J Psychiatr. 1990;147:401–8.
23. Sharp CW, Clark SA, Dunan JR, Blackwood DHR, Shapiro CM. Clinical presentation of anorexia nervosa in males: 24 new cases. Int J Eat Disord. 1994;15:125–34.
24. Madden S, Morris A, Zurynski YA, Kohn M, Elliot EJ. The burden of eating disorders in 5-13-year-old children in Australia. Med J Aust. 2009;190:410–4.
25. Nicholls DE, Lynn R, Viner RM. Childhood eating disorders: British national surveillance study. Br J Psychiatry. 2011;198:295–301.
26. Eddy KT, Thomas JT, Hastings E, Edkins K, Lamont E, et al. Prevalence of DSM-5 avoidant/restrictive food intake disorder in a pediatric gastroenterology healthcare network. Int J Eat Disord. 2014;48:464–70.
27. Bryant-Waugh R. Feeding and eating disorders in children. Curr Opin Psychiatry. 2013;26:537–42.
28. Hudson JI, Hiripi E, Pope HG, Kessler R. The prevalence and correlates of eating disorders in the national comorbidity survey replication. Biol Psychiatry. 2007;61:348–58.
29. Mitchison D, Mond JM. Epidemiology of eating disorders, eating disordered behaviour, and body image disturbance in males: a narrative review. J Eat Disord. 2015;3:20.

Chapter 2
Models of Body Image for Boys and Men

Tracy L. Tylka

Learning Objectives

1. Evaluate whether current models of body image can explain body concerns among boys and men.
2. Synthesize variables and pathways with empirical support to generate an integrated model.
3. Explore how this integrated model can direct future research and clinical/prevention work.

Key Points

- Three models of body image were explored in relation to boys' and men's body concerns: the tripartite influence model, objectification theory, and gender role endorsement.
- Elements (variables, pathways) of these three models with empirical support among samples of boys and men were synthesized into an integrated model.
- This integrated model can be used to direct the next generation of research on body image for boys and men, which can be useful to guide public health, clinical, and prevention efforts.

Body image is a multi-faceted construct that represents a person's "inside view" of their body—that is, their feelings, perceptions, and thoughts about their body, which collectively impact how they behave toward it [1]. Body image is often studied in conjunction with disordered eating behavior, and both have been stereotyped as concerns that largely affect white adolescent girls and young adult women [2–4]. This stereotype guided how body image and disordered eating were originally defined (i.e., motivation to become very thin), measured (i.e., scales developed to

T. L. Tylka (✉)
Department of Psychology, The Ohio State University, Columbus, OH, USA
e-mail: tylka.2@osu.edu

J. M. Nagata et al. (eds.), *Eating Disorders in Boys and Men*,
https://doi.org/10.1007/978-3-030-67127-3_2

assess this motivation), studied (i.e., samples were predominantly young white women, and others were excluded), and modeled (i.e., factors primarily relevant to thinness were integrated) [4]. Basing the study of body dissatisfaction and disordered eating on the experiences of young white women created an illusion that they had higher body dissatisfaction and disordered eating relative to other groups, without regard to considering or assessing others' different and diverse body and eating-related concerns [3, 4]. See Chaps. 15 and 16 for further discussion of racial and ethnic factors in relation to body image and disordered eating among boys and men.

More recently, research on body image and disordered eating has been expanded to reflect experiences from more diverse samples and has revealed the complexity of body image among boys and men [5]. Researchers have moved away from assuming that boys' and men's body concerns mirror girls' and women's body concerns (i.e., drive for thinness) and toward exploring their drive for muscularity [6], which has prompted additional studies that demonstrated that the body ideal for boys and men, or the "mesomorphic ideal," differs from the "thin ideal" for girls and women [4, 7–9]. The mesomorphic ideal combines well-developed musculature with low body fat (to showcase muscles) and features larger shoulders, chest, and biceps and a narrower yet still muscled midsection (i.e., "six-pack") [4, 8]. Measures focused on the drive for muscularity [6] as well as dissatisfaction with muscularity and body fat [4] have emerged and guided a new generation of research on boys' and men's body image (see Chap. 7 for a discussion of assessment instruments). Indeed, the importance of both muscularity *and* low body fat to boys' and men's body image has been supported in many samples [4, 6, 10, 11].

A recent meta-analysis has upheld gender differences in body concerns. This study revealed that girls and women consistently scored higher than boys and men on thinness-oriented body dissatisfaction with moderate-to-large effects, whereas boys and men scored higher than girls and women on muscularity-oriented body dissatisfaction with large effects [12]. Importantly, thinness-oriented body dissatisfaction decreased over time for girls and women, whereas drive for muscularity did not decrease over time for boys and men. The authors posited that body positive programming developed for girls and women may have promoted sociocultural shifts in their body acceptance, whereas such programming has not been developed to be able to effectively target boys' and men's body image concerns. This meta-analysis highlights the need for additional theory and research into the predictors and outcomes of body image and concerns in boys and men, which then could be used to guide more effective programming. Exploring predictors and outcomes within body image models, then, is an excellent starting point for this endeavor.

Thus, in this chapter, body image models are explored in terms of their theoretical and empirical relevance for boys and men. How these models have been modified to account for their body concerns, social identities, and adoption of gender roles is reviewed. An integrated conceptual model of boys' and men's body image is presented to guide research and clinical work.

Tripartite Influence Model

Originally developed to represent the experiences of girls and women, the tripartite influence model [13] specifies how appearance-related pressures from three social influences (media, peers, and parents) encourage girls and women to experience body dissatisfaction directly as well as indirectly through internalizing appearance ideals (i.e., adopting cultural beauty ideals, such as the thin ideal, as their own personal aspiration, e.g., "I should be thin") and body comparison (i.e., comparing their body size and shape with others' bodies). Body dissatisfaction in turn predicts disordered eating. This model has been studied and validated extensively with girls and women [e.g., 13–15] and has been more recently expanded and modified to more closely fit the experiences of boys and men [15–19]. This research is reviewed within the following subsections. While some studies also included girls or women, only the findings for boys and men are reported.

Social Influences

Findings support the importance of examining media, peer, and parental appearance-related influences on boys' and men's body dissatisfaction, and they emphasize the need to assess both social pressures to gain muscle and decrease body fat across cultures. Adolescent boys from varied cultural backgrounds report high pressure from media, parents, and peers to lose body fat, as well as high pressure from media, but lower pressure from peers and parents, to increase muscularity [20]. In Brazil, sources of appearance-related pressure and internalization of appearance ideals were strong predictors of adolescent boys' increased body dissatisfaction over a 1-year period [21] (see Chap. 16 for further discussion of body image and disordered eating in boys and men from Latin America). In China, appearance-related media pressure predicted disordered eating among young adult men over a 1-year period, and appearance comparison mediated this association [22]. Various sources of appearance-related pressures are discussed below.

Media influence Traditional forms of media showcase mesomorphic men and promulgate messages to boys and men that they should aspire to be muscular and lean. Indeed, meta-analyses have shown that media appearance-related pressure is significantly linked to boys' and men's body dissatisfaction, with small-to-moderate effects [23]. A recent experimental study found that depictions of the mesomorphic ideal on television (in comparison to music videos or still images of male models) may be particularly detrimental to boys' and men's body image, as these televised images appear to activate appearance comparisons [24]. Another experimental study also found that men who viewed television commercials featuring mesomorphic men experienced lower muscle satisfaction than those who viewed non-appearance commercials, with men high on appearance investment (i.e., placing more importance on appearance) more vulnerable to the effects [25]. Men high on appearance investment also compared themselves more to the mesomorphic men in the commercials, which then predicted their lower body satisfaction.

Certain social media platforms and practices also can contribute to body concerns in boys and men. Appearance-focused social media applications such as Instagram, Facebook, and Snapchat have been linked to sexual minority men's muscularity dissatisfaction, eating disorder symptoms, and thoughts about using anabolic steroids [26]. Viewing others' selfie posts and related likes and comments were positively related to adolescent boys' facial dissatisfaction, with internalization of social appearance ideals accounting for this association [27]. Interestingly, the more that boys appreciated their bodies, the less internalization related to facial dissatisfaction, suggesting that body appreciation may be a protective factor with regard to facial satisfaction when viewing selfies. Further, men who are more likely to digitally alter their selfies posted online and are more concerned with selecting and uploading their selfies to social media also report higher body dissatisfaction [28]. Although hypothesized as a potential protective factor, self-compassion was not found to moderate this link.

Dating-specific social networking applications also have been linked to men's body dissatisfaction. Men who use Tinder (a dating-specific social networking application geared toward finding sexual partners) have been found to report higher facial and body dissatisfaction, internalization, and appearance comparison compared to non-users [29]. Similarly, men who use Grindr (a dating-specific social networking application for gay, bisexual, and other men who have sex with men) perceived that these applications negatively impact their body image due to their promotion of weight stigma and objectification, as well as the encouragement of appearance comparison [30].

Other media sources that are not considered in the context of the tripartite influence model may be of relevance to boys' and men's body image. Pro-muscularity websites may also promote body dissatisfaction, disordered eating, and unhealthy muscularity-focused behaviors. Indeed, a systematic content analysis of pro-muscularity websites revealed that these websites espouse rigid dietary practices, rigid exercise rules, the marginalization of other areas of life, and the use of muscle-enhancing substances, as well as minimizing risks associated with these practices [31]. Additionally, pornography often displays men who are muscular and lean. Even after considering appearance-related pressures from other media, partners, family, and friends, the extent to which men viewed pornography uniquely contributed to their internalization of mesomorphic ideal, which was then linked to their muscularity and body fat dissatisfaction [32].

Peer influence Peers also reinforce media messages for boys and men to be muscular and lean to improve their performance (e.g., in sports) and appearance. Preadolescent boys often discuss sports with their peers, and sports help shape their appearance ideals related to being fit and muscular, as well as their athletic skills to obtain popularity and acceptance [33]. By adolescence, boys report distinct body concerns related to body fat and muscularity, which are linked to appearance-related conversations with their peers [11]. Indeed, boys' muscularity concerns were found to be related to more frequent muscle-building conversations, and weight concerns were associated with more frequent appearance conversations [11]. Men's appearance-related conversations with peers were found to focus on both muscularity and body fat, which were related to their body dissatisfaction, muscle dysmorphia, and disordered eating behaviors [34]. Further, peer pressure to be both muscular and lean was found to be related to higher muscularity dissatisfaction among men [16], and peer pressure to be lean was related to higher body fat dissatisfaction and disordered eating among gay men [17].

Parent influence Parents are an important influence on boys' body image. A systematic review revealed that mothers communicated more messages to their sons (compared to daughters) about the need to become more muscular, and these messages uniquely predicted boys' body image disturbance [35]. Adolescent boys' reports of parental teasing and negative parental attitudes toward their weight and appearance also were associated with their appearance-related rejection sensitivity and body dysmorphic symptoms [36]. College men's retrospective accounts of their parents' restrictive and critical eating messages were positively linked to their current body dissatisfaction and disordered eating and inversely linked to their body appreciation and intuitive eating [37]. Further, parental influences (i.e., messages from fathers and mothers about the importance of being muscular and losing weight) were more closely associated with adolescent boys' body dissatisfaction and body change strategies (i.e., behaviors geared toward increasing muscles and decreasing weight) compared to media and peer influences [38].

Partner influence While not included in the original tripartite influence model, research has suggested that partners may be an important influence on men's body image and body change behaviors. Pressures from partners to be muscular and lean were related to men's internalization of the mesomorphic ideal, body comparison, muscularity and body fat dissatisfaction, muscularity-related behaviors, and disordered eating [16, 17]. When examined alongside other sources of social influence, partner pressure to be mesomorphic was uniquely and directly related to men's disordered eating [16]. Further, among gay men, partner pressure to be muscular was uniquely related to internalization of the mesomorphic ideal and muscularity enhancement behaviors [17].

Gay community Certain gay communities that emphasize appearance and lean muscularity may also be a source of social influence impacting gay men's body image and body change behaviors. Indeed, men's regular involvement in gay culture has been found to be related to their internalization of the mesomorphic ideal, appearance comparison, and engagement in behaviors to enhance their muscularity; these relationships remained even when examined alongside other sources of social influence [17].

Mediating Variables Connecting Social Influences with Body Change Behaviors

A key feature of the tripartite influence model is its central "mediating" variables that connect the sources of social influence with disordered eating [13]. Variables in this central role in the original model include thin-ideal internalization, body comparison, and body dissatisfaction. Specifically, once the thin ideal is internalized, it is manifested in behaviors that help girls and women gauge the status of their bodies (body comparison). Because the vast majority of girls and women do not have a body type that is consistent with the "thin ideal," they are dissatisfied with their bodies if they have internalized this ideal and regularly engage in body comparison, which then may prompt them to engage in disordered eating.

For boys and men, the thin ideal is replaced with the mesomorphic ideal. Because the mesomorphic ideal focuses on muscularity and leanness, boys and men can become dissatisfied with their bodies on two dimensions: muscularity and body fat [11, 16]. Muscularity dissatisfaction may prompt muscularity enhancement behaviors, whereas body fat dissatisfaction may prompt disordered eating [16]. Many studies uphold the mediating roles of internalization of the mesomorphic ideal [16–19, 39, 40], body comparison [16, 18, 39, 40], muscularity dissatisfaction [16, 17, 19, 39], and body fat dissatisfaction [16, 17, 39] with men. A prospective study with adolescent boys revealed that internalization of the mesomorphic ideal predicted increased muscularity dissatisfaction, body fat dissatisfaction predicted increased disordered eating, and internalization of the mesomorphic ideal predicted increased use of muscularity enhancement behaviors across a 5-year period [41]. Therefore, many of the proposed pathways within the tripartite influence model are supported cross-sectionally as well as longitudinally.

Objectification Theory

Researchers have also used objectification theory as a model to study men's body image, albeit far less frequently than the tripartite influence model. Objectification theory [42] posits that the sexual objectification of women in the media and through interpersonal encounters (e.g., being touched or grabbed against their will, the target of catcalls and leering) places women at a higher risk for eating disorders, depression, and sexual dysfunction. This connection occurs due to a sequential process by which repeated exposure to instances of sexual objectification orients women to see themselves from an "observer's perspective" or focus more on their appearance and less on their internal experience (e.g., how they feel). This is referred to as self-objectification, which prompts women's body shame, appearance anxiety, and safety anxiety as well as disrupts their internal body experiences (e.g., feelings, hunger) and flow (i.e., ability to become absorbed in challenging tasks). These consequences of self-objectification then place women at higher risk for disordered eating, depression, and sexual dysfunction. The tenets of objectification theory have been upheld in diverse samples of women [43].

Generally, research has not supported most of the proposed objectification theory pathways in samples of straight men [44–46]. Of note, more support for objectification theory has been accrued for men who may personally experience being sexually objectified, such as sexual minority men [44, 47, 48] (for links between sexual objectification and gay community involvement, see [49]). Evidence for this assertion is that straight men report lower levels of objectification (both sexual and self) compared to gay men [44, 47], experimentally induced self-objectification does not increase body shame and restrained eating for straight men but it does for gay men [47], and sexual objectification is unrelated to self-objectification and self-objectification is unrelated to body shame in straight men [44, 48], although these links are significant in sexual minority men [44, 48]. Of note, gay men often experience minority stress, including both experienced and expected stigma for being gay and internalized homophobia, and these sources of minority stress are linked to their body dissatisfaction [50]. Researchers have examined whether objectification theory may be more relevant for straight men when measures of male body image (e.g., drive for muscularity) are included in the model. However, self-objectification is either not linked or weakly linked to body shame and drive for muscularity among predominantly straight men [45, 46, 51].

Bodybuilding may represent a subculture that fosters sexual objectification due to its heightened focus on appearance [52]. In a mixed sample of male bodybuilders, male weightlifters, and undergraduate men, bodybuilders reported higher levels of self-objectification and drive for muscularity than weightlifters and/or undergraduate men [52]. Additionally, self-objectification accounted for bodybuilders' higher drive for muscularity.

Overall, the question of whether objectification theory is relevant for men may depend on whether they are involved in a community that sexually objectifies their bodies. As originally proposed by objectification theory, sexual objectification is the catalyst to psychological distress underlying body image disturbance. Objectifying communities may foster appearance investment [53], which may be conceptually similar to self-objectification, but does prospectively predict men's internalization of appearance ideals and drive for muscularity [54]. Men who report higher levels of sexual objectification also report higher body shame [44, 46], and this link may be due to appearance investment and perhaps sexual objectification's threats to masculinity.

Gender Role Endorsement

The mesomorphic ideal is embodied masculinity, representing strength, power, control, and dominance [55]. Indeed, men's drive for muscularity, leanness, and fitness are related to their endorsement of traditional notions of masculinity [56] and gendered expectations that they need to be successful and powerful [57].

The threatened masculinity hypothesis [58] suggests that increasing gender equality leaves men with fewer ways they can assert themselves over women. For men who endorse traditional notions of masculinity, this can lead to an identity crisis, whereby they may experience a compensatory need to publicly display their masculinity, such as through striving toward muscularity. Therefore, the more that men endorse traditional notions of masculinity, the more likely they are to be dissatisfied with their muscularity and engage in muscularity enhancement behaviors in particular. In contrast, the more they endorse gendered notions of femininity, the more they are dissatisfied with their body fat and engage in restrictive eating practices [59]. Research has supported associations between masculinity, muscularity dissatisfaction, and harmful muscularity enhancement behaviors, as well as associations between femininity, body fat dissatisfaction, and severe restrictive eating [60]. Further, men's higher endorsement of masculinity was found to predict higher muscularity dissatisfaction and muscularity-oriented disordered eating (e.g., eating according to a "bulking" and "cutting" cycle that involves the overconsumption of protein and restriction of dietary fats and carbohydrates), and higher endorsement of femininity predicted higher muscularity dissatisfaction and thinness- and muscularity-oriented disordered eating [61].

Given these findings, researchers have suggested the need to consider boys' and men's gender role endorsement within the tripartite influence model [62, 63] and objectification theory [46]. Specifically, internalization of the mesomorphic ideal was found to account for the relationships between masculinity and both drive for leanness and drive for muscularity in men from the United States, Sweden, and Australia [62]. Further, media influences (i.e., images of muscular men), masculine physical attributes investment (i.e., importance of athletic and physical superiority), and social comparison have been found to be uniquely related to preadolescent boys' drive for muscularity [63]. Also supporting this integration, gender role endorsement has been found to be related to body shame [46].

Integrated Model and Future Research

Aspects of the tripartite influence model, objectification theory, and gender role endorsement can be represented in a conceptual model that integrates current theory and research findings on boys' and men's body image, as well as generates ideas for future research in this area (see Fig. 2.1). While this integrated model contains pathways (see blue arrows) between variable domains (rectangles) similar to those from the tripartite influence model, it expands the variables included and pinpoints the need to examine moderators of certain relationships (see red arrows).

This integrated model can be used to guide research efforts in many ways. First, it greatly expands the sources of social influence from the original tripartite influence model. Preliminary research supports these additional sources (e.g., partner influences, social media, sexually objectifying contexts, pornography, stigmatic messages, gender role socialization) as relevant for boys and men, but more research

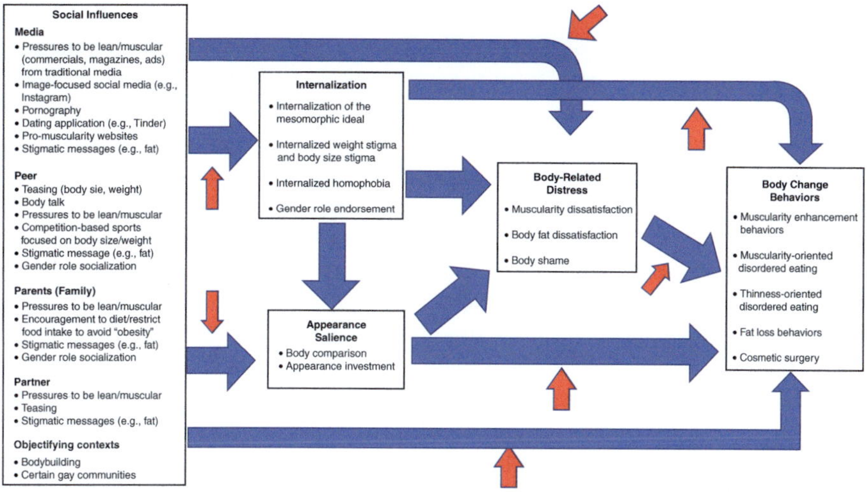

Fig. 2.1 Conceptual model, integrating elements of the tripartite influence model, objectification theory, and gender role endorsement to explain boys' and men's body image and body change behaviors. Blue arrows represent pathways connecting variables, and red arrows represent pathways that could be moderated by other variables, such as self-compassion, body appreciation, emotional regulation, body image flexibility, and social identities (e.g., sexual orientation, race/ethnicity, age, weight/body fat percentage). Stigmatic messages can include weight, but also other minority stress (e.g., stigma for being gay, racial stigma, etc.)

is needed to explore the mechanisms by which they impact boys' and men's body image and body change behaviors. Second, it expands the internalization domain to include gender role endorsement, which can represent the internalization of societal gender roles, as well as internalized weight stigma and internalized homophobia. Third, it includes body comparison within the broader domain of appearance salience (i.e., how much mental energy is devoted to appearance, encompasses body comparison and appearance investment). Fourth, it broadens body dissatisfaction by including muscularity dissatisfaction, body fat dissatisfaction, and body shame (which may be particularly relevant to sexually objectifying environments and appearance investment). Fifth, it includes muscularity-oriented disordered eating as well as cosmetic surgery alongside thinness-oriented disordered eating and non-eating-related muscularity enhancement behaviors in the body change behaviors domain. Sixth, it encourages the examination of moderators, which are variables that may influence the strengths of the pathways. For example, sexual orientation, age, ethnicity, and weight/body fat percentage may impact the strength of the model paths (e.g., the path from internalization of the mesomorphic ideal to body fat dissatisfaction may be stronger for men who have a higher percentage of body fat). Personality variables, such as maladaptive perfectionism and emotional regulation, may impact the strength of the variable pathways as well. It is important that researchers also explore potential resilience and protective factors as moderators in the model. Variables such as self-compassion, body appreciation, and body complexity (i.e., viewing the body as more than its appearance) could be potential candidates. For example, they may be able to offset maladaptive social influences, protecting men's body image from these influences. Overall, resilience variables have been understudied within the area of men's body image.

This model is conceptual, and thus it may not be feasible to examine the model in its entirety in one research study. Rather, researchers may want to examine specific pathways within the model to elucidate mechanisms of action (e.g., mediators), as well as examine whether certain pathways vary based on men's diverse social identities, experiences, personalities, and protective characteristics (e.g., moderators). In these investigations, variables within each domain (see bulleted terms) should be examined independently rather than combined into latent variables (e.g., body fat dissatisfaction and muscularity dissatisfaction should be treated as separate variables within the same analysis, given that they have been shown to be distinct facets of men's body image [16, 17]). While this suggestion does not apply to every case, it allows researchers to explore nuances between variables within the same domain. Further, the bulleted terms in Fig. 2.1 are examples that have research support, but they are not meant to be exhaustive. Researchers are encouraged to examine the ones provided and explore others that may be theoretically relevant to men's body image. For instance, there may be important positive social influences (e.g., unconditional body acceptance, non-appearance-related hobbies and sports, nature exposure) that prevent the development of negative body image and particularly harmful body change behaviors and thus need to be explored.

Conclusion

This chapter reviews three models of boys' and men's body image: the tripartite influence model, objectification theory, and gender role endorsement. Variables and pathways with empirical support were integrated into a unified model, which can direct the next generation of research on boys' and men's body image, shape public health and clinical efforts to prevent their body concerns, and guide clinical interventions with boys and men in eating disorder treatment. For example, pinpointing the sources of social influence that independently increase appearance investment and internalization of the mesomorphic ideal can inform public health and policy efforts to decrease the likelihood of these messages (e.g., removing pro-muscularity websites, changing public health messages to remove weight stigma). In addition, identifying personal variables that make boys less likely to internalize the mesomorphic ideal, invest their self-worth in their appearance, engage in body comparison, and/or experience body-related distress can be used to inform primary and secondary prevention programs. For example, if functionality appreciation is found to weaken the link between media sources and boys' internalization of the mesomorphic ideal, then prevention programs can design and incorporate interventions to increase their functionality appreciation. In clinical work, the model can be given to boys and men to generate discussion on how their body dissatisfaction and/or body change behaviors developed and are maintained. Interventions can also be designed to increase variables shown to weaken the links between model variables. For example, if body image flexibility weakens the link between body-related distress and muscularity-oriented eating disorders, then interventions building body image flexibility can be incorporated in eating disorder treatment with boys and men.

References

1. Cash TF. Body image: past, present, and future. Body Image. 2004;1:1–5. https://doi.org/10.1016/S1740-1445(03)00011-1.
2. Murnen SK, Karazsia BT. A review of research on men's body image and drive for muscularity. In: Levant RF, Wong YJ, editors. The psychology of men and masculinities. Washington, D.C.: American Psychological Association; 2017. p. 229–57.
3. Murray SB, Nagata JM, Griffiths S, Calzo JP, Brown TA, Mitchison D, et al. The enigma of male eating disorders: a critical review and synthesis. Clin Psychol Rev. 2017;57:1–11. https://doi.org/10.1016/j.cpr.2017.08.001.
4. Tylka TL, Bergeron D, Schwartz JP. Development and psychometric evaluation of the male body attitudes scale (MBAS). Body Image. 2005;2:161–75. https://doi.org/10.1016/j.bodyim.2005.03.001.
5. Griffiths S, Murray SB, Touyz S. Disordered eating and the muscular ideal. J Eat Disord. 2013;1:15. https://doi.org/10.1186/2050-2974-1-15.
6. McCreary DR, Sasse DK. An exploration of the drive for muscularity in adolescent boys and girls. J Amer Coll Health. 2000;48:297–304. https://doi.org/10.1080/07448480009596271.
7. Grogan S, Richards H. Body image: focus groups with boys and men. Men Masculinities. 2002;4:219–32. https://doi.org/10.1177/1097184X02004003001.
8. Ridgeway RT, Tylka TL. College men's perceptions of ideal body composition and shape. Psychol Men Masculinity. 2005;6:209–20. https://doi.org/10.1037/1524-9220.6.3.209.
9. Tiggemann M, Martins Y, Kirkbride A. Oh to be lean and muscular: body image ideals in gay and heterosexual men. Psychol Men Masculinity. 2007;8:15–24. https://doi.org/10.1037/1524-9220.8.1.15.
10. Bergeron D, Tylka TL. Support for the uniqueness of body dissatisfaction from drive for muscularity among men. Body Image. 2007;4:288–95. https://doi.org/10.1016/j.bodyim.2007.05.002.
11. Jones DC, Crawford JK. Adolescent boys and body image: weight and muscularity concerns as dual pathways to body dissatisfaction. J Youth Adolesc. 2005;34:629–36. https://doi.org/10.1007/s10964-005-8951-3.
12. Karazsia BT, Murnen SK, Tylka TL. Is body dissatisfaction changing across time? A cross-temporal meta-analysis. Psychol Bull. 2017;143:293–320. https://doi.org/10.1037/bul0000081.
13. Thompson JK, Coovert MD, Stormer SM. Body image, social comparison and eating disturbance: a covariance structure modeling investigation. Int J Eat Disord. 1999;26:43–53. https://doi.org/10.1002/(sici)1098-108x(199907)26:1%3C43::aid-eat6%3E3.0.co;2-r.
14. Keery H, van den Berg P, Thompson JK. An evaluation of the tripartite influence model of body image and eating disturbance with adolescent girls. Body Image. 2004;1:237–51. https://doi.org/10.1016/j.bodyim.2004.03.001.
15. Menzel JE, Sperry SL, Small B, Thompson JK, Sarwer DB, Cash TF. Internalization of appearance ideals and cosmetic surgery attitudes: a test of the tripartite influence model of body image. Sex Roles. 2011;65:469–77. https://doi.org/10.1007/s11199-011-9983-7.

16. Tylka TL. Refinement of the tripartite influence model for men: dual body image pathways to body change behaviors. Body Image. 2011;8:199–207. https://doi.org/10.1016/j.bodyim.2011.04.008.
17. Tylka TL, Andorka MJ. Support for an expanded tripartite influence model with gay men. Body Image. 2012;9:57–67. https://doi.org/10.1016/j.bodyim.2011.09.006.
18. Karazsia BT, Crowther JH. Social comparison and internalization: mediators of social influences on men's muscularity-oriented body dissatisfaction. Body Image. 2009;6:106–12. https://doi.org/10.1016/j.bodyim.2008.12.003.
19. Karazsia BT, Crowther JH. Sociocultural and psychological links to men's engagement in risky body change behaviors. Sex Roles. 2010;63:747–56. https://doi.org/10.1007/s11199-010-9802-6.
20. McCabe MP, Busija L, Fuller-Tyszkiewicz M, Ricciardelli L, Mellor D, Mussap A. Sociocultural influences on strategies to lose weight, gain weight, and increase muscles among ten cultural groups. Body Image. 2015;12:108–14. https://doi.org/10.1016/j.bodyim.2014.10.008.
21. Amaral ACS, Ferreira MEC. Body dissatisfaction and associated factors among Brazilian adolescents: a longitudinal study. Body Image. 2017;22:32–8. https://doi.org/10.1016/j.bodyim.2017.04.006.
22. Luo YJ, Jackson T, Niu GF, Chen H. Effects of gender and appearance comparisons on associations between media-based appearance pressure and disordered eating: testing a moderated mediation model. Sex Roles. 2020;82:293–305. https://doi.org/10.1007/s11199-019-01058-4.
23. Barlett CP, Vowels CL, Saucier DA. Meta-analyses of the effects of media images on men's body-image concerns. J Soc Clin Psychol. 2008;27:279–310. https://doi.org/10.1521/jscp.2008.27.3.279.
24. Allen A, Mulgrew KE. Differential media effects on male body satisfaction and mood. Aust J Psychol. 2020;72:3–10. https://doi.org/10.1521/jscp.2008.27.3.279.
25. Hargreaves DA, Tiggemann M. Muscular ideal media images and men's body image: social comparison processing and individual vulnerability. Psychol Men Masculinity. 2009;10:109–19. https://doi.org/10.1037/a0014691.
26. Griffiths S, Murray SB, Krug I, McLean SA. The contribution of social media to body dissatisfaction, eating disorder symptoms, and anabolic steroid use among sexual minority men. Cyberpsychol Behav Soc Netw. 2018;21:149–56. https://doi.org/10.1089/cyber.2017.0375.
27. Wang Y, Fardouly J, Vartanian LR, Lei L. Selfie-viewing and facial dissatisfaction among Chinese adolescents: a moderated mediation model of general attractiveness internalization and body appreciation. Body Image. 2019;30:35–43. https://doi.org/10.1016/j.bodyim.2019.05.001.
28. Lonergan AR, Bussey K, Mond J, Brown O, Griffiths S, Murray SB, Mitchison D. Me, my selfie, and I: the relationship between editing and posting selfies and body dissatisfaction in men and women. Body Image. 2019;28:39–43. https://doi.org/10.1016/j.bodyim.2018.12.001.
29. Strubel J, Petrie TA. Love me tinder: body image and psychosocial functioning among men and women. Body Image. 2017;21:34–8. https://doi.org/10.1016/j.bodyim.2017.02.006.
30. Filice E, Raffoul A, Meyer SB, Neiterman E. The influence of Grindr, a geosocial networking application, on body image in gay, bisexual and other men who have sex with men: an exploratory study. Body Image. 2019;31:59–70. https://doi.org/10.1016/j.bodyim.2019.08.007.
31. Murray SB, Griffiths S, Hazery L, Shen T, Wooldridge T, Mond JM. Go big or go home: a thematic content analysis of pro-muscularity websites. Body Image. 2016;16:17–20. https://doi.org/10.1016/j.bodyim.2015.10.002.
32. Tylka TL. No harm in looking, right? Men's pornography consumption, body image, and Well-being. Psychol Men Masculinity. 2015;16:97–107. https://doi.org/10.1037/a0035774.
33. Tatangelo GL, Ricciardelli LA. A qualitative study of preadolescent boys' and girls' body image: gendered ideals and sociocultural influences. Body Image. 2013;10:591–8. https://doi.org/10.1016/j.bodyim.2013.07.006.

34. Sladek MR, Engeln R, Miller SA. Development and validation of the male body talk scale: a psychometric investigation. Body Image. 2014;11:233–44. https://doi.org/10.1016/j.bodyim.2014.02.005.
35. Tatangelo G, McCabe M, Mellor D, Mealey A. A systematic review of body dissatisfaction and sociocultural messages related to the body among preschool children. Body Image. 2016;18:86–95. https://doi.org/10.1016/j.bodyim.2016.06.003.
36. Densham K, Webb HJ, Zimmer-Gembeck MJ, Nesdale D, Downey G. Early adolescents' body dysmorphic symptoms as compensatory responses to parental appearance messages and appearance-based rejection sensitivity. Body Image. 2017;23:162–70. https://doi.org/10.1016/j.bodyim.2017.09.005.
37. Kroon Van Diest AM, Tylka TL. The caregiver eating messages scale: development and psychometric investigation. Body Image. 2010;7:317–26. https://doi.org/10.1016/j.bodyim.2010.06.002.
38. Stanford JN, McCabe MP. Sociocultural influences on adolescent boys' body image and body change strategies. Body Image. 2005;2:105–13. https://doi.org/10.1016/j.bodyim.2005.03.002.
39. Rodgers RF, Ganchou C, Franko DL, Chabrol H. Drive for muscularity and disordered eating among French adolescent boys: a sociocultural model. Body Image. 2012;9:318–23. https://doi.org/10.1016/j.bodyim.2012.03.002.
40. Stratton R, Donovan C, Bramwell S, Loxton NJ. Don't stop till you get enough: factors driving men toward muscularity. Body Image. 2015;15:72–80. https://doi.org/10.1016/j.bodyim.2015.07.002.
41. Hoffmann S, Warschburger P. Prospective relations among internalization of beauty ideals, body image concerns, and body change behaviors: considering thinness and muscularity. Body Image. 2019;28:159–67. https://doi.org/10.1016/j.bodyim.2019.01.011.
42. Fredrickson BL, Roberts TA. Objectification theory: toward understanding women's lived experiences and mental health risks. Psychol Women Q. 1997;21:173–206. https://doi.org/10.1111/j.1471-6402.1997.tb00108.x.
43. Roberts TA, Calogero RM, Gervais SJ. Objectification theory: continuing contributions to feminist psychology. In: Travis CB, White JW, Rutherford A, Williams WS, Cook SL, Wyche KF, editors. APA handbook of the psychology of women: history, theory, and battlegrounds. Washington D.C.: American Psychological Association; 2018. p. 249–71.
44. Engeln-Maddox R, Miller SA, Doyle DM. Tests of objectification theory in gay, lesbian, and heterosexual community samples: mixed evidence for proposed pathways. Sex Roles. 2011;59:518–32. https://doi.org/10.1007/s11199-011-9958-8.
45. Daniel S, Bridges SK. The drive for muscularity in men: media influences and objectification theory. Body Image. 2010;7:32–8. https://doi.org/10.1016/j.bodyim.2009.08.003.
46. Davids CM, Watson LB, Gere MP. Objectification, masculinity, and muscularity: a test of objectification theory with heterosexual men. Sex Roles. 2019;80:443–57. https://doi.org/10.1007/s11199-018-0940-6.
47. Martins Y, Tiggemann M, Kirkbride A. Those speedos become them: the role of self-objectification in gay and heterosexual men's body image. Personal Soc Psychol Bull. 2007;33:634–7. https://doi.org/10.1177/0146167206297403.
48. Wiseman MC, Moradi B. Body image and eating disorder symptoms in sexual minority men: a test and extension of objectification theory. J Couns Psychol. 2010;57:154–66. https://doi.org/10.1037/a0018937.
49. Davids CM, Watson LB, Nilsson JE, Marszalek JM. Body dissatisfaction among gay men: the roles of sexual objectification, gay community involvement, and psychological sense of community. Psychol Sexual Orient Gender Diver. 2015;2:376–85. https://doi.org/10.1037/sgd0000127.
50. Kimmel SB, Mahalik JR. Body image concerns of gay men: the roles of minority stress and conformity to masculine norms. J Consult Clin Psychol. 2005;73:1185–90. https://doi.org/10.1037/0022-006X.73.6.1185.

51. Parent MC, Moradi B. His biceps become him: a test of objectification theory's application to drive for muscularity and propensity for steroid use in college men. J Couns Psychol. 2011;58:246–56. https://doi.org/10.1037/a0021398.
52. Hallsworth L, Wade T, Tiggemann M. Individual differences in male body image: an examination of self-objectification in recreational body builders. Br J Health Psychol. 2005;10:453–65. https://doi.org/10.1348/135910705X26966.
53. Cash TF. Cognitive-behavioral perspectives on body image. In: Cash TF, Smolak L, editors. Body image: a handbook of science, practice, and prevention. New York: Guilford; 2011. p. 39–47.
54. Kling J, Rodgers RF, Frisén A. Young men's endorsement and pursuit of appearance ideals: the prospective role of appearance investment. Body Image. 2016;16:10–6. https://doi.org/10.1016/j.bodyim.2015.10.001.
55. Hunt CJ, Gonsalkorale K, Murray SB. Threatened masculinity and muscularity: an experimental examination of multiple aspects of muscularity in men. Body Image. 2013;10:290–9. https://doi.org/10.1016/j.bodyim.2013.02.007.
56. Holmqvist Gattario K, Frisén A, Fuller-Tyszkiewicz M, Ricciardelli LA, Diedrichs PC, Yager Z, et al. How is men's conformity to masculine norms related to their body image? Masculinity and muscularity across Western countries. Psychol Men Masculinity. 2015;16:337–47. https://doi.org/10.1037/a0038494.
57. McCreary DR, Saucier DM, Courtenay WH. The drive for muscularity and masculinity: testing the associations among gender-role traits, behaviors, attitudes, and conflict. Psychol Men Masculinity. 2005;6:83–94. https://doi.org/10.1037/1524-9220.6.2.83.
58. Mishkind ME, Rodin J, Silberstein LR, Striegel-Moore RH. The embodiment of masculinity: cultural, psychological, and behavioral dimensions. Am Behav Scient. 1986;29:545–62. https://doi.org/10.1177/000276486029005004.
59. Murray SB, Touyz SW. Masculinity, femininity, and male body image: a recipe for future research. Int J Men Health. 2012;11:227–39. https://doi.org/10.3149/jmh.1103.227.
60. Murray SB, Rieger E, Karlov L, Touyz SW. Masculinity and femininity in the divergence of male body image concerns. J Eat Disord. 2013;1:11. https://doi.org/10.1186/2050-2974-1-11.
61. Griffiths S, Murray SB, Touyz S. Extending the masculinity hypothesis: an investigation of gender role conformity, body dissatisfaction, and disordered eating in young heterosexual men. Psychol Men Masculinity. 2015;16:108–14. https://doi.org/10.1037/a0035958.
62. Franko DL, Fuller-Tyszkiewicz M, Rodgers RF, Holmqvist Gattario K, Frisén A, Diedrichs PC, et al. Internalization as a mediator of the relationship between conformity to masculine norms and body image attitudes and behaviors among young men in Sweden, US, UK, and Australia. Body Image. 2015;15:54–60. https://doi.org/10.1016/j.bodyim.2015.05.002.
63. Smolak L, Stein JA. The relationship of drive for muscularity to sociocultural factors, self-esteem, physical attributes gender role, and social comparison in middle school boys. Body Image. 2006;3:121–9. https://doi.org/10.1016/j.bodyim.2006.03.002.

Chapter 3
Muscularity-Oriented Disordered Eating in Boys and Men

Mitchell L. Cunningham, Jason M. Nagata, and Stuart B. Murray

Learning Objectives

1. To understand the core tenets of the muscular body ideal among boys and men, the pursuit of which can precipitate muscle-oriented eating regimes and other associated medical concerns
2. To gain an appreciation of the special and potentially maladaptive muscle-oriented eating and exercise behaviors exhibited by boys and men wishing to be more muscular, and how these are distinct from thinness-oriented eating practices
3. To understand the issues associated with current "gold-standard" eating disorder assessment and treatment tools in the context of muscularity-oriented concerns and related eating pathology

Key Points

- This chapter synthesized the available literature to underscore what we currently understand about muscularity-oriented disordered eating among boys and men.
- The muscular body ideal is pursued by many boys and men, and attendant muscularity dissatisfaction appears to be common across various populations of boys and men.
- A broad and unique spectrum of ED pathologies closely accompany the pursuit of muscularity.
- Widely used ED assessment and treatment tools may need to be revised to be sensitive to, and adequately index, muscularity-oriented ED pathology.

M. L. Cunningham
School of Psychology, The University of Sydney, Sydney, NSW, Australia

J. M. Nagata
Division of Adolescent and Young Adult Medicine, Department of Pediatrics, University of California, San Francisco, San Francisco, CA, USA

S. B. Murray (✉)
Department of Psychiatry and Behavioral Sciences, USC Keck School of Medicine, University of Southern California, Los Angeles, CA, USA
e-mail: stuartmu@usc.edu

J. M. Nagata et al. (eds.), *Eating Disorders in Boys and Men*,
https://doi.org/10.1007/978-3-030-67127-3_3

Introduction

A prevailing misconception is that eating disorders (EDs) are rare among boys and men[1]. In fact, men are estimated to make up 25% of ED diagnoses; however, remarkably, they represent less than 1% of published empirical research related to EDs (namely, anorexia nervosa) [1, 2]. This lack of male-centric research has meant that our knowledge of ED-related cognitions, feelings, and behaviors in men largely stem from, and is obstensibly analogous to, that among females [1–3]. An overvaluation of weight and shape is a critical factor in the development and maintenance of ED pathology; yet, importantly, the idealized weight and shape for men and women often substantially differ [1, 2, 4]. That is, a key distinction between the sexes is that men often pursue a body characterized by lean and developed muscularity, which polarizes the overly thin body ideal typically valued by women [1, 2, 4]. Consequently, crucial qualitative differences likely exist in the maladaptive eating-related cognitions, feelings, and behaviors men and women each engage in (or experience) in the quest to reach their respective body ideals. Regrettably, to date, far richer empirical and clinical investigations have been devoted to exploring thinness-oriented ED pathology in women, findings and knowledge which may not extrapolate well or completely to men and their drive for muscularity.

The overarching aim of this chapter is to synthesize the available and cutting-edge literature to highlight our current understanding of muscularity-oriented disordered eating among men. In doing so, we first aim to provide the reader with an appreciation of specific and unique medical complications facing males pursuing overt muscularity. Second, we describe the muscular body ideal commonly preferred by males and the prevalence of concomitant body dissatisfaction in achieving such an unrealistic physique.

Third, we highlight the muscularity-oriented eating behaviors likely to accompany the drive for muscularity and in doing so demonstrate their clear distinction from thinness-oriented eating behaviors. Fourth, we consider issues with existing recognized and "gold-standard" ED assessment tools which are informative and useful in capturing thinness-oriented ED pathology, but may have limited utility in assessing muscularity concerns and related ED pathology. Finally, we close the chapter by advocating fruitful directions for future research.

Medical Considerations Associated with the Pursuit of Muscularity

Eating disorders in men can lead to medical consequences affecting every organ system in the body [5]. Further details can be found in the chapter "Medical Consequences of Eating Disorders." Males who present with muscularity-oriented disordered eating can develop medical instability, thus warranting urgent admission

[1] In this chapter, we use the terms males and boys/men interchangeably.

to the hospital [6]. In particular, greater hours of exercise per week and participation in team sports have been shown to be associated with bradycardia (heart rate < 50 beats per minute) among adolescents with anorexia nervosa and bulimia nervosa [7].

The female athlete triad has been long recognized as a medical consequence of sports participation. The triad consists of low energy availability with or without disordered eating, menstrual dysfunction, and low bone density [8]. However, this term has recently been updated to be called Relative Energy Deficiency in Sport (RED-S) [9], given that its health consequences can also be seen in male athletes.

Men may also use specific appearance- and performance-enhancing drugs (APEDs) and supplements to enhance muscularity. For example, sports supplement use among college athletes is associated with eating disorder symptoms [10]. Furthermore, adolescents who use dietary supplements for muscle building or weight loss had higher risk for severe adverse events and medical outcomes including death and hospitalization [11]. In particular, anabolic-androgenic steroid use is associated with cardiovascular, liver, kidney, neuropsychiatric, and endocrine toxicity [12]. A greater concern is that other APEDs may be available over the counter or online without regulation and are often mixed with harmful substances such as anabolic-androgenic steroids [13].

The Muscular Body Ideal

In contrast to the stereotypical female body ideal characterized primarily by thinness, men tend to exhibit a drive for a lean muscular physique [1, 4, 14–16]. Specifically, this body ideal is hallmarked by a mesomorphic shape consisting of upper-body muscularity, specifically a "well-developed chest and arm muscles, with wide shoulders tapering down to a narrow waist" (p. 30) [4], in conjunction with little/no body fat to ensure one's muscular stature is readily visible (i.e., to be "cut") [2, 17]. The strong proclivity toward this type of appearance ideal is unsurprising given that this male muscular physique is typically portrayed and celebrated in Western culture [4, 18], which continues to be permeated today through the widespread proliferation of social media messages, notably *fitspiration*-type content [19].

Like the overtly thin body ideal among women, a lean muscular physique is extraordinary difficult, if not impossible, for most boys and men to achieve. As such, the pursuit of this body ideal is likely to provoke significant body dissatisfaction among men when they fail to procure it. Tellingly, research points to the ubiquity of body dissatisfaction, namely, that associated with perceptions of being insufficiently muscular, among different male populations. For example, Frederick and colleagues [16] found that over 90% of college men in the USA reported a desire for enhanced muscularity, as well as high prevalences of men in both Ukraine (69%) and Ghana (49%) [16]. Among one large Internet panel survey of US adults, 27% of men were found to be somewhat-to-extremely dissatisfied with their muscle tone/size, while 10% reported as being very-to-extremely dissatisfied [20]. Muscularity dissatisfaction also appears to an extent in younger male populations. For instance, a recent nationwide study consisting of over 15,000 adolescent boys across the USA found that 29.6% reported attempts to gain weight (ostensibly in the form of greater muscle mass) – even among those in the *healthy* weight range (i.e., as judged through body mass index), where almost 40% of this group still engaged in efforts to put on size [21]. Of concern, preferences for muscularity have even been reported among boys as young as 6 years of age, with one study demonstrating that 32.6% of boys express the desire to be increasingly muscular, compared to 16.8% wishing to be less muscular or thinner (20.8%) (and 8.9% wanting to be larger-fatter) [22].

Muscularity-Oriented Disordered Eating

The drive for the lean muscular body ideal among men is likely to bring about a distinct profile of eating-related cognitions and behaviors aimed at bringing one closer to this ideal [1, 3, 23]. To more precisely conceptualize the qualitative nature of such behaviors, it is worthwhile underscoring two primary mechanisms (pathways) via which such behaviors can manifest – muscle growth/size and leanness [2, 3, 24]. The former relates to the growing of muscle mass, that is, increasing muscle volume and density (i.e., to "bulk" up), while the latter concerns the minimization of body adiposity so one's muscles are defined, are readily visible, and appear prominent. As such, different muscularity-oriented body change behaviors may manifest via through these two distinct muscle-change mechanisms [2, 24]. For example, those wanting to facilitate muscle *growth* may be inclined to intake surplus calories and macronutrients, particularly centered around the large and frequent consumption of protein-rich foods (i.e., the building blocks of muscle mass) [3, 25]. In partaking in this process, men may engage in other special eating practices that are alien to the layperson, for instance, adhering to a strict dietary regime centered on protein intake based on arbitrary rules, including the consumption of a certain amount of protein per day according to one's body weight (e.g., 3 grams per kilogram) [26, 27]. Some men may also feel coerced to continue eating despite reaching satiety, and indeed do so, to ensure their muscles are always "fed" with the necessary protein and macronutrients [26, 27], where some go to extreme efforts by liquefying foods into shakes to facilitate the ingestion of maximal calories [25]. There can also be a particular allure toward practices involving pre-planned food, or 'meal prep', to assist these men to not deviate from their strict dietary regimes by providing ongoing access to 'clean' high-protein meals and other foods with special macronutrient densities (e.g., to consume in situations where high-protein or healthier food options are not available) [23, 26, 27].

Conversely, the pursuit of *leanness* is likely to elicit a distinct spectrum of eating-related behaviors and practices aimed at enhancing muscularity indirectly, that is, facilitate fat loss so muscles appear more defined and unobscured [1–3]. This pursuit could manifest through traditional ED behaviors such as deliberate and extreme calorie restriction, periods of fasting, or binge-purging behaviors. Indeed, research indicates that men with an extreme pursuit of muscularity (i.e., muscle dysmorphia) exhibit high levels of dietary restraint (e.g., caloric restriction, fasting), shape concern, and weight concern compared to controls [28]. The pursuit of leanness may also be typified through meticulous attention to and acute restriction of the intake of dietary carbohydrates [26, 29], and also cardiovascular exercise to expedite fat loss while preserving muscle [27]. Although at first blush this can appear counterintuitive for an individual wishing to put on weight (i.e., muscle mass), this indicates that individuals with a desire for muscularity may at times use thinness-oriented ED behaviors to enhance leanness to better showcase their muscles [3]. However, the simultaneous pursuit of muscle *growth* and *leanness* can be conflicting and counterproductive (e.g., consumption of calorie surplus for muscle *growth* vs. calorie deficit for *leanness*) [2, 3]. Consequently, those motivated to enhance muscle size and maximally reduce body fat may engage in rigid and prolonged "bulk and cut" dieting, which consists of alternating cyclic periods of distinct eating practices to "bulk" muscle size and "cut" body fat [2, 3]. However, the process of "cutting" and sometimes the extreme reduction of calorie intake, while beneficial for muscle definition, may curtail muscle growth and therefore promote muscularity concerns (and vice versa for "bulking" in terms of eliciting body fat concerns by virtue of increased caloric intake and body adiposity), potentially perpetuating this cycle of bulk-cut type of dieting [3, 30].

Although a paucity of research has purposively examined muscularity-oriented eating and related behaviors such as weight-lifting exercise, the available evidence indicates they are prevalent among male adolescents and adults. An earlier study among adolescent boys found that greater than 90% engaged in special exercise, and almost 70% reported special eating practices, exclusively aimed at improving muscularity [31]. Moreover, the study found that close to 35% of the boys in the study consumed protein powder/shakes, 6% reported using anabolic steroids, and over 10% had used other muscle-enhancing substances to improve muscularity during the past year (e.g., creatine, amino acids, growth hormones) [31]. Consistent with these findings, Yager et al. [32] found that, among 235 undergraduate men, 41% reported using protein shakes/snacks/powders, 18% used creatine supplements, and 4% had used anabolic steroids, all of which are well-recognized muscle-seeking behaviors. Recently, findings among a large sample of US adults ($n = 14,891$) found that 22% of men engage in muscularity-oriented eating behaviors, including eating greater volumes and special foods as well as taking dietary supplements [33]. Moreover, the study found that 7% used supplements for the purposes of expediting muscle growth, and almost 3% engaged in anabolic steroid use [33]. In a sample of almost 19,000 adolescents across the USA, 29% of boys reported weight gain attempts (vs. 7% of girls), while 25% of boys reported engaging in muscle-enhancing behaviors (vs. 4% of girls) [34]. Alongside the muscularity dissatisfaction experienced by scores of men, this preliminary research indicates the proclivity to engage in potentially harmful muscularity-change eating behaviors in parallel.

And while engagement in behaviors and consumption of legal substances (e.g., protein powder, creatine) aimed at enhancing muscularity may appear benign, research suggests these behaviors may in some capacity act as a gateway to illicit APEDs (e.g., anabolic-androgenic steroids). For instance, earlier cross-sectional research has found links between the use of fat loss (e.g., caffeine, ephedra) and muscle gain (e.g., protein powder, creatine) dietary supplements and higher endorsement of the efficacy and safety of illicit APED use, which is in turn predictive of the actual use of these substances [35]. Emerging work by Nagata and colleagues [36] builds on these findings through an examination of the prospective relationship between legal performance-enhancing substances and later steroid use. At one wave of the study, over 14,000 US adults aged 18–26 years were asked if they had used legal performance-enhancing substances (e.g., creatine) over the past year. Men who had responded in the affirmative were over three times as likely to have engaged in illicit anabolic-androgenic steroid use at a 7-year follow-up (no such prospective relationship was found for women), even after controlling for important covariates (e.g., age, ethnicity, body mass index). Indeed, research suggests a significant number of men are at risk of engaging in such unhealthy and illicit substance use to address muscularity concerns. For example, through the analysis of large national datasets, Pope and colleagues [37] estimate that 2.9–4.0 million Americans (virtually all men) have engaged in anabolic-androgenic steroid use. Together, this research provides compelling insight into the perhaps hidden dangers of seemingly 'healthy' muscularity-oriented body change behaviors and dietary substances.

Another particularly interesting and nascent dietary concept in the context muscularity is the 'cheat meal'. A cheat meal is typically earmarked by an excessive intake of calorie-ridden food(s) in a discrete time period (e.g., up to 9000+ calories) [38, 39]. This concept has largely been promoted and conveyed through image-centric social media platforms, with a search on Instagram of *#cheatmeal* yielding over 4 million posts (as of 3 March 2021). Due to its extreme calorie count and often times association with prohibited "junk" foods (e.g., burgers, pizza, fries), these meals typically represent a very brief intermission of one's otherwise rigid and carefully calculated dietary schedule [39]. However, while these sporadic influxes of high calories may seem inconsistent with one's pursuit of muscular leanness, these binge-type episodes may actually confer a positive benefit; to temporarily provides the body a metabolic advantage and expedite lean muscle growth [3, 39]. Specifically, it is believed these deluges of large and high calorie meals trick the body into processing dietary fats as a primary source of energy, where they remain for some time during subsequent periods of restriction and accelerate fat loss during this period as a result [39, 40]. Consistent with this notion, *#cheatmeal* social media images are almost four times more likely to be associated with an overtly muscular body than a slender physique [38]. Cheat meals may also be used to satisfy psychological and physical food cravings (e.g., these have been found to be the most important motivations for consuming cheat meals [40]), portending a greater subsequent compliance with one's strict, and in many cases banal, muscle-oriented dietary practices, as well as thoroughly replenishing energy stores to support intensive exercise [38, 40]. A thematic analysis of social media (Instagram) content related to cheat meals also highlights this dietary practice bears semblance to objective binge eating episodes in the context of bulimia nervosa [38]; that is, through the overconsumption of a large amount of food(s), a sense of lack of control over eating these foods, and engagement in immediate compensatory measures in response to the consumption of the cheat meal (e.g., dietary restraint, exercise to expunge ingested calories) [38]. Indeed, this is supported empirically, with Murray and colleagues [40] finding that 84% of men reported engaging in strenuous exercise, 64% restricted food consumption, and 22% vomited or used laxatives/diuretics after consuming a cheat meal. However, unlike with objective binge episodes, we have only a very limited understanding about what factors trigger engagement in cheat meals (e.g., emotional distress) or whether engagement itself is associated with psychological distress and/or psychosocial impairment [3]. Preliminary research suggests that, although partaking in cheat meal consumption is associated with ED pathology in men, it does not appear to be associated with significant distress or impairment (i.e., poor mental health-related quality of life) [40]. Rather, an analysis of cheat meal images that were accompanied by textual captions suggest this eating practice is associated with the idealization of food and the normalization of binge eating, as well as 'inspiring' users to commit to strict rule-driven dietary and exercise regimes (e.g., '*no pain no gain*' style of messages) [38]. Considering that scores of images depicting these meals tend to be accompanied by idealized defined muscular physiques, it is easy to conceive how one with preoccupations about being inadequately muscular may be allured to engage in such eating practices. Further research into this overlooked phenomenon is required to ascertain its clinical relevance in the context of male muscularity.

Empirically Assessing and Indexing Muscularity Concerns and Related Eating Pathology

The emerging research reviewed to this point suggests that, like the pursuit of thinness eliciting thinness-oriented eating pathology, the pursuit of the muscular body ideal is likely to manifest through a distinct array of eating behaviors aimed at improving one's muscular stature. However, as poignantly alluded to earlier, most ED research to date has focused predominantly on the presentation of symptoms among women. Consequently, the ways in which EDs are often conceptualized extrapolate from a female-centric diagnostic framework [2]. As a testament to this, cognitive-behavioral models typically conceptualize the development and maintenance of ED pathology in relation to an excessive drive for thinness, manifesting through core symptoms such as an incessant desire to lose weight, intense fear of becoming fat, and extended periods of fasting, to name a few [2]. However, the assumption underpinning these ED models largely derives from empirical and clinical research using females for whom the overvalued ideal appearance is one hallmarked by excessive thinness [2]. It remains actively debated how well such conceptualizations of EDs consider and account for the unique and broad spectrum of ED pathology in men for whom an overvaluation of lean and overt muscularity is more relevant [2].

Cognizant of this, the question is begged as to whether current ED assessment and diagnostic tools are adequate in fully capturing muscularity concerns and related ED pathology in males. Arguably the most widely recognized and utilized self-report measure in the ED field, the Eating Disorder Examination Questionnaire (EDE-Q; [41]), gauges core tenets of ED psychopathology (e.g., dissatisfaction with, and overvaluation of, one's weight and shape, extreme caloric restriction, preoccupation with appearance or food) for use in both male and female populations. Nonetheless, and merely as a point of example, certain items in the EDE-Q may lack sensitivity among men and the concomitant pursuit of muscularity [25]. For instance, the item "Have you had a definite desire to have a totally flat stomach?" may not map well onto muscularity concerns in men and their attendant pursuit of a bulging 'six-pack' of abdominal muscles. Items related to weight, for example, "Have you had a definite fear that you might gain weight?" may not be applicable to men who actually desire weight gain in the form of lean muscle mass [4, 25]. Another example is "How much would it have upset you if you had been asked to weigh yourself once a week (no more, or less, often) for the next four weeks?" where men and women may show similar concerns about being weighed, but perhaps for entirely different reasons (e.g., women believing they weigh too much, men believing they weigh too little). As such, high scores on this item may conflate thinness-and muscularity-oriented concerns in some men. Items related to thinness-oriented eating, such as "Have you had a definite desire to have an empty stomach with the aim of influencing your shape or weight?", would not capture the 'bulking' eating practices men may wish to employ to boost muscle growth. Further, while we commend the inclusion of muscularity-oriented eating items in other self-report measures, such as the Drive for Muscularity Scale (e.g., "I drink weight-gain or protein shakes"; [42]) and Eating Pathology Symptoms Inventory (e.g., "I used muscle building supplements"; [43]), these are not exhaustive and do not account for the broad spectrum of muscle-change eating behaviors one may exhibit. As such, while bearing clinical utility from the perspective of thinness-oriented eating pathology, many current "gold-standard" and recognized ED assessment tools may not be adequately capturing muscularity-oriented ED psychopathology [3, 25].

The recent development and publication of the Muscularity Oriented Eating Test (MOET) is an important advancement in addressing this caveat in the literature [23]. The brief questionnaire (15 items) is the first purposive instrument designed to index cognitive, affective, and behavioral aspects of (potentially) disordered eating practices related to the pursuit of muscularity. Items assessing cognitive components of muscularity-oriented disordered eating pathology include "What I ate has influenced how I think about myself as a person" and "I cannot achieve my body ideal unless I exert complete control over everything I eat"; items assessing affective components include "I have felt less anxious about eating out if I knew the macro-nutrient content of the food at the restaurant." Items which tap into behavioral facets of muscularity-oriented eating include "I have continued eating despite feeling full, in attempting to influence my muscularity" and "I have recorded the macro-nutritional values of everything that I ate." The MOET has been validated for use among US college men and demonstrates sound psychometric properties, including convergent validity (through correlations with recognized muscle dysmorphic disorder symptomatology and drive for muscularity scales), providing a unitary measure of muscularity-oriented eating pathology [23].

Emerging research also depicts the development of the Eating for Muscularity Scale (EMS; [44]). This self-report measure asks participants to rate how often 27 statements related to muscularity-oriented attitudes and behaviors applied to them over the past 28 days (4 weeks), building upon the MOET by providing an increasingly nuanced examination of muscularity-oriented eating. Here, EMS items form nine subscales: preoccupation (e.g., "I gave a lot of time and thought to becoming more muscular"), diet gain (e.g., "I must eat mostly protein-based foods [e.g., red meat, fish, chicken, etc.]"), diet loss (e.g., "I have eaten a low fat diet"), dietary restraint (e.g., "I felt forced to stick to my diet regime even when I was full"), excessive attention (e.g., "I have attempted to follow definite rules about my eating"), functional impairment (e.g., "I have given up important social events to maintain my diet schedule"), health risk (e.g., "I have used dieting methods that I know are unhealthy"), compensatory exercise (e.g., "I added extra exercise into my normal regime if I had eaten too many carbohydrates"), and negative affect (e.g., "I was uncomfortable if I was not able to prepare my meals and snacks in advance"). The EMS has been validated for use among men and women and demonstrates sound psychometric properties [44]. As a result, both the MOET and EMS are critical advancements in allowing us to index and therefore better understand muscularity-oriented disordered eating. Such measures will facilitate empirical research in relevant clinical populations and, by doing so, contribute to the discussion about how we might modify traditional ED conceptualizations and treatment practices to better address this unique form of ED pathology.

Directions for Future Research

Given that the concept of muscularity-oriented disordered eating has only recently garnered empirical and clinical attention, this necessitates multiple important directions for future research to help us understand the experience and treatment of this clinical phenomenon. First, from a theoretical perspective, careful consideration needs to be given to how and when a muscularity-oriented eating belief or behavior should be considered "disordered" or maladaptive [2, 23]. We reiterate here that muscularity-oriented behaviors are not inherently disordered and, in fact, in certain contexts, may be integrated as part of a healthy lifestyle [2]. For instance, consuming protein and taking protein supplements is not necessarily unhealthy; however, becoming highly distressed upon the prospect of running out of or not consuming sufficient protein would be. Counting the macronutrients of the food one consumes is not an intrinsically unhealthy practice; however, becoming markedly upset and/or refusing to eat all foods for which one does not know the precise macronutrient makeup of may be. Maintaining a special diet aimed at enhancing muscularity is not necessarily maladaptive; however, neglecting important social events or work commitments because they would interfere with one's rigid diet schedule would be. As such, the extent to which muscularity-oriented eating practices should be considered disordered is proportional to the distress and/or functional impairment they are associated with [2, 23]. However, given the infancy of research in this domain, we do not yet have a precise understanding of what clinically relevant muscularity-oriented disordered eating may entail [23]. This will likely be informed through future research examining such measures as the MOET and EMS in relevant clinical populations. These findings will likely also contribute to the establishment of benchmarks for MOET and EMS scores that will aid the identification of individuals engaging in or at an exacerbated risk of exhibiting muscularity-oriented disordered eating and related psychopathologies, such as muscle dysmorphia (Chap. 8) [23]. A related consideration next regards how best to incorporate this knowledge and components of such instruments into current "gold-standard" ED assessment and treatment tools to not only ensure the pathology can be accurately identified but then addressed in an effective and timely manner.

Second, we currently lack a treatment evidence base to help us specifically address muscularity-oriented disordered eating in men. This may be due to the fact that we have only begun examining this phenomenon, which is in stark contrast to the clinical attention which has been devoted to thinness-oriented pathology over the years. Despite this, inspiration for what these treatments may entail can be drawn from other related psychiatric domains. For instance, in treating a young male meeting diagnostic criteria for muscle dysmorphia, research demonstrated that a program largely consistent with family-based therapy [45, 46] was useful. Here, Murray and Griffiths [47] facilitated a parental intervention to ensure the afflicted 15-year-old adolescent did not heavily scrutinize and restrict his diet to only high-protein and low-calorie foods, but also attenuate other muscularity-oriented eating practices (e.g., "seasoning" food with protein powder instead of salt, distress if he could not eat every 3 hours) [47]. Here, the parents directly intervened to ensure previously feared foods were no longer avoided at both home and school, as well as to prevent other disordered eating practices (e.g., cutting the fat out of meats before consumption). In conjunction, the parents established strict limits on the patient's excessive and compensatory exercise practices (e.g., 45 minutes of cardiovascular exercise each morning, up to 75 minutes lifting weights nightly, continuing workouts when physically injured), which would only be relaxed if his anxiety and fear about eating certain foods diminished. At discharge, it was reported that no disordered eating practices were detected over the months prior, that the patient had improved control over his eating and exercise regimes, and that his unhealthy preoccupation with muscularity significantly subsided [47]. Although promising at first glance, this treatment case study needs to be extended to larger clinical populations with more robust designs, and its utility considered in light of its (likely) limited use among boys and adolescent males still living with their families or primary caregivers.

Cunningham et al. [48] provided an overview of other potential treatment approaches for muscle dysmorphia which may also bear utility in addressing muscularity-oriented disordered eating. For example, cognitive restructuring techniques may be used to dismantle the belief that masculinity is exclusively synonymous with hyper-muscularity. Indeed, research points to a close link between masculinity and the drive for muscularity [49–52] and subsequent muscle dysmorphia symptoms [53, 54], as well as weight gain attempts and related behaviors (including eating more, consuming food supplements to bulk up) [55]. Therefore, the pursuit to feel or be perceived as increasingly 'manly' and 'larger than life' may to some extent be driving one's engagement in muscularity-oriented eating. Moreover, therapies which specifically address problems of emotion regulation, such as dialectical behavior therapy (DBT) [56], may also be useful, especially if muscularity-oriented eating is theorized to be precipitated by aversive emotional experiences and an inability to adaptively regulate them (i.e., poor emotion regulation), as found among thinness-oriented eating disorders (e.g., anorexia nervosa; [57]). However, this is just speculation at this early stage - to our knowledge, there have been no purposive studies on the treatment of muscularity-oriented disordered eating in men, and only limited research on related psychiatric conditions in men (e.g., muscle dysmorphia, other EDs) [3, 48]. It is therefore imperative that further research aims to elucidate the utility of the aforementioned approaches (as well as others) for muscularity-oriented disordered eating among men.

A further complicating issue is that thinness-focused disordered eating pathology may even transition or evolve into muscularity-oriented pathology. Murray, Griffiths, Mitchison, and Mond [58] present a clinical case study in which a 14-year-old boy presented for treatment with anorexia nervosa, reporting core thinness-oriented pathology including a relentless drive for weight loss, an extreme restrictive dietary regime, and laxative abuse. The patient was treated with family-based therapy, with positive outcomes demonstrable through a relaxation of his previously strict and restrictive diet, an allayed drive for weight loss, and sufficient restoration of a 'healthy' weight. However, in parallel with the refeeding process to address his anorexia nervosa, and unbeknownst to clinicians, the patient experienced a covert and intensified drive for muscularity. At 6-month follow-up, the patient described himself as "too small" and consumed a strict high-protein diet to support muscle growth, became markedly distressed if he could not adhere to this diet, and engaged in strenuous muscle-building workouts. Regrettably, this drive for muscularity further evolved into a severe preoccupation with gaining weight and muscularity-oriented disordered eating which also warranted specialized treatment. At this point, the patient described the intensity of his pursuit of muscularity as "100/100," while the intensity of his drive for thinness had seemingly diminished completely (being described as "0/100" by the patient) [58]. Together, these findings demonstrate the potential for thinness- and muscularity-oriented psychopathology to crossover, emphasizing the importance of continual monitoring of how the latter may evolve when assessing and treating the former (e.g., anorexia nervosa). With this in mind, it becomes even more crucial that ED treatment tools be adapted to better detect muscularity-oriented pathology and related eating practices.

Summary and Conclusion

To date, men have suffered a systemic inattention in the ED field. Consequently, our knowledge about the presentation of EDs in men largely derives from the research and treatment of EDs in women. However, men and women typically aspire to attain vastly different body types that are likely to beget distinct arrays of eating pathology. Specifically, men tend to be motivated to achieve an increasingly muscular body, which polarizes the overtly thin body ideal pursued by many women. Regrettably, the predominant empirical and clinical focus of ED research on women and the pursuit of thinness means we lack a comprehensive conceptualization of how ED behaviors manifest in men through the pursuit of muscularity.

This chapter synthesized the available literature to underscore what we currently understand about muscularity-oriented disordered eating among men. First, we describe the muscular ideal pursued by a diverse range of male populations and the levels of body (and muscle) dissatisfaction this pursuit is likely to engender. Second, we highlight the distinct profile of eating behaviors men may be likely to engage in to move themselves closer to reaching this muscular ideal, including frequent and excessive consumption of protein and rigid rules around eating (e.g., "meal prep"). Third, we highlight issues associated with current ED assessment tools in adequately gauging muscularity-oriented eating pathology, as most have been developed through the lens of thinness-oriented eating pathology. Fortunately, with the recent advent of dedicated and purposive muscularity-oriented eating measures [23, 44], we can advance the discussion about how existing ED measures and tools may be modified to better capture muscularity-related eating and pathology. We close this chapter with a call for future research to continue examining muscularity-oriented eating, in particular how it manifests in relevant clinical samples (e.g., individuals with muscle dysmorphia) and precisely how we might leverage emerging knowledge in this domain to update current best practice ED tools and efforts to address this clinical phenomenon.

References

1. Murray SB, Griffiths S, Mond JM. Evolving eating disorder psychopathology: conceptualising muscularity-oriented disordered eating. Br J Psychiatry. 2016;208(5):414–5.
2. Murray SB, Nagata JM, Griffiths S, Calzo JP, Brown TA, Mitchison D, et al. The enigma of male eating disorders: a critical review and synthesis. Clin Psychol Rev [Internet]. 2017;57:1–11. Available from: https://www.sciencedirect.com/science/article/pii/S027273581730137X
3. Lavender JM, Brown TA, Murray SB. Men, muscles, and eating disorders: an overview of traditional and muscularity-oriented disordered eating. Curr Psychiatry Rep. 2017;19(6):1.
4. Pope HG, Phillips KA, Olivardia R. The Adonis Complex: The secret crisis of male body obsession. New York: The Free Press; 2000.
5. Nagata JM, Golden NH. Sex differences in eating disorders. Adolesc Med State Art Rev. 2018;29:245–59.
6. Murray SB, Accurso EC, Griffiths S, Nagata JM. Boys, biceps, and bradycardia: the hidden dangers of muscularity-oriented disordered eating. J Adolesc Health. 2018;62(3):352–5. Available from: http://www.ncbi.nlm.nih.gov/pubmed/29241987.
7. Nagata JM, Carlson JL, Kao JM, Golden NH, Murray SB, Peebles R. Characterization and correlates of exercise among adolescents with anorexia nervosa and bulimia nervosa. Int J Eat Disord. 2017;50(12):1394–403. Available from: http://www.ncbi.nlm.nih.gov/pubmed/29112280.
8. in Sport IOCMCWGW. International Olympic Committee Medical Commission Position Stand on the Female Athlete Triad. 2005.
9. Mountjoy M, Sundgot-Borgen J, Burke L, Carter S, Constantini N, Lebrun C, et al. The IOC consensus statement: beyond the female athlete triad–relative energy deficiency in sport (RED-S). Br J Sports Med. 2014;48(7):491–7.
10. Nagata JM, Peebles R, Hill KB, Gorrell S, Carlson JL. Associations between erogenic supplement use and eating behaviors among university students. Eat Disord. 2020. Advanced online publication.
11. Or F, Kim Y, Simms J, Austin SB. Taking stock of dietary supplements' harmful effects on children, adolescents, and young adults. J Adolesc Heal Off Publ Soc Adolesc Med. 2019; 65(4):455–61.

12. Pope HG Jr, Wood RI, Rogol A, Nyberg F, Bowers L, Bhasin S. Adverse health consequences of performance-enhancing drugs: an Endocrine Society scientific statement. Endocr Rev. 2014;35(3):341–75.
13. Abbate V, Kicman AT, Evans-Brown M, Mcveigh J, Cowan DA, Wilson C, et al. Anabolic steroids detected in bodybuilding dietary supplements – a significant risk to public health. Drug Test Anal. 2015;7(7):609–18.
14. Cafri G, Thompson J, Ricciardelli L, Mccabe M, Smolak L, Yesalis C. Pursuit of the muscular ideal: physical and psychological consequences and putative risk factors. Clin Psychol Rev. 2005;25(2):215–39.
15. Leit RA, Gray JJ, Pope HG. The media's representation of the ideal male body: a cause for muscle dysmorphia? Int J Eat Disord. 2002;31(3):334–8.
16. Frederick DA, Buchanan GM, Sadehgi-Azar L, Peplau LA, Haselton MG, Berezovskaya A, et al. Desiring the muscular ideal: men's body satisfaction in the United States, Ukraine, and Ghana. Psychol Men Masculinity. 2007;8(2):103–17.
17. Ridgeway RT, Tylka TL. College men's perceptions of ideal body composition and shape. Psychol Men Masculinity. 2005;6(3):209–20.
18. Leit RA, Pope HG, Gray JJ. Cultural expectations of muscularity in men: the evolution of playgirl centerfolds. Int J Eat Disord. 2000;29(1):90–3.
19. Tiggemann M, Zaccardo M. 'Strong is the new skinny': a content analysis of #fitspiration images on Instagram. J Health Psychol. 2016;23(8):1003–11.
20. Frederick DA, Garcia JR, Gesselman AN, Mark KP, Hatfield E, Bohrnstedt G. The happy American body 2.0: predictors of affective body satisfaction in two U.S. national internet panel surveys. Body Image. 2020;32:70–84.
21. Nagata JM, Bibbins-Domingo K, Garber AK, Griffiths S, Vittinghoff E, Murray SB. Boys, bulk, and body ideals: sex differences in weight-gain attempts among adolescents in the United States. J Adolesc Health. 2019;64(4):450–3.
22. McLean SA, Wertheim EH, Paxton SJ. Preferences for being muscular and thin in 6-year-old boys. Body Image. 2018;26:98–102.
23. Murray SB, Brown TA, Blashill AJ, Compte EJ, Lavender JM, Mitchison D, et al. The development and validation of the muscularity-oriented eating test: a novel measure of muscularity oriented disordered eating. Int J Eat Disord. 2019;52(12):1389–98.
24. Tylka TL. Refinement of the tripartite influence model for men: dual body image pathways to body change behaviors. Body Image. 2011;8(3):199–207.
25. Griffiths S, Murray SB, Touyz S. Disordered eating and the muscular ideal. J Eat Disord. 2013;1(1):1.
26. Mosley PE. Bigorexia: bodybuilding and muscle dysmorphia. Eur Eat Disord Rev. 2009;17(3):191–8.
27. Murray SB, Rieger E, Touyz SW. Muscle dysmorphia symptomatology during a period of religious fasting: a case report. Eur Eat Disord Rev. 2011;19(2):162–8.
28. Murray SB, Rieger E, Hildebrandt T, Karlov L, Russell J, Boon E, et al. A comparison of eating, exercise, shape, and weight related symptomatology in males with muscle dysmorphia and anorexia nervosa. Body Image. 2012;9(2):193–200.
29. Murray SB, Maguire S, Russell J, Touyz SW. The emotional regulatory features of bulimic episodes and compulsive exercise in muscle dysmorphia: a case report. Eur Eat Disord Rev. 2012;20(1):68–73.
30. Gorrell S, Murray SB. Eating disorders in males. Child Adolesc Psychiatr Clin N Am. 2019;28:641–51.
31. Eisenberg MA, Wall M, Neumark-Sztainer D. Muscle-enhancing behaviors among adolescent girls and boys. Pediatrics. 2012;130(6):X4.
32. Yager Z, Gray T, Curry C, McLean SA. Body dissatisfaction, excessive exercise, and weight change strategies used by first-year undergraduate students: comparing health and physical education and other education students. J Eat Disord. 2017;3:5. Available from: https://www.ncbi.nlm.nih.gov/pmc/articles/PMC5376693/

33. Nagata JM, Murray SB, Bibbins-Domingo K, Garber AK, Mitchison D, Griffiths S. Predictors of muscularity-oriented disordered eating behaviors in U.S. young adults: a prospective cohort study. Int J Eat Disord. 2019;52(12):1380–8. Available from: https://www.ncbi.nlm.nih.gov/pubmed/31220361.
34. Nagata JM, Ganson KT, Griffiths S, Mitchison D, Garber AK, Vittinghoff E, Bibbins-Domingo K, Murray SB. Prevalence and correlates of muscle-enhancing behaviors among adolescents and young adults in the United States. Int J Adolesc Med Health. 2020. Advanced online publication.
35. Hildebrandt T, Harty S, Langenbucher JW. Fitness supplements as a gateway substance for anabolic-androgenic steroid use. Psychol Addict Behav. 2012;26(4):955–62.
36. Nagata JM, Ganson KT, Gorrell S, Mitchison D, Murray SB. Association between legal performance-enhancing substances and use of anabolic-androgenic steroids in young adults. JAMA Pediatrics. 2020;174(10):992–3.
37. Pope HG, Kanayama G, Athey A, Ryan E, Hudson JI, Baggish A. The lifetime prevalence of anabolic-androgenic steroid use and dependence in Americans: current best estimates. Am J Addict. 2014;23(4):371–7.
38. Pila E, Mond JM, Griffiths S, Mitchison D, Murray SB. A thematic content analysis of #cheatmeal images on social media: characterizing an emerging dietary trend. Int J Eat Disord. 2017;50(6):698–706.
39. Murray SB, Griffiths S, Hazery L, Shen T, Wooldridge T, Mond JM. Go big or go home: a thematic content analysis of pro-muscularity websites. Body Image. 2016;16:17–20.
40. Murray SB, Pila E, Mond JM, Mitchison D, Blashill AJ, Sabiston CM, et al. Cheat meals: a benign or ominous variant of binge eating behavior? Appetite. 2018;130:274–8. Available from: https://www.sciencedirect.com/science/article/pii/S0195666318306275
41. Fairburn CG, Beglin SJ. Assessment of eating disorders: interview or self-report questionnaire? Int J Eat Disord. 1994;16:363–70.
42. McCreary DR, Sasse DK. An exploration of the drive for muscularity in adolescent boys and girls. J Am Coll Heal. 2000;48(6):297–304.
43. Forbush KT, Wildes JE, Pollack LO, Dunbar D, Luo J, Patterson K, et al. Development and validation of the eating pathology symptoms inventory (EPSI). Psychol Assess. 2013;25(3):859–78.
44. Cooper M, Griffiths KM, Burns R. Getting shredded: development and validation of a measure of muscularity-oriented disordered eating. Psychol Assess. 2020;32(5):451–60.
45. Le Grange D, Lock J, Loeb K, Nicholls D. Academy for eating disorders position paper: the role of the family in eating disorders. Int J Eat Disord. 2009;43(1):1–5.
46. Lock J, Le Grange D. Treatment manual for anorexia nervosa : a family-based approach. New York: Guilford Press; 2015.
47. Murray SB, Griffiths S. Adolescent muscle dysmorphia and family-based treatment: a case report. Clin Child Psychol Psychiatry. 2014;20(2):324–30.
48. Cunningham ML, Griffiths S, Mitchison D, Mond JM, Castle D, Murray SB. Muscle dysmorphia: an overview of clinical features and treatment options. J Cogn Psychother. 2017;31(4):255–71.
49. Blashill AJ. Gender roles, eating pathology, and body dissatisfaction in men: a meta-analysis. Body Image. 2011;8(1):1–11.
50. Griffiths S, Murray SB, Touyz S. Extending the masculinity hypothesis: an investigation of gender role conformity, body dissatisfaction, and disordered eating in young heterosexual men. Psychol Men Masculinity. 2015;16(1):108–14.
51. Mishkind ME, Rodin J, Silberstein LR, Striegel-Moore RH. The embodiment of masculinity. Am Behav Sci. 1986;29(5):545–62.
52. Cunningham ML, Nagata JM, Frederick D, Rodgers RF, Lavender JM, Szabo M, Murray SB. Who's the 'bigger' man? Parsing the relationships between masculinity and men's muscularity dissatisfaction. Body Image. 2020;34:94–100.

53. Cunningham ML, Rodgers RL, Lavender JM, Nagata JM, Frederick D, Szabo M, Murray SB. 'Big boys don't cry': Examining the indirect pathway of masculinity discrepancy stress and muscle dysmorphia symptomatology through dimensions of emotion dysregulation. Body Image. 2020;34:209–14.
54. Murray SB, Rieger E, Karlov L, Touyz SW. Masculinity and femininity in the divergence of male body image concerns. J Eat Disord. 2013;1:1.
55. Nagata JM, Domingue BW, Darmstadt GL, Weber AM, Meausoone V, Cislaghi B, et al. Gender norms and weight control behaviors in U.S. adolescents: a prospective cohort study (1994–2002). J Adolesc Health. 2020;66(1):S34–41.
56. Linehan MM. Cognitive-behavioral treatment of borderline personality disorder. New York: Guilford Press; 1993.
57. Lavender JM, Wonderlich SA, Engel SG, Gordon KH, Kaye WH, Mitchell JE. Dimensions of emotion dysregulation in anorexia nervosa and bulimia nervosa: a conceptual review of the empirical literature. Clin Psychol Rev. 2015;40:111–22.
58. Murray SB, Griffiths S, Mitchison D, Mond JM. The transition from thinness-oriented to muscularity-oriented disordered eating in adolescent males: a clinical observation. J Adolesc Health. 2017;60(3):353–5.

Chapter 4
Epidemiology of Eating Disorders in Boys and Men

Nora Trompeter, Kay Bussey, and Deborah Mitchison

Learning Objectives

1. Understand the prevalence and distribution of eating disorders among men and how this differs to that of women.
2. Understand the shared and unique (e.g., stigma associated with identifying as a boy or man with an eating disorder) individual and community burden caused by eating disorders in men.
3. Recognize the complexity of comorbidity and treatment-seeking for an eating disorder, which is particularly relevant for men.

Key Points

- Eating disorders affect around 5–10% of adolescent boys and 2% of adult men.
- Eating disorders tend to be more common in adolescents and younger men, compared to older men; however, they can occur at any age.
- Men with eating disorders face significant impairment in terms of quality of life and comorbid psychological disorders, in particular anxiety and depression.
- Treatment-seeking among men with eating disorders is low and likely is related to stigmatization.

N. Trompeter · K. Bussey
Centre for Emotional Health, Department of Psychology, Macquarie University, Sydney, NSW, Australia

D. Mitchison (✉)
Centre for Emotional Health, Department of Psychology, Macquarie University, Sydney, NSW, Australia

Translational Health Research Institute, School of Medicine, Western Sydney University, Sydney, NSW, Australia
e-mail: deborah.mitchison@westernsydney.edu.au

J. M. Nagata et al. (eds.), *Eating Disorders in Boys and Men*,
https://doi.org/10.1007/978-3-030-67127-3_4

Introduction

This chapter aims to give an overview of the epidemiology of eating disorders as they occur in boys and men. Epidemiology includes information about the distribution, patterns, and outcomes of health conditions and is crucial in understanding these conditions. Furthermore, knowing the impact of health conditions, such as eating disorders, provides important information for evidence-based practice and public health policy-makers. Early research on eating disorders posed that eating disorders only affect young women from affluent societies [1]. However, research has now shown that this is not the case. It is clear that eating disorders affect men, as well as women [2, 3]. This chapter will cover how common eating disorders and eating disorder symptoms are in adolescent boys and men and how these disorders are distributed in terms of demographic characteristics [age, socioeconomic status (SES), ethnic groups, sexual orientation, and gender identity]. The burden and impairment of eating disorders will be discussed, in regard to impact on mental, physical, social, and occupational functioning, taking into account comorbidity with other mental health issues. Lastly, treatment-seeking among men with eating disorders will be summarized.

The chapter aims to highlight that eating disorders and eating disorder symptoms are not uncommon in boys and men, despite popular perceptions, and that the burden and impairment of these disorders are similar to that observed among women with these problems. Thus, while more women are affected by eating disorders, once eating disorders have developed, they do not discriminate in terms of impairment. Moreover, the epidemiology of muscularity concerns and associated sequelae and how this relates to eating disorders in boys and men will be explored. Where appropriate and the availability of literature allows, parallels and comparisons with girls and women will be drawn.

Prevalence

Prevalence refers to the proportion of a particular population, in this case men, who are affected by a health condition, in this case eating disorders. To better understand the prevalence of eating disorders among men, prevalence rates of both disordered eating symptoms and eating disorders are presented below.

Disorders

Eating disorders typically have an onset during late adolescence for both boys and girls [4], with anorexia nervosa having the earliest onset, while binge eating disorder has the latest onset for both sexes. Indeed, research on cumulative prevalence has found that among men, new incidents of anorexia nervosa and bulimia nervosa reach a plateau by 20–21 years of age [5], indicating that most men develop an eating disorder during adolescence or early adulthood. Among adolescents, findings have shown that around 5% of boys meet criteria for an eating disorder at any one time [6].

Anorexia Nervosa

Anorexia nervosa is rare among men, especially compared to women [7]. While some boys meet criteria for anorexia nervosa during early childhood [8], few adolescents or adults meet criteria for the disorder. However, it is unclear whether this discrepancy is due to pathological differences whereby men are unlikely to develop anorexia nervosa or whether differences might be due to gender biases in diagnostic criteria. It is only in the most recent version of the *Diagnostic and Statistical Manual of Mental Disorders* (DSM) that the criterion for amenorrhea, for instance, was dropped, which had complicated application of the diagnosis among boys and men [11]. Thus, population-based research using the DSM-IV may have underestimated the rate of anorexia nervosa among men. Indeed, applying DSM-5 criteria as opposed to DSM-IV among adults more broadly was observed to lead to a 12% increase in anorexia nervosa prevalence in recent research comparing the two classification versions [12]. However, research looking at differences in diagnostic criteria among adolescent boys found no difference between the versions in regard to anorexia nervosa, as neither version detected any boys meeting criteria in the sample used [10, 13].

Bulimia Nervosa

Bulimia nervosa has been found to affect around 1–2% of men [3, 4, 14]. These rates are fairly consistent across studies and across age groups, with adolescent boys reporting similar prevalence rates of bulimia nervosa to that of adult men [3, 6].

Binge Eating Disorder

Compared to other major eating disorders, research on the whole suggests that men are most likely to meet criteria for binge eating disorder. Among adults binge eating disorder affects around 0.4% of men at any one time [15], with a lifetime prevalence of 2% [4]. Binge eating disorder has only been added to the DSM-5 in its most recent version, having previous been classified as an "Eating disorder not otherwise specified" (EDNOS) [16]. Thus population-based studies prior to the release of

DSM-5 may have underestimated the prevalence of eating disorders among men or failed to capture the prevalence of binge eating disorder in men, if this was only captured alongside other eating disorders that fall under the EDNOS umbrella.

Otherwise Specified Feeding/Eating Disorders and Unspecified Feeding/Eating Disorder

Alongside the major disorders, the DSM-5 includes residual diagnostic categories to capture clinical cases that do not quite fit the criteria for the major listed mental disorders. However, while this category is meant for residual cases, most men with an eating disorder are diagnosed with Otherwise specified feeding/eating disorders (OSFED) [16, 17], which encompass a range of syndromes that classifies people who experience symptoms of a major eating disorder, but do not meet the full criteria for diagnosis of these disorders [11]. Prior to 2013, this was previously classified as EDNOS in the DSM-IV, leading to fewer prevalence studies using the updated diagnostic criteria. A recent prevalence study with Australian adolescents (see Fig. 4.1), however, revealed that 8.5% of adolescent boys meet criteria for OSFED, most commonly for night eating syndrome (4.8%) [3]. Similarly, among adolescents accessing treatment for an eating disorder, 62% are diagnosed with OSFED [17]. However, more prevalence data is needed on these disorders to fully assess their prevalence among boys and men.

Another understudied eating disorder in regard to prevalence is unspecified feeding/eating disorder (UFED), an eating disorder that is characterized by significant disordered eating and body image concerns, which are not captured in any other disorder or syndrome [10]. Among Australian adolescents, 1.3% of boys meet criteria for UFED [3].

Muscle Dysmorphia

Muscle dysmorphia is a fairly new disorder in the eating disorder field, which is being regarded as particularly relevant for boys and men and is currently included as a subtype of body dysmorphic disorder in the DSM-5 [11]. However, due to its similarity to eating disorders in regard to concerns about overall body shape and weight and extreme dietary and exercise behaviors [18], there is a debate that it should be included as an eating disorder [2]. No nationally representative studies have investigated the prevalence of muscle dysmorphia. However, an epidemiological study among young men in South America found that almost half (42.37%) of men were classified as "at risk" for muscle dysmorphia, compared with only 3.8% of men who were classified as "at risk" for an eating disorder [19]. Furthermore,

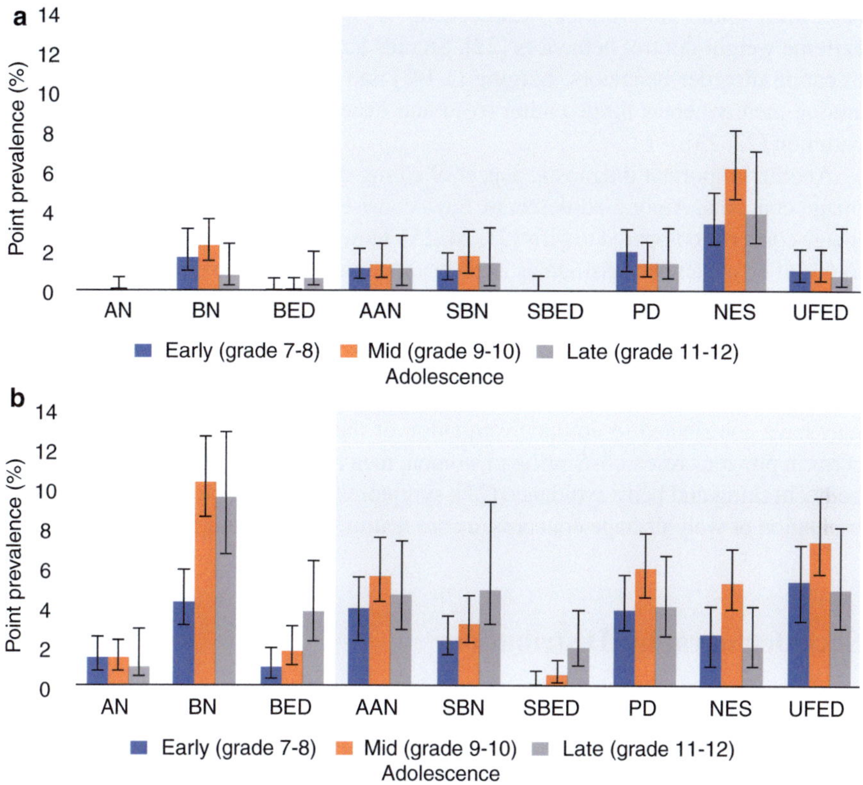

Fig. 4.1 Point prevalence of DSM-5 eating disorders in adolescent (**a**) boys and (**b**) girls. Shaded area indicates other specified and unspecified feeding and eating disorders. AN, anorexia nervosa; BN, probable bulimia nervosa; BED, probable binge eating disorder; AAN, atypical anorexia nervosa; SBN, subthreshold bulimia nervosa; SBED, subthreshold binge eating disorder; PD, purging disorder; NES, night eating syndrome; UFED, unspecified feeding or eating disorder. (Source: Reprinted with permission from Mitchison D, Mond J, Bussey K, Griffiths S, Trompeter N, Lonergan A, et al. (2019), p. 6, Fig. 4.1)

research in adolescents found that of the 1.8% of boys who met criteria for body dysmorphic disorder, 44% reported primary appearance concerns regarding their muscularity [20].

Disordered Eating Symptoms

In regard to disordered eating symptoms (e.g., dietary restraint, purging, binge eating, excessive exercise), boys less commonly exhibit disordered eating symptoms compared to girls, with the exception of driven exercise [21]. Similar differences have been found among men; however, up to 30% of men frequently engage in extreme weight-control behaviors [22]. Studies have typically shown that in regard to eating disorder behaviors, purging (1.1%) and dietary restraint (3.4%) are rare among men, whereas binge eating (6%) and excessive exercise (20.7%) are more common [22, 23].

Another important diagnostic aspect of eating disorder psychopathology is body image concerns. Among adolescents, boys consistently report lower levels of body image concerns compared to girls [21, 24, 25]. However, despite these differences, up to 6% of boys can be classified as experiencing clinical levels of body image disturbances by age 22 [26]. Importantly, while body image concerns in girls are typically centered around a drive for thinness, boys are more typically concerned with a drive for muscularity [27]. Thus, while fewer men might report issues regarding a drive for thinness, they could instead experience issues with a drive for muscularity, which may have contributed to an underestimation of the prevalence of body image concerns in previous research. Similar to women, men have also been found to engage in body checking and body avoidance [27], symptoms that commonly indicate an overevaluation of weight/shape concerns, a core feature of most eating disorders [11].

Sociodemographic Distribution

As is the case for women, the characteristics of men with eating disorders are broader than once thought in terms of demographic diversity. The sections below examine eating disorders among boys and men in regard to differences in age, SES, and ethnicity. Furthermore, as recent research has highlighted that eating disorders may be more common in sexual minority men as opposed to heterosexual men, as well as transgender men compared to cisgender men [28], the distribution of eating disorders related to sexual orientation and gender non-conforming boys and men will be discussed.

Age

Eating disorders commonly have an onset during late adolescence and tend to affect younger men more commonly than older men [4]. Anorexia nervosa tends to have the earliest onset compared to other eating disorders [4], with boys aged 15–19 years of age reporting the highest incidences compared to other age groups [28]. During adolescence, there is a steady increase in risk of eating disorders with disordered eating behaviors increasing linearly from younger to older boys [29].

While eating disorders tend to peak in early adulthood [30], they typically run a long and protracted course and occur throughout the lifespan [4]. They have been found to affect 0.02% of older (i.e., >40 years) men [31].

See Chap. 21 for further discussion on eating disorders and body image concerns among men across the lifespan.

SES

Research on binge eating disorder has found no significant differences in prevalence rates of the disorder between low-income and high-income countries [15]. This is in line with research on binge eating more broadly, which found that men who engage in regular binge eating did not differ from those who did not binge eat in terms of education status [32]. However, research among Australian adults found that men with binge eating disorder did have lower incomes than men without an eating disorder [33]. Looking at eating disorders more broadly, Australian prevalence research among adolescents found no effect of SES on current eating disorder status, when controlling for age, gender, and BMI status [3]. As a modifiable demographic factor, it is conceivable that SES status may also be influenced by the eating disorder itself (e.g., through loss of capacity to study or work). Longitudinal studies investigating the personal economic burden of eating disorders are required to examine this further.

Considering eating disorders more broadly across the Australian population (including men), research has found that household income was not related to eating disorder symptoms [34]. However, this study did not examine the effects on men separately. On the other hand, a recent study in Switzerland has found that young men at risk for disordered eating were more likely to come from a lower socioeconomic background than their peers [35]. More international research is required to examine the distribution of eating disorders and disordered eating across SES in men.

Ethnicity

Prevalence rates of eating disorders in different ethnic groups generally show similar patterns among men in the United States (USA) [9, 14, 36, 37]. Moreover, research among ethnically diverse American men showed that ethnicity was not related to eating disorder prevalence [36]. Less is known about the role of ethnicity in non-Western countries and developing countries nor eating disorders among indigenous men from different world regions. Research among American Indian/Native American adults suggests that there were no differences in terms of disordered eating symptoms between American Indian/Native American men and white men [38]. On the other hand, recent research among Australian adolescents suggests that First Australians have higher rates of eating disorders compared to other Australians. However, much more research is needed in this area, especially in regard to Indigenous populations within other world regions.

See Chap. 15 for further discussion on racial and ethnic considerations regarding eating disorders and body image concerns among men.

Sexual Orientation

Increasing research shows that homosexual and bisexual men have higher levels of body image concerns and are at greater risk for eating disorders compared to heterosexual men [39, 40]. More specifically, a recent US study revealed that 0.55% of cisgender heterosexual men report having an eating disorder in the past year, whereas 2.06% of cisgender sexual minority men reported an eating disorder within the previous year [40]. Moreover, homosexual and bisexual men report greater objectification and appearance-based social comparisons than heterosexual men [41], key risk factors for increased body dissatisfaction and hence eating disorders.

See Chap. 17 for further discussion on eating disorders and body image concerns among sexual minority men.

Gender Identity

Research among transgender men has further pointed to this population being at increased risk for eating disorders. Transgender men have been found to have higher rates of eating disorders compared to cisgender men [40, 42]. Among adolescents, transmasculine youth prevalence rates of eating disorders were six times higher compared to cisgender adolescent boys [43]. Additionally, disordered eating behaviors may functionally serve as a mechanism to disrupt unwanted biological gender expression (e.g., breast development) in transgender boys and men [44]. While little research has been conducted in this area, there is evidence to suggest that body image concerns among transgender boys may be mitigated by puberty suppression and gender reassignment [45].

See Chap. 18 for further discussion on gender identity in relation to eating disorders and body image concerns.

Impairment/Burden

Within epidemiology, impairment refers to the impact on functioning and quality of life of a health condition (i.e., eating disorders), whereas burden describes the impact of the health condition on society more broadly by taking into account both prevalence and impairment. Thus, information on impairment of eating disorders on men gives insight into the personal impact of the disorder/symptoms on daily functioning and quality of life, as well as how this impacts society as a whole.

Disorders

Eating disorders are associated with significant impairment for individuals, mostly relating to their quality of life. Research has consistently shown that men with eating disorders report poorer health-related quality of life than men without eating disorders [46]. Specifically, whereas 97.8% of men without eating disorders reported being satisfied with life, only 87.1% of men with eating disorders reported being satisfied with life [7].

Eating disorders are further associated with increased societal burden, whereby OSFED disorders have been shown to have the highest burden among Australian men [47]. This burden on society can in part be explained by the impairment of eating disorders on daily functioning. For example, research consistently shows that men with eating disorders have more sick days than their peers (e.g., 2.3 vs 1.8 days/year for men who binge eat vs those who do not) [32, 33]. Furthermore, these disorders often require extensive treatment leading to increased service use [46]. Men have been found to receive less treatment compared to women and thus have lower treatment costs; however, this likely contributes to a more protracted illness and increased personal burden, and treatment costs were still found to be higher than that of certain other mental health disorders [48].

Eating disorders are generally associated with an increased mortality risk [49, 50] due to both medical complications and suicide [51, 52]. Research among adults with eating disorders found a crude mortality of around 4% among patients with anorexia nervosa, whereas patients with bulimia nervosa had the lowest mortality rate [49]. Indeed, men with eating disorders are typically at higher risk for suicide attempts (up to 7.4 times) compared to men without eating disorders [30]. No studies have compared the mortality associated with eating disorders between men and women.

Disordered Eating Symptoms

Eating disorders and symptoms cause affected individuals serious distress [21, 53] and are associated with significant impairment to those individuals [23, 32]. In terms of eating disorder symptoms, research among adolescents has found that disordered eating was associated with negative physical and mental health outcomes [20, 51]. Similar findings have emerged for body dissatisfaction [23]. Importantly, these studies have shown that genders do not differ in terms of impairment. Among adults, disordered eating has been linked to functional impairment, in regard to both personal activities and work activities [23, 32].

This impairment of individuals adds a significant burden to society as a whole. For example, in 2012, Deloitte reported that in Australia, eating disorders had a total annual socioeconomic cost of $ 69.7 billion Australian dollars [54].

Comorbidity

Men with eating disorders often experience other mental health concerns as well. One common comorbidity in men with eating disorders is anxiety [7, 17, 55]. While the overlap between anxiety and eating disorders is well-established [4], research suggests that men, in particular, may be at risk for anxiety disorders if they also experience an eating disorder [56]. In particular, men with obsessive-compulsive disorder nervosa have a 37 times higher risk of having a comorbid diagnosis of anorexia nervosa compared to those without obsessive-compulsive disorder. Moreover, men with eating disorders are more likely to experience depression than their peers (14.5% vs 5.0% of lifetime diagnosis) [7]. Similarly, among treatment-seeking boys with an eating disorder, 18.6% also presented with a comorbid mood disorder [17]. Furthermore, prospective research has shown that men who experience eating disorder symptoms, especially those with thinness concerns and bulimic behaviors, were at risk for subsequent depressive symptoms [57].

Men who experience muscularity concerns are also at an increased risk for drug use [19, 26, 57], including substances that will increase muscularity, such as anabolic steroids, but also other illicit drugs. Alarmingly, this has also been found in adolescent boys, with 3.2% of adolescent boys reporting "often" (and a further 6.8% "sometimes") taking steroids or other muscle-enhancing substances to build muscle mass [58]. This type of drug use is particularly relevant for men, as body image concerns typically center around issues with muscularity, rather than thinness [57]. Importantly, these substances have been linked with serious health problems (e.g., liver damage, gastrointestinal distress), whereby using supplements for muscle building or weight loss is associated with almost three times the risk for severe medical events when compared with using vitamins [59, 60].

The exact cause of these comorbidities is unknown. Thus, other mental health concerns may precede eating disorder onset, they could be a cause of the eating disorder, or the disorders could share a common vulnerability. While much research points toward a shared vulnerability model [61, 62], most studies, being cross-sectional in nature, have been unable to investigate this fully.

Treatment-Seeking

Treatment-seeking for eating disorders is generally low [63] and especially low for men [64–66]. Men report significantly lower rates of both wanting treatment (2%) and accessing treatment (1%) compared to women [67]. Similarly, among adolescents only 6.8% boys reported seeking help for an eating disorder [68]. This is significantly lower compared to other mental health disorders, such as depression (36.5%) or anxiety (14.5%) [64].

This lack of treatment-seeking may be due to both lower mental health literacy among individuals and gender biases within treatment settings [69, 70]. Mental health literacy research has shown that people generally associate eating disorders with women and men might be less likely than women to identify themselves as having an eating disorder [71, 72]. Furthermore, public health campaigns and treatment services are often aimed at women and girls, leaving men underrepresented [70]. This leads to a "double burden" of stigma given the documented stigma associated with eating disorders in general, which act alongside other more practical issues as a further barrier to treatment-seeking (e.g., stigma, cost) [73].

Conclusion

This chapter highlighted that eating disorders are a serious concern for men, especially adolescent boys and young adult men. Estimates of prevalence are highest when considering the full spectrum of typical, atypical, and muscularity-oriented eating disorder presentations. Eating disorders and eating disorder symptoms cause men significant impairment, including increased risk for other mental health and substance use problems, for which they rarely receive adequate treatment. Thus, governments and other stakeholders should prioritize the allocation of resources toward the prevention and treatment of these disorders – which carry a significant burden for the population of boys and men (as well as girls and women). Further, clinicians and general practitioners should screen for eating disorders among boys and men as they would among girls and women.

These issues have important implications for clinical settings, in which it is important to enable treatment-seeking among men from various backgrounds by gearing treatment services toward these groups. Furthermore, public health campaigns should be mindful of the prevalence of eating disorders occurring in boys and men to increase mental health literacy of eating disorders. This might be particularly relevant for school-based programs, as they are able to provide valuable information to adolescents and simultaneously reduce the stigma around eating disorders.

References

1. Anderson W. Eating disorders: obesity, anorexia nervosa and the person within. Soc Sci Med. 1974;8(4):213.
2. Murray SB, Nagata JM, Griffiths S, Calzo JP, Brown TA, Mitchison D, et al. The enigma of male eating disorders: a critical review and synthesis [Internet]. Vol. 57, Clinical Psychology Review. Pergamon; 2017 [cited 2019 Oct 28]. p. 1–11. Available from: https://www.sciencedirect.com/science/article/pii/S027273581730137X?via%3Dihub.
3. Mitchison D, Mond J, Bussey K, Griffiths S, Trompeter N, Lonergan A, et al. DSM-5 full syndrome, other specified, and unspecified eating disorders in Australian adolescents: prevalence and clinical significance. Psychol Med. 2019:1–10.

4. Hudson JI, Hiripi E, Pope HG, Kessler RC. The prevalence and correlates of eating disorders in the National Comorbidity Survey Replication. Biol Psychiatry. 2007;61(3):348–58.
5. Nagl M, Jacobi C, Paul M, Beesdo-Baum K, Höfler M, Lieb R, et al. Prevalence, incidence, and natural course of anorexia and bulimia nervosa among adolescents and young adults. Eur Child Adolesc Psychiatry. 2016;25(8):903–18.
6. Hammerle F, Huss M, Ernst V, Bürger A. Thinking dimensional: prevalence of DSM-5 early adolescent full syndrome, partial and subthreshold eating disorders in a cross-sectional survey in German schools. BMJ Open. 2016;6(5):1–7.
7. Woodside DB, Garfinkel PE, Lin E, Goering P, Kaplan AS, Goldbloom DS, et al. Comparisons of men with full or partial eating disorders, men without eating disorders, and women with eating disorders in the community. Am J Psychiatry [Internet]. 2001 Apr 1;158(4):570–4. Available from: https://doi.org/10.1176/appi.ajp.158.4.570.
8. Nicholls DE, Lynn R, Viner RM. Childhood eating disorders: British national surveillance study. Br J Psychiatry [Internet]. 2011 Apr 2 [cited 2019 Oct 27];198(4):295–301. Available from: https://www.cambridge.org/core/product/identifier/S0007125000254792/type/journal_article
9. Chen H, Jackson T. Prevalence and sociodemographic correlates of eating disorder endorsements among adolescents and young adults from China. Eur Eat Disord Rev [Internet]. 2008 Sep 1;16(5):375–85. Available from: https://doi.org/10.1002/erv.837.e
10. Swanson SA, Crow SJ, Le Grange D, Swendsen J, Merikangas KR. Prevalence and correlates of eating disorders in adolescents: results from the national comorbidity survey replication adolescent supplement. Arch Gen Psychiatry. 2011;68(7):714–23.
11. American Psychiatric Association. Diagnostic and statistical manual of mental disorders. 5th ed. Washington,D.C.: Author; 2013.
12. Mancuso SG, Newton JR, Bosanac P, Rossell SL, Nesci JB, Castle DJ. Classification of eating disorders: comparison of relative prevalence rates using DSM-IV and DSM-5 criteria. Br J Psychiatry [Internet]. 2015 Jun 2 [cited 2019 Nov 13];206(6):519–20. Available from: https://www.cambridge.org/core/product/identifier/S0007125000279178/type/journal_article.
13. Allen KL, Byrne SM, Oddy WH, Crosby RD. DSM-IV-TR and DSM-5 eating disorders in adolescents: prevalence, stability, and psychosocial correlates in a population-based sample of male and female adolescents. J Abnorm Psychol. 2013;122(3):720–32.
14. Alegria M, Woo M, Cao Z, Torres M, Meng X, Striegel-Moore R. Prevalence and correlates of eating disorders in Latinos in the United States. Int J Eat Disord [Internet]. 2007 Nov 1;40(S3):S15–21. Available from: https://doi.org/10.1002/eat.20406.
15. Erskine HE, Whiteford HA. Epidemiology of binge eating disorder. Curr Opin Psychiatry [Internet]. 2018;31(6). Available from: https://journals.lww.com/co-psychiatry/Fulltext/2018/11000/Epidemiology_of_binge_eating_disorder.7.aspx.
16. Le Grange D, Swanson SA, Crow SJ, Merikangas KR. Eating disorder not otherwise specified presentation in the US population. Int J Eat Disord. 2012;45(5):711–8.
17. Kinasz K, Accurso EC, Kass AE, Le Grange D. Does sex matter in the clinical presentation of eating disorders in youth? J Adolesc Heal [Internet]. 2016 Apr 1 [cited 2019 Nov 13];58(4):410–6. Available from: https://www.sciencedirect.com/science/article/pii/S1054139X15006709?via%3Dihub.
18. Murray SB, Rieger E, Hildebrandt T, Karlov L, Russell J, Boon E, et al. A comparison of eating, exercise, shape, and weight related symptomatology in males with muscle dysmorphia and anorexia nervosa. Body Image [Internet]. 2012 Mar 1 [cited 2020 Jan 6];9(2):193–200. Available from: https://www.sciencedirect.com/science/article/pii/S1740144512000125.
19. Compte EJ, Sepulveda AR, Torrente F. A two-stage epidemiological study of eating disorders and muscle dysmorphia in male university students in Buenos Aires. Int J Eat Disord. 2015;48(8):1092–101.
20. Schneider SC, Mond J, Turner CM, Hudson JL. Sex differences in the presentation of body dysmorphic disorder in a community sample of adolescents. J Clin Child Adolesc Psychol

[Internet]. 2019 May 4;48(3):516–28. Available from: https://doi.org/10.1080/15374416.2017.1321001.
21. Bentley C, Gratwick-Sarll K, Harrison C, Mond J. Sex differences in psychosocial impairment associated with eating disorder features in adolescents: a school-based study. Int J Eat Disord. 2015;48(6):633–40.
22. Anderson CB, Bulik CM. Gender differences in compensatory behaviors, weight and shape salience, and drive for thinness. Eat Behav [Internet]. 2004 Jan 1 [cited 2019 Oct 28];5(1):1–11. Available from: https://www.sciencedirect.com/science/article/pii/S1471015303000606?via%3Dihub.
23. Mond JM, Hay PJ. Functional impairment associated with bulimic behaviors in a community sample of men and women. Int J Eat Disord [Internet]. 2007 Jul 1;40(5):391–8. Available from: https://doi.org/10.1002/eat.20380.e
24. Griffiths S, Murray SB, Bentley C, Gratwick-Sarll K, Harrison C, Mond JM. Sex differences in quality of life impairment associated with body dissatisfaction in adolescents. J Adolesc Health. 2017;61(1):77–82.
25. Calzo JP, Sonneville KR, Haines J, Blood EA, Field AE, Austin SB. The development of associations among body mass index, body dissatisfaction, and weight and shape concern in adolescent boys and girls. J Adolesc Heal [Internet] 2012;51(5):517–523. Available from: https://doi.org/10.1016/j.jadohealth.2012.02.021.
26. Calzo JP, Horton NJ, Sonneville KR, Swanson SA, Crosby RD, Micali N, et al. Male eating disorder symptom patterns and health correlates from 13 to 26 years of age. J Am Acad Child Adolesc Psychiatry [Internet]. 2016 Aug 1 [cited 2019 Oct 28];55(8):693–700.e2. Available from: https://www.sciencedirect.com/science/article/pii/S0890856716302131?via%3Dihub.
27. Striegel-Moore RH, Rosselli F, Perrin N, DeBar L, Wilson GT, May A, et al. Gender difference in the prevalence of eating disorder symptoms. Int J Eat Disord [Internet]. 2009 Jul 1;42(5):471–4. Available from: https://doi.org/10.1002/eat.20625.
28. Gammelmark C, Jensen SOW, Plessen KJ, Skadhede S, Larsen JT, Munk-Jørgensen P. Incidence of eating disorders in Danish psychiatric secondary healthcare 1970–2008. Aust New Zeal J Psychiatry [Internet]. 2015 Feb 3;49(8):724–30. Available from: https://doi.org/10.1177/0004867414567758.
29. Mond J, Hall A, Bentley C, Harrison C, Gratwick-Sarll K, Lewis V. Eating-disordered behavior in adolescent boys: Eating disorder examination questionnaire norms. Int J Eat Disord [Internet]. 2014 May 1;47(4):335–41. Available from: https://doi.org/10.1002/eat.22237.
30. Zerwas S, Larsen JT, Petersen L, Thornton LM, Mortensen PB, Bulik CM. The incidence of eating disorders in a Danish register study: associations with suicide risk and mortality. J Psychiatr Res. 2015;65:16–22.
31. Reas DL, Stedal K. Eating disorders in men aged midlife and beyond [Internet]. Vol. 81, Maturitas. Elsevier; 2015 [cited 2019 Oct 28]. p. 248–55. Available from: https://www.sciencedirect.com/science/article/pii/S0378512215004661.
32. Striegel RH, Bedrosian R, Wang C, Schwartz S. Why men should be included in research on binge eating: results from a comparison of psychosocial impairment in men and women. Int J Eat Disord [Internet]. 2012 Mar 1;45(2):233–40. Available from: https://doi.org/10.1002/eat.20962.
33. Hay P, Mitchison D, Collado AEL, González-Chica DA, Stocks N, Touyz S. Burden and health-related quality of life of eating disorders, including avoidant/restrictive food intake disorder (ARFID), in the Australian population. J Eat Disord. 2017;5(1)
34. Mulders-Jones B, Mitchison D, Girosi F, Hay P, Jiménez-Murcia S. Socioeconomic correlates of eating disorder symptoms in an Australian population-based sample. PLoS One. 2017;12(1):e0170603.
35. Ammann S, Berchtold A, Barrense-Dias Y, Akre C, Surís J-C. Disordered eating: the young male side. Behav Med [Internet]. 2018 Oct 2;44(4):289–96. Available from: https://doi.org/10.1080/08964289.2017.1341383.

36. Nicdao EG, Hong S, Takeuchi DT. Prevalence and correlates of eating disorders among Asian Americans: results from the national Latino and Asian American study. Int J Eat Disord [Internet]. 2007 Nov 1;40(S3):S22–6. Available from: https://doi.org/10.1002/eat.20450.
37. Taylor JY, Caldwell CH, Baser RE, Faison N, Jackson JS. Prevalence of eating disorders among blacks in the national survey of American life. Int J Eat Disord [Internet]. 2007 Nov 1;40(S3):S10–4. Available from: https://doi.org/10.1002/eat.20451.
38. Striegel-Moore RH, Rosselli F, Holtzman N, Dierker L, Becker AE, Swaney G. Behavioral symptoms of eating disorders in Native Americans: Results from the add health survey wave III. Int J Eat Disord [Internet]. 2011 Sep 1;44(6):561–6. Available from: https://doi.org/10.1002/eat.20894.
39. Feldman M, Meyer I. Eating disorders in diverse lesbian, gay, and bisexual populations. Int J Eat Disord. 2007;40(3):218–26.
40. Diemer EW, Grant JD, Munn-Chernoff MA, Patterson DA, Duncan AE. Gender identity, sexual orientation, and eating-related pathology in a national sample of college students. J Adolesc Health [Internet]. Elsevier; 2015 [cited 2019 Dec 17]. p. 144–9. Available from: https://www.sciencedirect.com/science/article/pii/S1054139X15000877?via%3Dihub.
41. Frederick DA, Essayli JH. Male body image: the roles of sexual orientation and body mass index across five national U.S. studies. Psychol Men Masculinity. 2016;17(4):336–51.
42. Feder S, Isserlin L, Seale E, Hammond N, Norris ML. Exploring the association between eating disorders and gender dysphoria in youth. Eat Disord [Internet]. 2017 Aug 8;25(4):310–7. Available from: https://doi.org/10.1080/10640266.2017.1297112.
43. Becerra-Culqui TA, Liu Y, Nash R, Cromwell L, Flanders WD, Getahun D, et al. Mental health of transgender and gender nonconforming youth compared with their peers. Pediatrics [Internet]. 2018 May 1;141(5):e20173845. Available from: http://pediatrics.aappublications.org/content/141/5/e20173845.abstract.
44. Coelho JS, Suen J, Clark BA, Marshall SK, Geller J, Lam P-Y. Eating disorder diagnoses and symptom presentation in transgender youth: a scoping review. Curr Psychiatry Rep [Internet]. 2019;21(11):107. Available from: https://doi.org/10.1007/s11920-019-1097-x.
45. De Vries ALC, McGuire JK, Steensma TD, Wagenaar ECF, Doreleijers TAH, Cohen-Kettenis PT. Young adult psychological outcome after puberty suppression and gender reassignment. Pediatrics. 2014;134(4):696–704.
46. Ágh T, Kovács G, Supina D, Pawaskar M, Herman BK, Vokó Z, et al. A systematic review of the health-related quality of life and economic burdens of anorexia nervosa, bulimia nervosa, and binge eating disorder. Eat Weight Disord. 2016;21(3):353.
47. Le LK-D, Mihalopoulos C, Engel L, Touyz S, González-Chica DA, Stocks N, et al. Burden and health state utility values of eating disorders: results from a population-based survey. Psychol Med [Internet]. 2019 Oct 31 [cited 2019 Dec 3];1–8. Available from: https://www.cambridge.org/core/product/identifier/S0033291719003064/type/journal_article.
48. Striegel-Moore RH, Leslie D, Petrill SA, Garvin V, Rosenheck RA. One-year use and cost of inpatient and outpatient services among female and male patients with an eating disorder: evidence from a national database of health insurance claims. Int J Eat Disord [Internet]. 2000 May 1;27(4):381–9. Available from: https://doi.org/10.1002/(SICI)1098-108X(200005)27:4%3C381::AID-EAT2%3E3.0.CO.
49. Fichter MM, Quadflieg N. Mortality in eating disorders – results of a large prospective clinical longitudinal study. Int J Eat Disord. 2016;49(4):391–401.
50. Quadflieg N, Strobel C, Naab S, Voderholzer U, Fichter MM. Mortality in males treated for an eating disorder—a large prospective study. Int J Eat Disord. 2019;52:1365.
51. Jáuregui-Garrido B, Jáuregui-Lobera I. Sudden death in eating disorders. Vasc Health Risk Manag [Internet]. 2012/02/15. 2012;8:91–8. Available from: https://www.ncbi.nlm.nih.gov/pubmed/22393299.
52. Arcelus J, Mitchell AJ, Wales J, Nielsen S. Mortality rates in patients with anorexia nervosa and other eating disorders: a meta-analysis of 36 studies. Arch Gen Psychiatry [Internet]. 2011 Jul 1;68(7):724–31. Available from: https://doi.org/10.1001/archgenpsychiatry.2011.74.

53. Madden S, Morris A, Zurynski YA, Kohn M, Elliot EJ. Burden of eating disorders in 5–13-year-old children in Australia. Med J Aust [Internet]. 2009 Apr 1;190(8):410–4. Available from: https://doi.org/10.5694/j.1326-5377.2009.tb02487.x.
54. Butterfly Foundation. Paying the price: the economic and social impact of eating disorders [Internet]. Melbourne; 2012. Available from: www.thebutterflyfoundation.org.au/about-us/information-and-resources/paying-the-price.
55. Keski-Rahkonen A, Mustelin L. Epidemiology of eating disorders in Europe: prevalence, incidence, comorbidity, course, consequences, and risk factors. Curr Opin Psychiatry. 2016;29:340.
56. Cederlöf M, Thornton LM, Baker J, Lichtenstein P, Larsson H, Rück C, et al. Etiological overlap between obsessive-compulsive disorder and anorexia nervosa: a longitudinal cohort, multigenerational family and twin study. World Psychiatry. 2015;14(3):333–8.
57. Field AE, Sonneville KR, Crosby RD, Swanson SA, Eddy KT, Camargo Jr CA, et al. Prospective associations of concerns about physique and the development of obesity, binge drinking, and drug use among adolescent boys and young adult men. JAMA Pediatr [Internet]. 2014 Jan 1;168(1):34–9. Available from: https://doi.org/10.1001/jamapediatrics.2013.2915.
58. Eisenberg ME, Wall M, Neumark-Sztainer D. Muscle-enhancing behaviors among adolescent girls and boys. Pediatrics. 2012;130(6):1019–26.
59. Or F, Kim Y, Simms J, Austin SB. Taking stock of dietary supplements' harmful effects on children, adolescents, and young adults. J Adolesc Heal [Internet]. 2019 Oct 1 [cited 2020 Jan 7];65(4):455–61. Available from: https://www.sciencedirect.com/science/article/pii/S1054139X19301636.
60. Guyda HJ. Use of dietary supplements and hormones in adolescents: a cautionary tale. Paediatr Child Health [Internet]. 2005 Dec 1;10(10):587–90. Available from: https://doi.org/10.1093/pch/10.10.587.
61. Pallister E, Waller G. Anxiety in the eating disorders: understanding the overlap. Clin Psychol Rev. 2008;28(3):366–86.
62. Wolfe WL, Maisto SA. The relationship between eating disorders and substance use: moving beyond co-prevalence research. Clin Psychol Rev [Internet]. 2000 Aug 1 [cited 2019 Dec 12];20(5):617–31. Available from: https://www.sciencedirect.com/science/article/pii/S0272735899000094.
63. Hart LM, Granillo MT, Jorm AF, Paxton SJ. Unmet need for treatment in the eating disorders: a systematic review of eating disorder specific treatment seeking among community cases. Clin Psychol Rev. 2011;31:727–35.
64. Merikangas KR, He JP, Burstein M, Swendsen J, Avenevoli S, Case B, et al. Service utilization for lifetime mental disorders in U.S. adolescents: results of the national comorbidity survey Adolescent supplement (NCS-A). J Am Acad Child Adolesc Psychiatry. 2011;50(1):32–45.
65. Forrest LN, Smith AR, Swanson SA. Characteristics of seeking treatment among U.S. adolescents with eating disorders. Int J Eat Disord. 2017;50(7):826–33.
66. Merikangas KR, He JP, Burstein M, Swanson SA, Avenevoli S, Cui L, et al. Lifetime prevalence of mental disorders in U.S. adolescents: results from the national comorbidity survey replication-adolescent supplement (NCS-A). J Am Acad Child Adolesc Psychiatry [Internet]. 2010 Oct 1 [cited 2019 Nov 14];49(10):980–9. Available from: https://www.sciencedirect.com/science/article/pii/S0890856710004764?via%3Dihub.
67. Lewinsohn PM, Seeley JR, Moerk KC, Striegel-Moore RH. Gender differences in eating disorder symptoms in young adults. Int J Eat Disord [Internet]. 2002 Dec 1;32(4):426–40. Available from: https://doi.org/10.1002/eat.10103.
68. Fatt SJ, Mond J, Bussey K, Griffiths S, Murray SB, Lonergan A, et al. Help-seeking for body image problems among adolescents with eating disorders: findings from the EveryBODY study. Eat Weight Disord [Internet]. 2019 Aug. Available from: https://doi.org/10.1007/s40519-019-00759-9.

69. Dearden A, Mulgrew KE. Service provision for men with eating issues in Australia: an analysis of organisations', practitioners', and men's experiences. Aust Soc Work [Internet]. 2013 Dec 1;66(4):590–606. Available from: https://doi.org/10.1080/0312407X.2013.778306.
70. Robinson KJ, Mountford VA, Sperlinger DJ. Being men with eating disorders: Perspectives of male eating disorder service-users. J Health Psychol [Internet]. 2012;18(2):176–86. Available from: https://doi.org/10.1177/1359105312440298.
71. Cibralic S, Conti JE. "I'm More Acknowledged": a qualitative exploration of men's positioning of their body image, eating, and exercise concerns. J Constr Psychol [Internet]. 2018 Apr 3;31(2):186–205. Available from: https://doi.org/10.1080/10720537.2017.1304298.
72. Thapliyal P, Hay PJ. Treatment experiences of males with an eating disorder: a systematic review of qualitative studies. Transl Dev Psychiatry [Internet]. 2014 Jan 1;2(1):25552. Available from: https://doi.org/10.3402/tdp.v2.25552.
73. Regan P, Cachelin FM, Minnick AM. Initial treatment seeking from professional health care providers for eating disorders: a review and synthesis of potential barriers to and facilitators of "first contact." Int J Eat Disord 2017.

Part II
Assessment and Diagnosis

Chapter 5
Assessing and Diagnosing Eating Disorders in Boys and Men: An Overview

Brittany K. Bohrer and Joseph M. Donahue

Learning Objectives
1. Describe the diagnostic criteria for core eating disorders and how they can present differently in boys and men.
2. Recognize disparities in eating disorder research and diagnostic prevalence rates in boys and men.
3. Identify specific considerations for assessing eating disorder psychopathology in boys and men.

Key Points
- The current diagnostic criteria for eating disorders may not accurately and comprehensively capture the full spectrum of eating disorder symptomatology in boys and men.
- There are specific diagnostic considerations to take into account for boys and men with eating disorders.
- The recognition of eating disorder symptoms in boys and men, both by the individual himself and by healthcare providers, may be influenced by the broader misperception that eating disorders are "female issues."

Generally speaking, diagnosis is an important part of both clinical and research endeavors for several reasons, including that it (1) provides means of communication, (2) may serve to validate a person's experience, and (3) can inform treatment for the disease/condition for which it provides a name. Undoubtedly, diagnostic communication is the bedrock of a multidisciplinary approach to patient care. A proper diagnosis can facilitate communication among providers, between providers

B. K. Bohrer (✉) · J. M. Donahue
Department of Psychiatry, UC San Diego Health Eating Disorders Center for Treatment and Research, San Diego, CA, USA
e-mail: bbohrer@health.ucsd.edu; jdonahue@health.ucsd.edu

J. M. Nagata et al. (eds.), *Eating Disorders in Boys and Men*,
https://doi.org/10.1007/978-3-030-67127-3_5

and patients/their families, and with insurance companies. Perhaps most importantly, a diagnosis communicates to patients that what they are experiencing has a name and has been investigated and that there may be evidence-based interventions for their problem. Indeed, numerous evidence-based treatments have been developed and refined for eating disorders (e.g., family-based therapy for anorexia nervosa [1]; enhanced cognitive behavioral therapy for eating disorders [2]). However, evidence suggests that certain eating disorder diagnoses may respond better to specific treatments (e.g., bulimia nervosa and cognitive behavioral therapy for eating disorders [3]). Accordingly, it is imperative for clinicians to utilize appropriate diagnostic tools and best practices when diagnosing eating disorders.

A crucial first step to providing a diagnosis is understanding the diagnostic criteria and how they apply to persons with eating disorders. Furthermore, there are important considerations to be made when applying these diagnoses to boys and men with eating disorders. Historically, eating disorders have been "gendered" in that they have been thought to almost exclusively affect girls and women; this is evidenced in the relative paucity of eating disorder research in boys and men, the low percentage of boys and men present in eating disorder treatment facilities, and the stigma that exists regarding who "can" or "should" have an eating disorder. Today, researchers in the field recognize that the diagnostic criteria for eating disorders were created to describe a female-centric eating disorder experience [4]. As such, the diagnostic criteria may not fully or accurately capture the experience and expression of eating disorders in boys and men, which is problematic for many reasons (see Fig. 5.1 for a summary).

The *Diagnostic and Statistical Manual of Mental Disorders, Fifth Edition* (*DSM-5*) [5] featured changes to the eating disorder diagnostic criteria and categories that were aimed to more accurately capture the experience of the wider population of persons with eating disorders. For example, amenorrhea (i.e., absence of menstruation) was removed as a diagnostic criterion for anorexia nervosa. Further, binge eating disorder was recognized as its own disorder, rather than a variant of the "not otherwise classified" category, and the diagnosis of avoidant/restrictive food intake disorder (ARFID) was introduced. Additional forms of eating disorder psychopathology, such as atypical anorexia nervosa and purging disorder, are also now explicitly recognized as examples of other specified feeding or eating disorders (OSFED). Researchers also have begun to document and characterize "muscularity-oriented" disordered eating [6]. Although boys and men can and do develop symptoms of traditionally defined eating disorders (e.g., anorexia nervosa), recent evidence suggests that symptoms can often also present as "muscularity-oriented" based on body ideals specific to boys and men [7]. As such, there is a growing call for broadening conceptualizations of eating disorders to better capture muscularity-oriented eating disorder presentations [8].

Importantly, research highlights that boys and men have a higher likelihood of having an undiagnosed eating disorder [9], suggesting that both past and current diagnostic criteria for eating disorders may not fully account for the eating disorder experiences of boys and men. Fortunately, there has been an increase in research

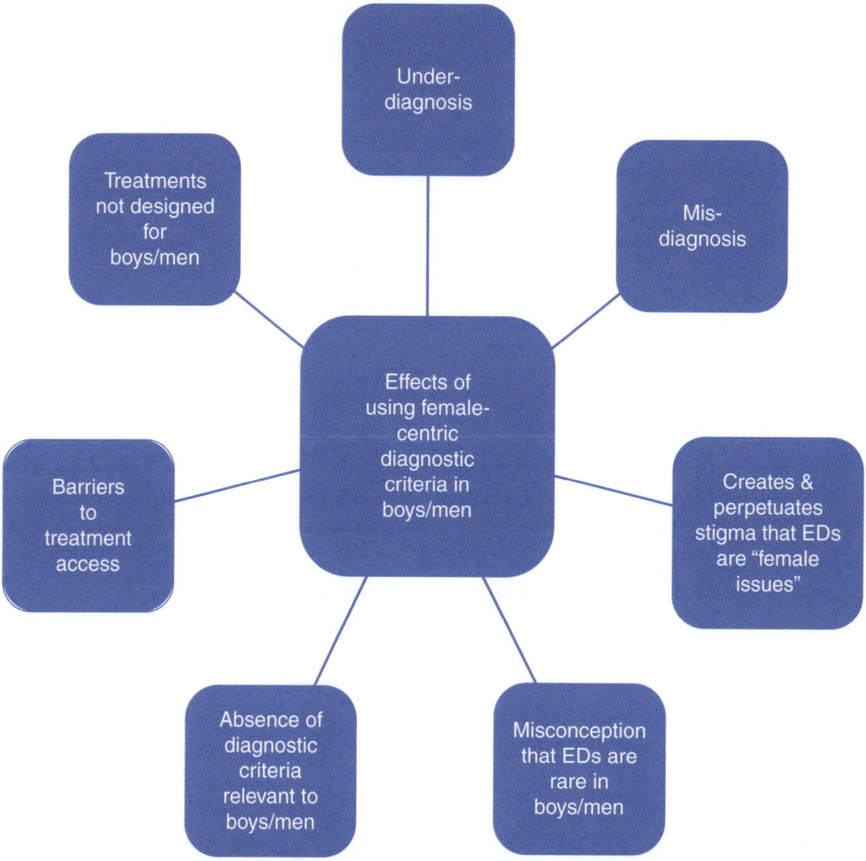
Under-
diagnosis
Treatments
not designed
for
boys/men
Mis-
diagnosis
Effects of
using female-
centric
diagnostic
criteria in
boys/men
Barriers
to
treatment
access
Creates &
perpetuates
stigma that EDs
are "female
issues"
Absence of
diagnostic
criteria
relevant to
boys/men
Misconception
that EDs are
rare in
boys/men

Fig. 5.1 Potential consequences of applying female-centric diagnostic criteria to diagnose eating disorders (EDs) in boys and men

exploring eating disorders among boys and men in recent years, and sustained attention will help improve the applicability and utility of diagnostic frameworks for eating disorders in this population.

Eating Disorder Diagnoses

Within the *DSM-5* [5], anorexia nervosa, bulimia nervosa, and binge eating disorder could be considered the "primary" eating disorders, given that they have been recognized and specifically named within multiple versions of the *DSM*. In addition, there are two "residual" diagnostic categories for presentations that do not fit the diagnostic criteria for the primary disorders: OSFED and unspecified feeding or eating disorder. The present chapter will focus on the three primary eating disorders and OSFED; the following chapter in this section (Chap. 6) focuses specifically on the newer diagnosis of ARFID.

Anorexia nervosa The three diagnostic criteria for anorexia nervosa [5] can be somewhat confusing, and careful attention must be paid to these criteria to ensure accurate diagnosis. *Criterion A* can be thought of as the "low body weight" criterion. It states that energy intake must be restricted relative to the person's requirements based on considerations, such as their age, sex, developmental trajectory, etc., and that this failure to meet energy requirements results in a significantly low body weight (i.e., less than what is considered "normal" or expected). Previous versions of the *DSM* gave suggestions for body mass index (BMI) cutoffs; however, these recommendations were often interpreted literally, and, as a result, some individuals with anorexia nervosa were misdiagnosed and/or denied treatment because of an insufficiently low BMI. As such, the *DSM-5* defines "significantly low body weight" as less than what is considered "normal" or expected for that person. *Criterion B* states that one or more of the following must be present: fear of weight gain *or* fear of becoming "fat" *or* persistent behaviors that interfere with weight gain (e.g., excessive exercise). *Criterion C* involves body image disturbance, overvaluation of weight and/or shape, or denial of the seriousness of the low body weight. There are two anorexia nervosa subtypes: anorexia nervosa binge eating/purging subtype, in which the person regularly engages in binge eating *and/or* purging behaviors, and anorexia nervosa restricting subtype, in which the person does not regularly engage in either binge eating *or* purging behaviors.

Bulimia nervosa Bulimia nervosa is characterized by recurrent binge eating episodes (*Criterion A*) *and* inappropriate compensatory behaviors (*Criterion B*), each of which must occur at least once per week, on average, for a duration of at least 3 months (*Criterion C*) [5]. *Binge eating* involves a subjective sense of loss of control over eating what most people would consider an unusually large amount of food in a discrete period of time. *Inappropriate compensatory behaviors* may include purging behaviors (e.g., self-induced vomiting, misuse of laxatives, diuretics, etc.) and may also include non-purging behaviors, such as dietary restriction or excessive exercise. Another diagnostic feature of bulimia nervosa is *overvaluation of weight and/or shape* (*Criterion D*), which is typically exhibited as a person's weight and/or shape having a large influence on that person's self-evaluation. Consider an example: Many people without eating disorders may evaluate themselves based on their familial relationships or work performance; persons with eating disorders may also use these metrics for self-evaluation, but to a lesser degree than they use their body weight or shape to evaluate whether they perceive themselves to be a "good" or "bad" person. Finally, in order to diagnose bulimia nervosa, the person may not be at a low body weight (i.e., the presentation would be better accounted for by anorexia nervosa; *Criterion E*).

Binge eating disorder Persons with binge eating disorder engage in recurrent *binge eating episodes* (*Criterion A*) at least once per week, on average, for duration of 3 months (*Criterion D*), but in contrast to those with bulimia nervosa, persons with binge eating disorder *do not* engage in inappropriate compensatory behaviors. The binge eating episodes also must be associated with at least three of five *specified features* (e.g., eating alone because one is embarrassed by the amount of food consumed; *Criterion B*) and *marked distress* related to the binge eating (*Criterion C*). Persons with binge eating disorder may not be at a low body weight (i.e., the presentation would be better accounted for by anorexia nervosa) and may not regularly engage in inappropriate compensatory behaviors (i.e., the presentation would be better accounted for by bulimia nervosa; *Criterion E*). It is important to note that persons with binge eating disorder need not fall in the medical categories of "overweight" or "obesity," although higher weight status is often associated with binge eating disorder. Furthermore, although overvaluation of weight and/or shape is not a diagnostic criterion for binge eating disorder, it is commonly associated with the diagnosis and may indicate a more severe presentation [10] and should thus be considered.

Other specified feeding or eating disorder The OSFED diagnostic category is designated to describe persons with clinically significant eating pathology whose presentation does not fit the criteria of the other core feeding and eating disorder diagnoses. It is imperative to note that OSFED is no less serious or deadly than other eating disorders [11] and is, in fact, the most common eating disorder [12]. As female-centric conceptualizations of primary eating disorder diagnoses do not sufficiently address the ways in which eating disorders typically present in boys and men (e.g., muscularity-oriented disordered eating), boys and men with eating pathology in particular are often placed into residual diagnostic categories [13, 14].

The *DSM-5* names five examples of OSFED [5], and detailed discussion of each is beyond the scope of the present chapter. Three of the most common types of OSFED are "bulimia nervosa (of low frequency and/or limited duration)," "binge eating disorder (of low frequency and/or limited duration)," and "atypical anorexia nervosa." The former two can be thought of as "subthreshold" forms of bulimia nervosa and binge eating disorder, respectively. A person may be diagnosed with these forms of OSFED if their eating disorder behaviors (e.g., binge eating, inappropriate compensatory behaviors) do not meet or exceed the frequency criterion (i.e., they happen less than once per week, on average) or if they do not meet or exceed the duration criterion (i.e., symptoms for less than 3 months). Furthermore, for persons who may otherwise be diagnosed with bulimia nervosa, lack of overvaluation of weight/shape may warrant a diagnosis of "bulimia nervosa (of low frequency and/or duration)."

Sometimes an individual may exhibit all features of anorexia nervosa, except their body weight is not significantly low; this presentation is consistent with "atypical anorexia nervosa." Oftentimes such persons are on a weight-loss trajectory that is concerning due to the amount of weight lost in a relatively short amount of time, and if not interrupted, that trajectory could eventually lead to significantly low body weight (i.e., meeting diagnostic criteria for anorexia nervosa). Importantly, even in the absence of a currently low body weight, substantial weight loss, particularly over a short timeframe, also may be associated with clinically significant malnutrition and other medical complications [15, 16].

Diagnostic Considerations for Boys and Men

Overview Overall, current findings provide evidence that more boys and men are affected by eating disorders than historical prevalence statistics suggested, particularly those based on data derived from specialty treatment settings. Moreover, data suggests that distress and impairment related to eating disorder symptoms are comparable across genders and that certain eating disorder behaviors are increasing at faster rates among boys and men [14]. A number of factors may help account for the apparent increase in rates of eating disorders and related symptoms among boys and men. First, the release of *DSM-5* [5] reflects a progression in the detection and assessment of eating disorders in general, including among boys and men, and may in part explain higher rates of these issues more recently detected in this population. Specifically, the *DSM-5* expanded and refined eating disorder diagnostic criteria in such a way that allows more boys and men to fit primary eating disorder diagnoses (e.g., with the removal of amenorrhea as a criterion of anorexia nervosa and increased flexibility with the weight criterion). Binge eating disorder, which had previously been included as a provisional diagnosis encompassed within the residual "eating disorder not otherwise specified" category, is also included as a distinct diagnosis. Moreover, the required frequency of binge eating and duration of symptoms were also reduced, thus now capturing those who would have previously been diagnostically subthreshold.

Importantly, traditional eating disorder assessment measures (e.g., the Eating Attitudes Test, the Eating Disorder Inventory) were originally developed, validated, and normed in samples consisting predominantly or completely of girls and/or women [17]. As men and women often report distinct body image concerns and related manifestations of eating pathology (e.g., desired body weights and shapes; [18]), it is likely that previous research did not accurately describe and quantify these issues in men. In addition to affecting reported prevalence rates, this gap in the eating disorder literature has likely contributed to under-diagnosis and under-treatment of eating disorders in boys and men. Further, although recent data suggest that eating disorders are more common among boys and men than previously believed, the prevalence of most eating disorders does still appear to be higher in girls and women (e.g., [5, 19]), and as such there are certain clinical implications to consider. First, eating disorder prevalence rates have a considerably higher skewed sex distribution in comparison with other mental health concerns [20], which may sustain the misconception that eating disorders in particular are "female issues." This may lead to biases that could interfere with clinicians recognizing, detecting, and even considering whether to assess these issues in boys and men. In addition, there still remains a significant social stigma for men with eating disorders that is compounded by the lower rates of help seeking for mental health problems in general that have been found among men [21]. As such, boys and men can face unique barriers to seeking treatment for an eating disorder [9].

Body image concerns and fear of weight gain Historically, a diagnosis of bulimia nervosa (and anorexia nervosa, to some degree) was conceptualized as arising from a desire for a smaller body size or shape (i.e., "drive for thinness"), which in turn can be associated with fear of weight gain, desire for weight loss, and/or behaviors aimed to facilitate changes in body mass (e.g., dietary restriction). However, recent work has also recognized that traditional "thin-ideal" conceptualizations of eating disorders do not adequately capture the experiences of boys and men, as the body ideal often held by boys and men is one of lean muscularity [8, 22]. For example, a study of undergraduate men with eating disorders found that they reported greater concern for muscle tone and less concern for weight loss/fear of weight gain as compared to undergraduate women [23].

Boys and men with eating disorders may endorse either the traditional thin body ideal, muscularity-oriented ideals, or some combination, which can impact eating disorder presentation and symptomatology. A comparison of men with muscle dysmorphia and anorexia nervosa found the differences in eating disorder symptoms were largely related to contrasting body ideals (i.e., thin versus muscular) being pursued; however, there were also numerous symptomatic similarities related to disturbed body image, disordered eating, and exercise behaviors across diagnoses [24]. Pursuit of contrasting body ideals may also confer risk for additional negative outcomes. A large, epidemiological study of adolescent boys found that boys who reported concerns related to both muscularity and thinness were more likely than their peers to abuse drugs [25]. Importantly, this study demonstrated that body image concerns experienced by boys were heterogeneous and collectively associated with poor outcomes (e.g., depression, binge drinking, drug use), thus highlighting the need for careful attention and assessment of such concerns in boys.

Lavender and colleagues [6] described how muscularity-oriented eating disorder symptoms are more common than previously understood – especially among men – which may partly account for the lower rates of traditionally defined eating disorders among this population. An extensive epidemiological study provided additional evidence for the link between muscularity-oriented body concerns and eating pathology in boys and men from 13 to 26 years of age, citing prevalent disordered eating behaviors often driven by muscularity concerns [7]. In addition, muscularity-oriented body concerns were associated with an elevated risk for nonprescription drug abuse. Calzo and colleagues [7] suggested that these muscularity-oriented body concerns may be as prevalent in boys and men as are traditional eating disorder symptoms (e.g., drive for thinness) in girls and women and are associated with similar negative physical and psychosocial outcomes.

Thus, the experience of certain diagnostic criteria among some boys and men may differ from the typical experience of girls and women, including in their experience and expression of body image and weight concerns. As such, careful attention must be paid to these symptoms in order to guide a diagnosis that most accurately describes the individual's experiences.

Compensatory behaviors Men with eating disorders, bulimia nervosa in particular, are more likely to engage in non-purging compensatory behaviors (i.e., excessive exercise, dietary restriction) than purging behaviors such as self-induced vomiting [26, 27]. Furthermore, exercise is more common among boys and men than in girls and women with anorexia nervosa and has been documented to serve as an affect regulation strategy more often in boys and men than in girls and women with anorexia nervosa. Additionally, boys and men with anorexia nervosa tend to employ more rigid exercise habits than girls and women [28].

A unique and potentially pathological cyclical pattern of eating and exercise behaviors salient to pursuit of the lean and muscular body ideal has been termed "bulking" (e.g., consuming a calorie-dense meal plan, weightlifting/resistance training to gain muscle mass) and "cutting" (i.e., diet and exercise aimed at reducing fat mass so that muscularity built during the "bulking" phase is emphasized). In particular, the dietary restriction (often involved in the "cutting" phase) oriented toward pursuit of a lean body mass in order to highlight muscularity may be a diagnostic feature for a number of eating disorder diagnoses [8]. Another related but distinct and potentially pathological behavior that is clinically relevant to eating disorder psychopathology in boys and men is the use of appearance- and performance-enhancing substances (e.g., anabolic-androgenic steroids). Motivations for the use of such substances are heterogeneous, but may often be related to body image disturbance and/or muscularity-oriented concerns [25, 29]. Use of these substances may be associated with negative outcomes, such as risk for eating disorders, substance use disorders, and body dysmorphic disorder [25, 30], thus warranting their consideration in the assessment and diagnosis process.

Binge eating As with the other diagnostic criteria for eating disorders, the operationalization of binge eating was based predominantly on the experience of girls and women; as such, the current definition of binge eating may not fully capture the experiences of boys and men, and there are several factors regarding binge eating to consider when assessing for eating disorders in boys and men.

Binge eating can occur in any eating disorder diagnosis, and the size of the binge eating episode must be considered. To be classified as objective binge eating, the amount of food consumed must be larger than what most people would consume under similar circumstances[1]. The size threshold for food consumed during binge eating episodes in boys and men may be higher than for girls and women [31, 32],

[1] Subjective binge eating is similar to objective binge eating with respect to loss of control over eating, but the amount of food consumed in a subjective binge eating episode is not larger than what most people would consume under similar circumstances (i.e., a small or normal amount of food). Persons with any eating disorder diagnosis can experience subjective binge eating; objective binge eating is required to diagnose bulimia nervosa or binge eating disorder.

and boys and men are less likely to report distress associated with binge eating [33]. Cultural and social standards must be considered as well. For example, it may be culturally normative for men to eat more than women. It should not be automatically assumed that because the amount of food a man consumes is larger than what a woman may consume – and is expected to be so culturally – the amount of food cannot be considered objectively large. Additionally, the caloric needs of boys and men are on average larger than those of girls and women. Careful assessment of the types and amounts of foods consumed during the binge eating episode is important for accurate diagnosis and clinical conceptualization.

A second consideration is related to the subjective experience of loss of control. In order for an eating episode to be considered binge eating, the person must report having experienced a subjective sense of loss of control over their eating. This could present in the form of feeling that they cannot control the types or amounts of food consumed, or that they could not stop eating once they started, or that it was inevitable that they would eat the amount of food consumed. Notably, boys and men are less likely than girls and women to endorse loss of control over their eating [27, 33]. In addition, cultural and societal norms for boys, men, and masculinity may influence one's perceptions of or willingness to endorse loss of control. As such, careful assessment of loss of control that includes multiple example descriptions and alternative terminologies that capture the construct is warranted.

Another important consideration related to caloric overconsumption is the concept of "cheat meals," "cheat days," and other planned eating episodes wherein large volumes of food are consumed, typically after prolonged periods of comparative caloric restriction. This may accompany a broader pattern of "bulking and cutting" as described above and may be employed by boys and men pursuing muscularity-oriented body image goals [34]. As such, these discrete periods of eating high volumes of calorie-dense food are often followed by compensatory behaviors such as strict dietary restraint and excessive exercise [35]. Accordingly, these "cheat meal" episodes share many of objective clinical characteristics of binge eating, although the overeating during "cheat" episodes is subjectively distinct in that it is typically perceived positively in the context of working toward one's muscularity-oriented goals. Conversely, binge eating involves a sense of loss of control that is most often associated with distress, shame, and guilt. Further research on the consequences of engaging in "cheat" episodes is needed, as the clinical significance of this behavior is not yet fully understood [34].

Shame and psychosocial impairment It is crucial to consider the potential shame, embarrassment, and denial that may accompany eating disorder symptomatology in boys and men in particular, given the female-centric nature of these diagnoses and the sociocultural depictions that sustain the idea that eating disorders are "female issues." Shame may be associated with symptom denial and/or lack of symptom recognition in boys and men [36], particularly among those who more strongly prioritize adherence to traditional masculine norms. Providing psychoeducation on the prevalence of eating disorder symptoms in boys and men (i.e., it is a myth that eating disorders only affect girls and women) and on the ways in which symptoms may be experienced differently among boys and men may have clinical utility. In addition, enhancing mental health literacy about eating disorders among healthcare providers, particularly those in primary care settings, may be beneficial [37]. Finally, eating disorders are no less impairing for boys or men with eating disorders compared to girls and women [38, 39], and as such it is important to assess general psychosocial functioning and to further assess for impairment related to eating disorder symptoms.

Conclusion

Although diagnostic presentations of eating disorders in boys and men can be similar to those observed in girls and women, there are unique considerations that must be taken into account when assessing and diagnosing eating disorders in boys and men. Research initiatives must strive for greater inclusion of boys and men with eating disorders, including in epidemiological research with community samples. Treatment-focused research is needed to evaluate the efficacy and effectiveness of novel and existing interventions in samples of boys and men with eating disorders. In sum, greater refinement of the diagnostic criteria for eating disorders with regard to boys and men, outreach initiatives designed to combat stigma and educate healthcare providers about eating disorders, and treatment development specific to this population will allow for better understanding of eating disorders in boys and men.

References

1. Lock J, Le Grange D. Treatment manual for anorexia nervosa: a family-based approach. Guilford Publications; New York, NY, USA. 2015.
2. Fairburn CG, Cooper Z, Shafran R, Wilson GT. Eating disorders: A transdiagnostic protocol. In: Barlow DH, editor. Clinical handbook of psychological disorders: A step-by-step treatment manual. The Guilford Press: New York City. 2008, pp. 578–614.
3. Wilson GT, Shafran R. Eating disorders guidelines from NICE. Lancet. 2005;365(9453):79–81.
4. Mond JM, Mitchison D, Hay P. Eating disordered behavior in men: prevalence, impairment in quality of life, and implications for prevention and health promotion. Current findings on males with eating disorders, New York, NY, USA. 2013. pp. 209–231.
5. American Psychiatric Association. Diagnostic and statistical manual of mental disorders (DSM-5®). American Psychiatric Pub; Arlington, VA, USA. 2013.
6. Lavender JM, Brown TA, Murray SB. Men, muscles, and eating disorders: an overview of traditional and muscularity-oriented disordered eating. Curr Psychiatry Rep. 2017;19(6):32.
7. Calzo JP, Horton NJ, Sonneville KR, Swanson SA, Crosby RD, Micali N, Eddy KT, Field AE. Male eating disorder symptom patterns and health correlates from 13 to 26 years of age. J Am Acad Child Adolesc Psychiatry. 2016;55(8):693–700.
8. Murray SB, Griffiths S, Mond JM. Evolving eating disorder psychopathology: conceptualising muscularity-oriented disordered eating. Br J Psychiatry. 2016;208(5):414–5.
9. Griffiths S, Mond JM, Li Z, Gunatilake S, Murray SB, Sheffield J, Touyz S. Self-stigma of seeking treatment and being male predict an increased likelihood of having an undiagnosed eating disorder. Int J Eat Disord. 2015;48(6):775–8.

10. Grilo CM, Masheb RM, White MA. Significance of overvaluation of shape/weight in binge-eating disorder: comparative study with overweight and bulimia nervosa. Obesity. 2010;18(3):499–504.
11. Crow SJ, Peterson CB, Swanson SA, Raymond NC, Specker S, Eckert ED, Mitchell JE. Increased mortality in bulimia nervosa and other eating disorders. Am J Psychiatr. 2009;166(12):1342–6.
12. Hay P, Girosi F, Mond J. Prevalence and sociodemographic correlates of DSM-5 eating disorders in the Australian population. J Eat Disord. 2015;3(1):19.
13. Le Grange D, Swanson SA, Crow SJ, Merikangas KR. Eating disorder not otherwise specified presentation in the US population. Int J Eat Disord. 2012;45(5):711–8.
14. Mitchison D, Mond J, Slewa-Younan S, Hay P. Sex differences in health-related quality of life impairment associated with eating disorder features: a general population study. Int J Eat Disord. 2013;46(4):375–80.
15. Garber AK, Cheng J, Accurso EC, Adams SH, Buckelew SM, Kapphahn CJ, Kreiter A, Le Grange D, Machen VI, Moscicki AB, Saffran K. Weight loss and illness severity in adolescents with atypical anorexia nervosa. Pediatrics. 2019;144(6):e20192339.
16. Whitelaw M, Lee KJ, Gilbertson H, Sawyer SM. Predictors of complications in anorexia nervosa and atypical anorexia nervosa: degree of underweight or extent and recency of weight loss? J Adolesc Health. 2018;63(6):717–23.
17. Yager J, Powers PS, editors. Clinical manual of eating disorders. American Psychiatric Pub; Washington, D.C., USA. 2008.
18. Furnham A, Badmin N, Sneade I. Body image dissatisfaction: gender differences in eating attitudes, self-esteem, and reasons for exercise. J Psychol. 2002;136(6):581–96.
19. Raevuori A, Keski-Rahkonen A, Hoek HW. A review of eating disorders in males. Curr Opin Psychiatry. 2014;27(6):426–30.
20. Pedersen CB, Mors O, Bertelsen A, Waltoft BL, Agerbo E, McGrath JJ, Mortensen PB, Eaton WW. A comprehensive nationwide study of the incidence rate and lifetime risk for treated mental disorders. JAMA Psychiat. 2014;71(5):573–81.
21. Räisänen U, Hunt K. The role of gendered constructions of eating disorders in delayed help-seeking in men: a qualitative interview study. BMJ Open. 2014;4(4):e004342.
22. Pope H, Phillips KA, Olivardia R. The Adonis complex: how to identify, treat and prevent body obsession in men and boys. Touchstone; New York, NY, USA 2002.
23. Ousley L, Cordero ED, White S. Eating disorders and body image of undergraduate men. J Am Coll Heal. 2008;56(6):617–22.
24. Murray SB, Rieger E, Hildebrandt T, Karlov L, Russell J, Boon E, Dawson RT, Touyz SW. A comparison of eating, exercise, shape, and weight related symptomatology in males with muscle dysmorphia and anorexia nervosa. Body Image. 2012;9(2):193–200.
25. Neumark-Sztainer D, Eisenberg ME. Body image concerns, muscle-enhancing behaviors, and eating disorders in males. JAMA. 2014;312(20):2156–7.
26. Lavender JM, De Young KP, Anderson DA. Eating disorder examination questionnaire (EDE-Q): norms for undergraduate men. Eat Behav. 2010;11(2):119–21.
27. Striegel-Moore RH, Rosselli F, Perrin N, DeBar L, Wilson GT, May A, Kraemer HC. Gender difference in the prevalence of eating disorder symptoms. Int J Eat Disord. 2009;42(5):471–4.
28. Murray SB, Griffiths S, Rieger E, Touyz S. A comparison of compulsive exercise in male and female presentations of anorexia nervosa: what is the difference?. Advances in eating disorders: theory, research. Practice. 2014;2(1):65–70.
29. Olivardia R, Pope HG Jr, Borowiecki JJ III, Cohane GH. Biceps and body image: the relationship between muscularity and self-esteem, depression, and eating disorder symptoms. Psychol Men Masculinities. 2004;5(2):112–20.
30. Piacentino D, Kotzalidis GD, Longo L, Pavan A, Stivali L, Stivali G, Ferracuti S, Brugnoli R, Frati P, Fineschi V, Girardi P. Body image and eating disorders are common among professional and amateur athletes using performance and image enhancing drugs: a cross-sectional study. J Psychoactive Drugs. 2017;49(5):373–84.

31. Forney KJ, Holland LA, Joiner TE, Keel PK. Determining empirical thresholds for “definitely large” amounts of food for defining binge-eating episodes. Eat Disord. 2015;23(1):15–30.
32. Arikian A, Peterson CB, Swanson SA, Berg KC, Chartier L, Durkin N, Crow SJ. Establishing thresholds for unusually large binge eating episodes. Int J Eat Disord. 2012;45(2):222–6.
33. Lewinsohn PM, Seeley JR, Moerk KC, Striegel-Moore RH. Gender differences in eating disorder symptoms in young adults. Int J Eat Disord. 2002;32(4):426–40.
34. Murray SB, Nagata JM, Griffiths S, Calzo JP, Brown TA, Mitchison D, Blashill AJ, Mond JM. The enigma of male eating disorders: a critical review and synthesis. Clin Psychol Rev. 2017;57:1–1.
35. Connan, F. Machismo nervosa: An ominous variant of bulimia nervosa. Eur Eat Disord Rev. 1998;6(3),154–9. https://doi.org/10.1002/(SICI)1099-0968(199809)6:3<154::AID-ERV257>3.0.CO;2-S.
36. Griffiths S, Mond JM, Murray SB, Touyz S. The prevalence and adverse associations of stigmatization in people with eating disorders. Int J Eat Disord. 2015;48(6):767–74.
37. MacCaughelty C, Wagner R, Rufino K. Does being overweight or male increase a patient's risk of not being referred for an eating disorder consult? Int J Eat Disord. 2016;49(10):963–6.
38. Bentley C, Gratwick-Sarll K, Harrison C, Mond J. Sex differences in psychosocial impairment associated with eating disorder features in adolescents: a school-based study. Int J Eat Disord. 2015;48(6):633–40.
39. Bentley C, Mond J, Rodgers B. Sex differences in psychosocial impairment associated with eating-disordered behavior: what if there aren't any? Eating Behav. 2014;15(4):609–14.

Chapter 6
Avoidant/Restrictive Food Intake Disorder

Jessie E. Menzel and Tana Luo

Learning Objectives
1. Describe overall prevalence rates of ARFID and review available findings on the prevalence of ARFID in boys and men.
2. Provide recommendations for the assessment of ARFID.
3. Summarize the current evidence base for psychotherapeutic and pharmacological interventions for ARFID.

Key Points
- Emerging evidence suggests ARFID may be as prevalent as other eating disorders and prevalence rates of ARFID may be similar across boys and girls, although boys and, particularly, men are still underrepresented in published samples.
- Selective eating and/or low appetite presentations of ARFID tend to be associated with boys.
- Individuals with ARFID are at risk for significant medical and psychiatric comorbidities and sequelae.
- Assessment of ARFID should include a physical examination, relevant medical work-up, evaluation of psychosocial impairment, and standardized measures of ARFID symptoms.
- Several psychotherapeutic and pharmacological interventions show initial promise in the treatment of ARFID.

J. E. Menzel (✉) · T. Luo
Department of Psychiatry, University of California, San Diego, San Diego, CA, USA
e-mail: jmenzel@health.ucsd.edu

J. M. Nagata et al. (eds.), *Eating Disorders in Boys and Men*,
https://doi.org/10.1007/978-3-030-67127-3_6

Introduction

Avoidant/restrictive food intake disorder (ARFID) is one of the newest eating disorders to be described in the fifth edition of the *Diagnostic and Statistical Manual of Mental Disorders* [1]. Replacing the old diagnostic category of Feeding Disorders of Infancy and Childhood, ARFID captures a wide range of restrictive and avoidant eating behaviors that present across the lifespan. Unlike anorexia nervosa (AN), individuals with ARFID have disordered eating behaviors that are not motivated by a desire to lose weight or a fear of gaining weight, and they may not necessarily exhibit significantly low body weight. Rather, ARFID is characterized by significantly limited volume (amount) and/or variety (range) of food intake resulting from sensitivity to the sensory properties of food, specific fears related to the outcomes of eating, and a lack of interest in eating or poor appetite.

Epidemiology

Large-scale, epidemiological studies of ARFID are currently lacking. Estimates of ARFID prevalence are beginning to emerge from targeted, population-based studies; these studies currently estimate the population prevalence of ARFID to be between 0.3% [2] and 3.2% [3]. The range of this estimate reflects the age range of the samples studied, with a higher prevalence of ARFID reported in a school-aged sample (ages 8–13) and a lower prevalence reported in an adult, community sample. These prevalence rates indicate that ARFID may be as prevalent as AN and bulimia nervosa (BN). However, unlike AN and BN, which show higher prevalence among girls and women, rates of ARFID appear to be similar across genders in both child and adult populations [2, 3].

Prevalence rates of ARFID are higher in samples drawn from specialist medical settings, such as eating disorder, feeding disorder, and gastroenterology clinics. Among patients referred to child and adult gastroenterology clinics, the rate of ARFID is estimated to be between 1.5% and 6.3% [4, 5]. Prevalence rates for ARFID are even higher in both feeding and eating disorder-specific settings. Studies of children referred to hospital-based feeding disorder clinics estimate the prevalence of ARFID to be between 32% and 64%, depending on the inclusion or exclusion of children who have comorbid medical conditions [6, 7]. Studies from eating disorder treatment programs have provided a range of prevalence estimates, from 9.2% [8] on the low end to 44% [9] on the high end.

Similar to findings from population-based studies, the frequency of ARFID diagnoses in eating disorder treatment settings varies depending on the age of the treatment sample. Estimates of ARFID prevalence rates are lowest in adult treatment settings (9.2%) [8] and higher in child and adolescent programs. Rates of ARFID in a combined child and adolescent day treatment program were reported to be 24.5% based on retrospective chart review [10]. Another specialist child eating disorder program (ages 6–12) reported that 44% of patients admitted after the ARFID diagnosis was published in DSM-5 met criteria for a primary diagnosis of ARFID [9]. The distribution of ARFID diagnoses across genders within these traditional eating disorder settings is difficult to discern. No men were included in the study from an adult eating disorder treatment setting [8]. The child and adolescent samples, however, reported a significant proportion of boys, with higher rates in the exclusively child setting (67% [9] vs. 19.7% [10]). Traditional eating disorder settings may underrepresent the proportion of boys and men suffering from ARFID; however, these estimates may change as the diagnosis gains more recognition.

Symptoms and Presentation

ARFID presents with a great deal of symptom heterogeneity, and patients with the disorder may endorse a wide range of symptoms and behaviors including food avoidance, reduced portion sizes, acute onset of eating problems, chronic eating and feeding problems, reduced variety of food intake, "picky" or "fussy" eating, gagging, all liquid diets, food neophobia (i.e., fear of trying new foods), nausea and other functional gastrointestinal symptoms (e.g., vomiting, constipation, abdominal pain), generalized anxiety, specific fears, lack of appetite, early satiety, compulsions, extended mealtimes, over-chewing food or packing food in cheeks or along the gum line, and use of nutritional supplements. These symptoms have been documented in numerous studies or clinical descriptions of ARFID patients [11–14]. Despite this heterogeneity, experts in the fields of feeding and eating disorders have characterized three general patterns of food avoidance: (1) selective eating due to sensory sensitivity, (2) avoidance due to the fear of aversive outcomes related to eating, and (3) lack of interest in eating or poor appetite (Fig. 6.1) [1, 15–17].

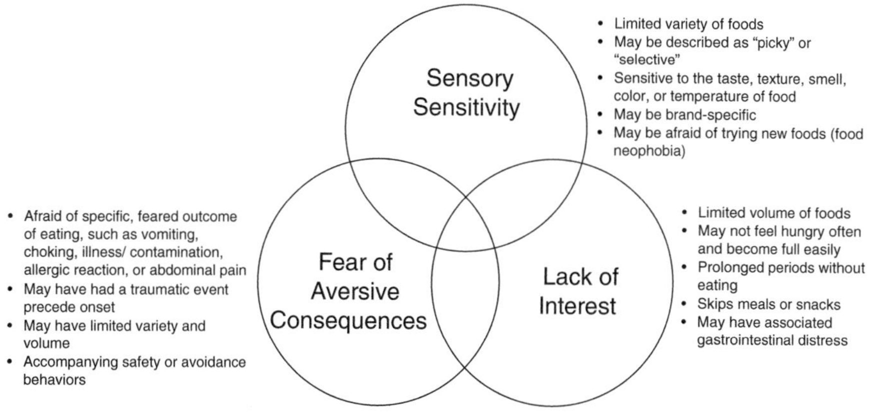

Fig. 6.1 Description of ARFID symptom profiles

Selective eating due to sensory sensitivity is often characterized by limitation of the variety of foods consumed and may be based on taste, texture, color, temperature, or brand. There may also be significant fear of trying new or novel foods, otherwise known as food neophobia. Individuals with this presentation are commonly referred to as "picky" or "selective" eaters. A fear of the aversive consequences of eating is typically associated with a specific, negative feared outcome. Commonly reported fears include fear of vomiting, choking, illness/contamination, allergic reaction, or abdominal pain. A triggering, traumatic event may or may not precede the onset of the specific food-related fear. In addition to avoiding specific foods associated with the fear, these individuals may also engage in a number of other safety or avoidance behaviors related to eating, such as prolonged chewing of food, taking extremely small bites of food, checking or reading food labels and expirations dates, eating in isolation, seeking reassurance, and excessive hand washing. Finally, lack of interest in eating or poor appetite is associated with early satiety, going prolonged periods without eating, skipping meals or snacks, and possibly other functional gastrointestinal complaints such as stomach discomfort, constipation, fullness, or nausea.

As the result of identifying these three patterns of food avoidance, researchers and clinical providers working in the field of ARFID have described "subtypes" of ARFID. Two studies within eating disorder treatment settings (tertiary care [18] and day treatment [19]) have examined the existence of such ARFID subtypes, and approximately a quarter of each sample was represented by boys. Both studies found that it was possible to assign ARFID patients to specific diagnostic subtypes. Findings from these samples generally supported that the fear of aversive consequences subtype was the most common presentation in a specialty eating disorder treatment setting and that this subtype was the most likely to present with acute onset and weight loss and require inpatient hospital admission. Girls were also more likely to present with fear of aversive consequences, and this subtype was associated with less psychiatric comorbidity [19]. However, other reports have found an increased odds of a lifetime anxiety disorder individuals with fear of aversive consequences [20]. While the least common subtype in both studies was the sensory sensitivity or selective eating subtype, individuals with this subtype were more likely to include boys and less likely to have poor growth or weight loss. Furthermore, sensory sensitivity is associated with increased odds of a current lifetime neurodevelopmental disorder [20].

Despite the emergence of some between-group differences, there remains a great deal of overlap among the putative ARFID subtypes. In a study examining the most commonly reported clinical features of ARFID, over half of all ARFID patients report restricting portion sizes (96.4%), a specific onset or trigger for their eating disturbance (71.4%), avoiding specific foods (64.3%), nausea (60.7%), early satiety (57.1%), and abdominal pain (50%) [11]. Several of these features could be endorsed across all three subtypes. Indeed, Norris and colleagues indicated in their study that 22% of patients presented with features of more than one subtype [18]. Furthermore, in a study by Zickgraf and colleagues, a fourth subtype of ARFID was identified that consisted of a group of patients who presented with shared features of both the sensory sensitivity and lack of interest subtypes, which was referred to as "co-primary" ARFID [19]. This study also found evidence that the co-primary group was associated with a higher proportion of boys, poorer growth, and a significantly longer duration of ARFID symptoms compared to the other three subtypes. Other studies that have examined overlap in subtypes have found that approximately half of ARFID patients meet criteria for multiple presentations [9, 21].

Due to the degree of overlap among ARFID presentations, Thomas and colleagues have proposed an alternative system for describing the presentations of ARFID patients [17]. Rather than a categorical subtyping system, they suggest that patterns of ARFID symptoms may represent distinct, but not mutually exclusive, domains of dysfunction. These domains each map onto possible underlying neurobiological mechanisms. Selective eating due to sensory sensitivity may be the result of hypersensitivity in perceptual systems relevant to eating, such as taste, smell, and texture. Lack of interest in eating may be related to a low homeostatic drive to eat, as well as disturbances in neurobiological and hormonal systems relevant to appetite regulation and processing of interoceptive signals. Finally, fears related to the aversive consequences of eating may be caused by vulnerabilities to physiological reactivity and hyperactivation of neurobiological threat systems. Conceptualizing ARFID symptoms from this perspective allows for the creation of unique profiles of symptoms for each individual with ARFID and reduces the need to characterize these complex patients by applying a single subtype. Furthermore, understanding the underlying mechanisms that may broadly contribute to the eating disturbances in ARFID will facilitate the creation of more targeted, effective treatments.

Course and Outcomes

Medical Sequelae and Comorbidity Patients with ARFID are at risk for severe medical consequences due to lack of adequate intake and/or nutrition. The majority of pediatric ARFID patients who present for treatment tend to be significantly underweight or have failed to gain weight at an expected rate, with up to one quarter requiring hospitalization due to low weight and/or unstable vital signs [22]. While ARFID patients who have had an acute onset are the most likely to require hospitalization, research indicates that those with a chronic course have the lowest body mass index (BMI) [21]. Compared to patients with AN, patients with ARFID have been found to have significantly lower bone mineral density, with 25% of patients falling in the osteoporotic range [22]. ARFID patients are also at risk for bradycardia, hypotension, prolonged QT interval on electrocardiogram, anemia, amenorrhea, electrolyte imbalances (e.g., hypokalemia, hypophosphatemia), and elevated liver enzymes [23–25]. Furthermore, patients with ARFID are also more likely than those with AN and BN to be diagnosed with a co-occurring medical condition [24, 26]. Gastrointestinal diseases and symptoms identified in samples of ARFID patients include gastroesophageal reflux disease, eosinophilic esophagitis (EOE), gastroparesis, nausea, abdominal pain, constipation, and irritable bowel syndrome

[19, 23, 27]. Individuals with ARFID are also more likely to suffer from food allergies [28]. Finally, nutritional disease is a major concern for individuals with ARFID, particularly those with selective eating due to sensory sensitivities. Three case reports have detailed severe, adverse medical events – blindness, optic neuropathy, and spinal cord degeneration – in adolescent boys the result of vitamin deficiencies resulting from ARFID [29–31].

Psychiatric Comorbidity The prevalence of current psychiatric comorbidities in patients with ARFID is estimated to be 45%, while the lifetime prevalence is estimated to be 54% [20]. In those patients receiving treatment at higher levels of care, psychiatric comorbidity has been reported to be as high as 74% [21]. Associated comorbidities include anxiety disorders, mood disorders, neurodevelopmental disorders (e.g., autism spectrum disorder), attention-deficit disorders, conduct disorders, and suicidality [9, 20, 24, 26, 28, 32, 33]. In comparison to patients with other eating disorders, patients with ARFID appear to have a higher rate of comorbid anxiety disorders and a lower rate of comorbid mood disorders [26, 28, 33]. Among anxiety disorders, generalized anxiety disorder appears to be most common, followed by panic disorder and social anxiety disorder [20].

Course of Illness Compared to patients with AN, those with ARFID tend to have a longer course of illness and earlier onset of eating disturbances prior to presenting to treatment [10, 26, 34]. Among children and adolescents treated for ARFID, some parents report eating problems beginning in infancy, often with breastfeeding or transition to solid foods [9]. Selective eating behaviors, in particular, emerge at young ages, and for a subset of these individuals, the pattern of restrictive eating persists into late childhood and adolescence [35, 36]. Preschool-aged children identified as moderate to severe selective eaters had a greater risk of developing anxiety, depression, and other psychosocial impairment at 2-year follow-up [37]. There are few long-term treatment outcomes studies of ARFID. One follow-up study of adolescent patients with ARFID (30% boys) from a day treatment program indicated that at 1-year post-treatment, the majority of patients were still receiving outpatient treatment and were continuing to take psychotropic medication [33]. Another study examined long-term psychiatric and psychosocial outcomes of patients with ARFID who received eating disorder treatment before the age of 13 [38]. Patients were evaluated an average of 15.9 years after treatment; at follow-up, 26.3% had a current ARFID diagnosis, 26.3% had another psychiatric diagnosis, and 47.4% did not meet criteria for any psychiatric diagnosis. Those who had a current eating disorder diagnosis all met criteria for ARFID, suggesting diagnostic stability. Compared with patients without a current eating disorder diagnosis, patients with ARFID were less likely to be earning a living through paid employment or enrolled as a student. It should be noted that ARFID diagnoses in this study were assigned retroactively, as the ARFID diagnosis had not been developed at the time of treatment for the sample. Furthermore, the majority of this sample were women (95%) and thus may not be reflective of long-term outcomes for ARFID patients who are boys and/or men.

Studies of adults with ARFID may also inform understanding of the potential long-term outcomes of individuals with the disorder. Adult patients with ARFID in Australia ($n = 10$) had poorer mental health-related quality of life compared to other eating disorders (with the exception of binge eating disorder; BED) and healthy individuals [2]. They also had more non-functional days than healthy individuals, meaning days in which they could not work or go to school. ARFID in adults has been associated with psychopathology, particularly obsessive-compulsive disorder, depressive symptoms, and lower quality of life, on par with other adults with disordered eating pathology [39]. Thus, the limited data we have on long-term outcomes for ARFID suggests that if left untreated, ARFID may place individuals at risk for other forms of psychopathology and serious impairments in psychosocial functioning. Therefore, it is imperative that mental health and medical professionals properly identify and treat ARFID.

Assessment

ARFID can be diagnosed at any age when an individual presents with restrictive eating behavior that persistently fails to meet nutritional and/or energy needs as evidenced by at least one of the four major associated complications (DSM-5 Criterion A) [1]: (1) weight loss or failure to grow as expected (i.e., faltering growth), (2) nutritional deficiency, (3) dependence on nutritional supplements or enteral (i.e., tube) feedings, or (4) psychosocial impairment. The restrictive eating should not be better attributed to cultural practices (e.g., observing dietary restrictions associated with a particular religion) or socioeconomic limitations (e.g., food insecurity; Criterion B). The restrictive eating should also not exist solely within the context of body image disturbance, a desire to lose weight, or a fear of gaining weight (Criterion C). Finally, the restrictive eating should not be better accounted for by a medical condition (Criterion D).

While best practices have yet to be established for the assessment and treatment of ARFID, it is generally agreed that assessment should include, at a minimum, a physical exam and a psychosocial interview to evaluate medical stability and criteria for a diagnosis [40]. While ARFID is less likely to result in hospitalization in comparison with AN, hospitalization may be required in cases with acute onset and associated rapid weight loss [19, 22, 24]. A physical exam and review of weight history by a physician can determine underweight status or failure to achieve expected growth. For adults, it is reasonable to use the same criteria for defining underweight status as is used in AN (i.e., BMI < 18.5) [40]. For children and adolescents, guidelines for determining underweight status such as those outlined by the Society for Adolescent Health and Medicine may be used [41]. Failure to achieve expected weight or height or “growth stunting” may be determined by examining individual growth curves.

Evaluation by a physician may also aid in determining whether or not criteria are met for nutritional deficiency. Individuals with ARFID who abstain from eating whole food groups or who eat a limited number of items infrequently from a specific food group are at risk for developing nutritional diseases, such as anemia, scurvy, and rickets, as well as other vitamin-specific deficiencies. Recent data show that individuals with full or subthreshold ARFID consume significantly fewer fruits, vegetables, and proteins compared to healthy same-aged peers and are more at risk for vitamin K and vitamin B12 deficiencies [42]. Nutritional deficiencies can be confirmed via bloodwork, and food monitoring records or a food frequency questionnaire may further be used to evaluate nutritional risk.

Psychosocial impairment as the result of restrictive eating may manifest in several ways. This criterion may refer to an inability to eat at school or in the workplace, an inability to eat outside of the home (e.g., avoidance of restaurants, avoidance of foods prepared by others), and avoidance of social events such as parties or family gatherings where food is served. A significant body of literature exists documenting the stress that selective eating behaviors may place on families [43–46]. Either in response to picky eating or as the result of picky eating, parents report that meal times can be highly emotional, with parents and children struggling over food intake [45]. Alternatively, parents may attempt to avoid conflict by catering to children's preferences and cooking alternative meals. High parental anxiety is frequently associated with selective eating styles, and the family's functioning may be negatively impacted as a result (e.g., avoidance of family vacations due to fear that child will not eat) [46]. The result of any of these limitations may be increased family stress, social isolation, loneliness, and embarrassment, all of which may contribute to the subsequent development of depression or social anxiety.

A thorough assessment of ARFID should also consider the appropriateness of referrals to specialist providers, as there are a number of medical conditions that may influence the course of ARFID treatment or partially account for the difficulty eating. Referrals to gastroenterology may be indicated for patients presenting with functional abdominal complaints such as diarrhea, constipation, pain, frequent vomiting, reflux, and effortful swallowing. While a significant portion of ARFID patients present with food allergies, others may present with probable food allergies and associated avoidance due to fear of an allergic reaction. Those with diagnosed food allergies may also broadly avoid foods due to the potential presence of an allergic contaminant. A consultation with a rheumatologist or allergist is important to determine the sensitivity of an allergy and/or to confirm the presence of additional food allergies. In other cases, patients with a history of eczema, asthma, or a family history of food allergy are at risk for developing food allergies, and an undiagnosed allergy or intolerance may be driving food avoidance. Finally, sensory sensitivities and oral-motor skills deficits may contribute to food avoidance and restriction. Consider referrals to occupational therapists for those patients who have sensitivities to tastes and textures and aversion to other sensory input, such as brushing teeth, cutting nails, and tags on clothing. Individuals who over-chew foods, pack foods along the gum line or in cheeks, have messy chewing, or require water to swallow may have an oral-motor skills deficit and should be referred to a speech pathologist for evaluation.

Finally, the assessment process should seek to characterize the reasons for or function of food avoidance or restriction. Several standardized assessment options are now available to help diagnose ARFID and/or provide a profile of the three symptom categories identified in DSM-5. The Pica, ARFID, and Rumination Disorder Interview (PARDI), the ARFID module of the Eating Disorder Examination (EDE), and the computerized Eating Disorder Assessment (EDA-5) are all semi-structured interviews that aid in the diagnosis of ARFID. The EDA-5 allows for the diagnosis of ARFID (along with other DSM-5 eating disorders); however, the interview does not provide information on symptom profiles and is only available for use in ages 8 and up [47]. The PARDI and the ARFID module of the EDE both provide symptom profile information. To date, the ARFID module of the EDE has only been piloted in children ages 8–13 [48]. Furthermore, the EDE does provide both a child and parent version to allow for multi-informant assessment, an important feature when assessing eating disorders in children. The PARDI currently has the broadest applicability and is the only structured ARFID assessment that can assess for ARFID across the lifespan [49]. The PARDI has self-informant versions for children as young as age 8 and parent-informant versions for children as young as age 2. In addition to providing information on diagnosis and symptom profiles, the PARDI also provides severity ratings for each symptom profile and includes an assessment of clinical impairment. It is currently the only ARFID assessment that provides this impairment index. Both the PARDI and the EDE have demonstrated good interrater reliability and the ability to distinguish ARFID from other restrictive eating disorders [48, 49].

Finally, a few short, self-report measures of ARFID are available that could serve as screening tools, although no clinical cutoffs or norms are yet available. The Eating Disorder in Youth Questionnaire (EDY-Q) is a 14-item self-report tool that provides information on the different symptom variants of ARFID. The questionnaire has been evaluated in a large sample of youth aged 8–13 years and provides guidelines (scoring suggestions) for the "probable" existence of ARFID "subtypes" [50]. The subtypes identified by the EDY-Q are selective eating, functional dysphagia, and Food Avoidance Emotional Disorder (FAED), which map onto the DSM-5 symptom profiles: selective eating with sensory sensitivity, functional dysphagia with fear of aversive consequences, and FAED with lack of interest/poor appetite. The EDY-Q also has one item each for the screening of pica and rumination and two items for the screening of weight and shape concerns. The other screening tool available is the Nine Item ARFID Scale (NIAS) [51]. The NIAS has now been validated in individuals aged 8–65 years, making it the most broadly applicable ARFID screening tool [51, 52]. It also provides subscale scores that map onto the DSM-5 ARFID symptom profiles and has demonstrated good psychometric properties (Table 6.1).

Table 6.1 Summary of measures that assess ARFID

Measure name	Measure type	Ages	Used for diagnosis	Symptom profiles	Features
Pica, ARFID, and Rumination Disorder Interview (PARDI)	Structured interview, self-report, and parent report	2 years to adult	Yes	Yes	Includes severity ratings and clinical impairment index; available in multiple languages [48]
Eating Disorder Examination, ARFID Supplement (EDE-ARFID)	Structured interview, self-report, and parent report	8 years to adult[a]	Yes	Yes	Assesses four ARFID symptom profiles, including Food Avoidance Emotional Disorder (FAED)
Eating Disorder Assessment for DSM-5 (EDA-5)	Computerized semi-structured interview, self-report	8 years to adult	Yes	No	Available in English, Spanish, Norwegian, and Turkish [47]
Nine Item ARFID Screen (NIAS)	Self-report questionnaire	8–65	No	Yes	Generates a total ARFID score and 3 subscale scores
Eating Disorders in Youth Questionnaire (EDY-Q)	Self-report questionnaire	8–13	No	Yes	Includes suggested clinical cutoffs; items to assess for weight/shape distortion and presence of pica and rumination disorder

[a]The EDE-ARFID assessment was designed to be used in ages 8 to adult; the assessment has only thus far been evaluated in ages 8–13 years [48]

Treatment

Information on the treatment of ARFID is rapidly expanding. Multiple single case studies and small case series are now available detailing the treatment of ARFID in specific presentations. A treatment manual for ARFID and a separate guide for ARFID caregivers/loved ones are now published and widely available [54, 55]. One randomized controlled trial on a brief, intensive treatment for ARFID has been published, and data are available on the outcomes of hospital-based ARFID treatments from two larger cohorts. Two additional randomized controlled trials to evaluate specific ARFID treatments are underway, and one large-scale effectiveness study is in progress.

While ARFID as a diagnosis may be new, those with the symptoms of the disorder are not. Patients who formally received the diagnosis of Feeding Disorder of Infancy and Childhood (FDIC) have been treated for years in the context of hospital-based and outpatient feeding clinics. The efficacy of the programs and techniques has largely been reported in small, case series reports and has included predominantly children in toddlerhood, late preschool, and early school ages [56]. The vast majority of techniques utilized in these clinics include behavioral interventions and aim to increase both the intake and variety of solid foods, often in children with developmental disabilities or on prolonged tube feedings. Interventions consistently include techniques such demand fading to increase tolerance of volume and new tastes/textures, effective prompting, escape extinction, and contingent reinforcement. Some programs also include elements aimed at improving parent-child dynamics, such as parent-child interaction therapy. Most feeding therapies are performed on an individual basis and include the involvement of a team of professionals, such as psychologists, gastroenterologists, dietitians, speech and language pathologists (SLP), occupational therapists (OT), and nurses. The techniques used in feeding therapies are reported to be generally effective, but quality data from large-scale studies and randomized controlled trials is lacking [56]. Furthermore, the participants included in these studies do not generalize well to typically developing older children, adolescents, and adults.

The only published randomized trial for ARFID to date was conducted within the context of a pediatric feeding clinic. This pilot study evaluated the efficacy of a 5-day intensive day treatment program for the treatment of severe, chronic food refusal in children ages 13–72 months (1–6 years) [57]. Twenty children (12 boys) and their parents were included in the trial. The treatment consisted of a manualized, behavioral intervention (reinforcement, escape extinction, and meal-time structure) delivered in the context of 40 meals. Parents were also provided with training in behavior management procedures. In comparison to a wait-list control, participants in the trial showed an increase in bite acceptance, a decrease in mealtime disruptions, an increase in grams consumed, and an increase in percent of median BMI-for-age percentile (%MBMI). These results are consistent with outcomes reported from other single case studies and case series using similar interventions. As is consistent with other treatment literature in children with feeding disorders, this study sample was very young and had a high comorbidity of medical problems and dependence on tube feeding, making the outcomes difficult to generalize to older and more typically developing children with ARFID.

Similar data are also available for the treatment of ARFID within the context of traditional, hospital-based eating disorder programs. Two studies, one from a child and adolescent day treatment program and one from an inpatient children's medical center, evaluated treatment outcomes for patients with ARFID in comparison to patients with AN. A retrospective chart review of 318 patients hospitalized for acute medical instability revealed that most patients hospitalized with ARFID ($n = 41$, 11% boys and/or men) achieved the target weight gain goal of 0.2 kg per day [25]. However, patients with ARFID required longer hospital stays on average and required more frequent enteral (i.e., tube feeding) supplementation to achieve their nutritional goals. In a day treatment program for children ages 8–18, patients with ARFID ($n = 32$, 18.7% boys) significantly increased their %MBMI throughout the course of their treatment stay and showed a significant decrease in self-reported anxiety [10]. In this study, children with ARFID had, on average, a shorter duration of treatment compared to their counterparts with anorexia. Importantly, increases in %MBMI were maintained in the ARFID group at 1-year follow-up [33].

Two other major types of interventions for ARFID have been proposed, and versions of these interventions are currently being evaluated in randomized controlled trials. First, family-based treatments for ARFID have received considerable attention, primarily due to the efficacy of Family-Based Treatment for Anorexia (FBT-AN) and the young average presentation of patients with ARFID. One case series from an ongoing trial of FBT-AN adapted for ARFID (FBT-ARFID) has been published to illustrate the consistencies and changes between the two treatments [58]. All three cases from this trial showed improvement in PARDI symptom severity at the end of treatment, although all lacked complete resolution of ARFID diagnostic criteria. Other case series and examples have also been published illustrating family-based treatments for ARFID. One case illustrated the success of an adapted form of FBT-AN combined with the Unified Protocol for Emotional Disorders in Children (UP-C) to treat the case of a young 9-year-old girl with weight loss and fears of choking and abdominal pain [59]. While not considered to be family-based, others have published on the usefulness of parenting-only interventions, particularly with school-aged children with selective eating due to sensory sensitivity [14, 60].

The second type of intervention proposed for use with ARFID is cognitive-behavior therapy (CBT). Several variations of CBT-based therapies have been described in case studies, and the only published manual for the treatment of ARFID is Cognitive-Behavior Therapy for Avoidant/Restrictive Food Intake Disorder (CBT-AR) [54]. Unlike family-based and behavioral feeding therapies, CBT-AR was written for children (ages 10+) and adults with ARFID. It has two versions, one family-supported for children, adolescents, and young adults who are underweight and one that is in individual format for those who are normal weight or more motivated older adults. Currently, it is the only comprehensive ARFID treatment that provides specific, targeted modules to address the unique symptoms profiles of ARFID. Results from case studies and case series suggest that a cognitive-behavioral approach to the treatment of ARFID may be successful [61–63]. Interventions in these studies generally emphasize exposure principles (to both food and fear cues), psychoeducation, and other skills such as cognitive restructuring, relaxation training, behavioral experiments, and relapse prevention. Cases have been illustrated across gender and among adolescents and adults with ARFID. One cognitive-behavioral intervention has been developed specifically for children presenting with the symptoms of poor appetite and lack of interest in eating and includes elements of acceptance-based treatments. The Feelings and Body Investigators (FBI) program, ARFID Division, provides psychoeducation on the overlap between emotions and body feelings, combined with interoceptive exposure, to reduce discomfort with feelings of fullness and abdominal pain and improve tolerance of eating [64].

Finally, several medications have been used to augment hospital-based treatments and psychotherapy. Olanzapine, selective-serotonin reuptake inhibitors, and mirtazapine have all been associated with increased weight gain, increased rate of weight gain, and reduction in anxious and depressive symptoms of ARFID in small case series [65–67]. One double-blinded, placebo-controlled feasibility trial in 20 children (18 months to 6 years) used d-cycloserine to enhance extinction of severe feeding aversion during behavioral treatment, improving rapid swallowing and decreasing mealtime disruptions [68]. Retrospective chart reviews have also revealed positive effects on feeding tolerance with the use of cyproheptadine in children younger than 6 years [69, 70]. Research on medication treatment for ARFID is still in early stages, and larger, well-controlled trials are needed.

Conclusion

ARFID is a complex eating disorder characterized by extremely selective food intake due to the sensory properties of foods, fears related to the aversive outcomes of eating, and lack of interest in eating. A growing body of data suggests that ARFID may be as prevalent and serious as other eating disorders and of particular concern for boys and/or men, as they may represent nearly half of all ARFID cases. To date, boys seem to comprise the majority of patients with the sensory sensitivity presentation of ARFID. However, boys and men are underrepresented in many published ARFID samples, particularly from clinical settings, and future research should seek to better understand potential gender differences in ARFID and their impact on treatment and illness outcomes. Furthermore, improved understanding of the unique symptom profiles in ARFID, and the neurobiological etiologies that underlie them, will be essential for developing effective therapies for ARFID. For now, several promising treatment options are under study and available to those who suffer.

References

1. American Psychiatric Association. Diagnostic and statistical manual of mental disorders. 5th ed. Washington, DC: Author; 2013.
2. Hay P, et al. Burden and health-related quality of life of eating disorders, including avoidant/restrictive food intake disorder (ARFID), in the Australian population. J Eat Disord. 2017;5:21.
3. Kurz S, et al. Early-onset restrictive eating disturbances in primary school boys and girls. Eur Child Adolesc Psychiatry. 2015;24(7):779–85.
4. Eddy KT, et al. Prevalence of DSM-5 avoidant/restrictive food intake disorder in a pediatric gastroenterology healthcare network. Int J Eat Disord. 2015;48(5):464–70.
5. Murray HB, et al. Prevalence and characteristics of avoidant/restrictive food intake disorder in adult neurogastroenterology patients. Clin Gastroenterol Hepatol. 2020;18(9):1995–2002.e1.
6. Williams K, et al. Implications of avoidant/restrictive food intake disorder (ARFID) on children with feeding problems. Child Health Care. 2015;44:307–21.
7. Krom H, et al. Health related quality of life of infants and children with avoidant restrictive food intake disorder. Int J Eat Disord. 2019;52(4):410–8.
8. Nakai Y, et al. Characteristics of avoidant/restrictive food intake disorder in a cohort of adult patients. Eur Eat Disord Rev. 2016;24(6):528–30.
9. Reilly EE, et al. Exploring the cooccurrence of behavioural phenotypes for avoidant/restrictive food intake disorder in a partial hospitalization sample. Eur Eat Disord Rev. 2019;27(4):429–35.
10. Ornstein RM, et al. Treatment of avoidant/restrictive food intake disorder in a cohort of young patients in a partial hospitalization program for eating disorders. Int J Eat Disord. 2017;50(9):1067–74.

11. Cooney M, et al. Clinical and psychological features of children and adolescents diagnosed with avoidant/restrictive food intake disorder in a pediatric tertiary care eating disorder program: a descriptive study. J Eat Disord. 2018;6:7.
12. Bloomfield BS, et al. Treatment of food selectivity in a child with avoidant/restrictive food intake disorder through parent teleconsultation. Behav Anal Pract. 2019;12(1):33–43.
13. Lopes R, et al. A case of choking phobia: towards a conceptual approach. Eat Weight Disord. 2014;19(1):125–31.
14. Murphy J, Zlomke KR. A behavioral parent-training intervention for a child with avoidant/restrictive food intake disorder. Clin Pract Pediatr Psychol. 2016;4(1):23–34.
15. Bryant-Waugh R, et al. Feeding and eating disorders in childhood. Int J Eat Disord. 2010;43(2):98–111.
16. Kreipe RE, Palomaki A. Beyond picky eating: avoidant/restrictive food intake disorder. Curr Psychiatry Rep. 2012;14(4):421–31.
17. Thomas JJ, et al. Avoidant/restrictive food intake disorder: a three-dimensional model of neurobiology with implications for etiology and treatment. Curr Psychiatry Rep. 2017;19(8):54.
18. Norris ML, et al. Building evidence for the use of descriptive subtypes in youth with avoidant restrictive food intake disorder. Int J Eat Disord. 2018;51(2):170–3.
19. Zickgraf HF, et al. Further support for diagnostically meaningful ARFID symptom presentations in an adolescent medicine partial hospitalization program. Int J Eat Disord. 2019;52(4):402–9.
20. Kambanis PE, et al. Prevalence and correlates of psychiatric comorbidities in children and adolescents with full and subthreshold avoidant/restrictive food intake disorder. Int J Eat Disord. 2020;53(2):256–65.
21. Duncombe Lowe K, et al. Youth with avoidant/restrictive food intake disorder: examining differences by age, weight status, and symptom duration. Nutrients. 2019;11(8):1955.
22. Norris ML, et al. Exploring avoidant/restrictive food intake disorder in eating disordered patients: a descriptive study. Int J Eat Disord. 2014;47(5):495–9.
23. Makhzoumi SH, et al. Hospital course of underweight youth with ARFID treated with a meal-based behavioral protocol in an inpatient-partial hospitalization program for eating disorders. Int J Eat Disord. 2019;52(4):428–34.
24. Keery H, et al. Attributes of children and adolescents with avoidant/restrictive food intake disorder. J Eat Disord. 2019;7:31.
25. Strandjord SE, et al. Avoidant/restrictive food intake disorder: illness and hospital course in patients hospitalized for nutritional insufficiency. J Adolesc Health. 2015;57(6):673–8.
26. Fisher MM, et al. Characteristics of avoidant/restrictive food intake disorder in children and adolescents: a "new disorder" in DSM-5. J Adolesc Health. 2014;55(1):49–52.
27. Robson J, et al. Avoidant/restrictive food intake disorder in diet-treated children with eosinophilic esophagitis. J Pediatr Gastroenterol Nutr. 2019;69(1):57–60.
28. Nicely TA, et al. Prevalence and characteristics of avoidant/restrictive food intake disorder in a cohort of young patients in day treatment for eating disorders. J Eat Disord. 2014;2(1):21.
29. Harrison R, et al. Blindness caused by a junk food diet. Ann Intern Med. 2019;171(11):859–61.
30. Chandran JJ, et al. Subacute combined degeneration of the spinal cord in an adolescent male with avoidant/restrictive food intake disorder: a clinical case report. Int J Eat Disord. 2015;48(8):1176–9.
31. Chiarello F, et al. Optic neuropathy due to nutritional deficiency in a male adolescent with avoidant/restrictive food intake disorder: a case report. Eat Weight Disord. 2018;23(4):533–5.
32. Norris ML, et al. Characteristics and clinical trajectories of patients meeting criteria for avoidant/restrictive food intake disorder that are subsequently reclassified as anorexia nervosa. Eur Eat Disord Rev. 2020;28(1):26–33.
33. Bryson AE, et al. Outcomes of low-weight patients with avoidant/restrictive food intake disorder and anorexia nervosa at long-term follow-up after treatment in a partial hospitalization program for eating disorders. Int J Eat Disord. 2018;51(5):470–4.

34. Becker KR, et al. Co-occurrence of avoidant/restrictive food intake disorder and traditional eating psychopathology. J Am Acad Child Adolesc Psychiatry. 2020;59(2):209–12.
35. Taylor CM, Hays NP, Emmett PM. Diet at age 10 and 13 years in children identified as picky eaters at age 3 years and in children who are persistent picky eaters in a longitudinal birth cohort study. Nutrients. 2019;11(4):807.
36. Mascola AJ, Bryson SW, Agras WS. Picky eating during childhood: a longitudinal study to age 11 years. Eat Behav. 2010;11(4):253–7.
37. Zucker N, et al. Psychological and psychosocial impairment in preschoolers with selective eating. Pediatrics. 2015;136(3):e582–90.
38. Lange CRA, et al. Long-term follow-up study of low-weight avoidant restrictive food intake disorder compared with childhood-onset anorexia nervosa: psychiatric and occupational outcome in 56 patients. Int J Eat Disord. 2019;52(4):435–8.
39. Zickgraf HF, Franklin ME, Rozin P. Adult picky eaters with symptoms of avoidant/restrictive food intake disorder: comparable distress and comorbidity but different eating behaviors compared to those with disordered eating symptoms. J Eat Disord. 2016;4:26.
40. Eddy KT, et al. Radcliffe ARFID Workgroup: toward operationalization of research diagnostic criteria and directions for the field. Int J Eat Disord. 2019;52(4):361–6.
41. Society for Adolescent Health and Medicine, et al. Position paper of the Society for Adolescent Health and Medicine: medical management of restrictive eating disorders in adolescents and young adults. J Adolesc Health. 2015;56(1):121–5.
42. Harshman SG, et al. A diet high in processed foods, total carbohydrates and added sugars, and low in vegetables and protein is characteristic of youth with avoidant/restrictive food intake disorder. Nutrients. 2019;11(9):2013.
43. Trofholz AC, Schulte AK, Berge JM. How parents describe picky eating and its impact on family meals: a qualitative analysis. Appetite. 2017;110:36–43.
44. Fishbein M, Benton K, Struthers W. Mealtime disruption and caregiver stress in referrals to an outpatient feeding clinic. J Parenter Enter Nutr. 2016;40(5):636–45.
45. Wolstenholme H, et al. Childhood fussy/picky eating behaviours: a systematic review and synthesis of qualitative studies. Int J Behav Nutr Phys Act. 2020;17(1):2.
46. Cole NC, et al. Correlates of picky eating and food neophobia in young children: a systematic review and meta-analysis. Nutr Rev. 2017;75(7):516–32.
47. The Columbia Center for Eating Disorders. Eating disorder assessment for DSM-5 (EDA-5). n.d. [2020, May 15]. Available from: https://eda5.org/.
48. Schmidt R, et al. Interview-based assessment of avoidant/restrictive food intake disorder (ARFID): a pilot study evaluating an ARFID module for the Eating Disorder Examination. Int J Eat Disord. 2019;52(4):388–97.
49. Bryant-Waugh R, et al. Development of the Pica, ARFID, and Rumination Disorder Interview, a multi-informant, semi-structured interview of feeding disorders across the lifespan: a pilot study for ages 10-22. Int J Eat Disord. 2019;52(4):378–87.
50. Kurz S, et al. Variants of early-onset restrictive eating disturbances in middle childhood. Int J Eat Disord. 2016;49(1):102–6.
51. Zickgraf HF, Ellis JM. Initial validation of the Nine Item Avoidant/Restrictive Food Intake disorder screen (NIAS): a measure of three restrictive eating patterns. Appetite. 2018;123:32–42.
52. Zickgraf HF, Elkins A. Sensory sensitivity mediates the relationship between anxiety and picky eating in children/adolescents ages 8-17, and in college undergraduates: a replication and age-upward extension. Appetite. 2018;128:333–9.
53. Bryant-Waugh R, Higgins C. Avoidant restrictive food intake disorder in childhood and adolescence: a clinical guide. New York: Routledge; 2020.
54. Thomas JJ, Wons OB, Eddy KT. Cognitive-behavioral treatment of avoidant/restrictive food intake disorder. Curr Opin Psychiatry. 2018;31(6):425–30.
55. Bryant-Waugh R. ARFID avoidant restrictive food intake disorder: a guide for parents and carers. 1st ed. New York: Routledge; 2020.

56. Sharp WG, et al. A systematic review and meta-analysis of intensive multidisciplinary intervention for pediatric feeding disorders: how standard is the standard of care? J Pediatr. 2017;181:116–124.e4.
57. Sharp WG, et al. Intensive, manual-based intervention for pediatric feeding disorders: results from a randomized pilot trial. J Pediatr Gastroenterol Nutr. 2016;62(4):658–63.
58. Lock J, et al. Applying family-based treatment (FBT) to three clinical presentations of avoidant/restrictive food intake disorder: similarities and differences from FBT for anorexia nervosa. Int J Eat Disord. 2019;52(4):439–46.
59. Eckhardt S, et al. An ARFID case report combining family-based treatment with the unified protocol for Transdiagnostic treatment of emotional disorders in children. J Eat Disord. 2019;7:34.
60. Dahlsgaard KK, Bodie J. The (extremely) picky eaters clinic: a pilot trial of a seven-session group behavioral intervention for parents of children with avoidant/restrictive food intake disorder. Cogn Behav Pract. 2019;26(3):492–505.
61. Fischer AJ, Luiselli JK, Dove MB. Effects of clinic and in-home treatment on consumption and feeding-associated anxiety in an adolescent with avoidant/restrictive food intake disorder. Clin Pract Pediatr Psychol. 2015;3(2):154–66.
62. Dumont E, et al. A new cognitive behavior therapy for adolescents with avoidant/restrictive food intake disorder in a day treatment setting: a clinical case series. Int J Eat Disord. 2019;52(4):447–58.
63. King LA, Urbach JR, Stewart KE. Illness anxiety and avoidant/restrictive food intake disorder: cognitive-behavioral conceptualization and treatment. Eat Behav. 2015;19:106–9.
64. Zucker NL, et al. Feeling and body investigators (FBI): ARFID division-an acceptance-based interoceptive exposure treatment for children with ARFID. Int J Eat Disord. 2019;52(4):466–72.
65. Brewerton TD, D'Agostino M. Adjunctive use of olanzapine in the treatment of avoidant restrictive food intake disorder in children and adolescents in an eating disorders program. J Child Adolesc Psychopharmacol. 2017;27(10):920–2.
66. Spettigue W, et al. Treatment of children and adolescents with avoidant/restrictive food intake disorder: a case series examining the feasibility of family therapy and adjunctive treatments. J Eat Disord. 2018;6:20.
67. Gray E, et al. Mirtazapine and weight gain in avoidant and restrictive food intake disorder. J Am Acad Child Adolesc Psychiatry. 2018;57(4):288–9.
68. Sharp WG, et al. Successful pharmacotherapy for the treatment of severe feeding aversion with mechanistic insights from cross-species neuronal remodeling. Transl Psychiatry. 2017;7(6):e1157.
69. Sant'Anna AM, et al. Use of cyproheptadine in young children with feeding difficulties and poor growth in a pediatric feeding program. J Pediatr Gastroenterol Nutr. 2014;59(5):674–8.
70. Merhar SL, et al. A retrospective review of cyproheptadine for feeding intolerance in children less than three years of age: effects and side effects. Acta Paediatr. 2016;105(8):967–70.

Chapter 7
Using Eating Disorder and Body Image Assessment Questionnaires with Boys/Men

Jason M. Lavender

Learning Objectives

1. Discuss how the history of the eating disorders field has impacted the development of the most commonly used questionnaires.
2. Describe core psychometric properties of questionnaires and related considerations for selection.
3. Summarize questionnaires that measure traditional eating disorder symptoms, that are specific to or inclusive of boys/men, and that assess related constructs of particular relevance to boys/men.
4. Identify overall options for the approach to selecting eating disorder questionnaires to use with samples of boys/men.

Key Points

- Many traditional eating disorder questionnaires were developed in the context of conceptualizations focused on symptom presentations in girls/women.
- Core psychometrics properties to consider are reliability and validity, particularly in samples reflecting the population of interest (i.e., boys/men).

J. M. Lavender (✉)
Department of Medicine, Military Cardiovascular Outcomes Research (MiCOR) Program, Uniformed Services University of the Health Sciences, Bethesda, MD, USA

The Metis Foundation, San Antonio, TX, USA
e-mail: jason.lavender.ctr@usuhs.edu

J. M. Nagata et al. (eds.), *Eating Disorders in Boys and Men*,
https://doi.org/10.1007/978-3-030-67127-3_7

- A variety of questionnaires have emerged that are specific to boys/men or that were inclusive of boys/men in the measurement development process.
- Overall options include using traditional questionnaires, using traditional questionnaires with modified items, utilizing newer questionnaires, or using a combination.

Introduction

Measures that provide scores with good psychometric properties are crucial for both research and clinical endeavors, including appropriately identifying the form and severity of symptoms, tracking symptoms over time either naturalistically or in response to interventions, and investigating relationships with other constructs that are theoretically salient to symptom onset, maintenance, and recovery. In particular, evidence of adequate reliability and validity of scores on a measure derived from samples similar to the group or individual to which that measure is to be administered is key. Importantly, the first step during the process of developing any measure is to identify and operationalize the construct that it will assess [1]. As such, if a construct is operationalized from a limited, biased, or non-inclusive perspective, then assessments that are developed to measure that construct will have the same limitations as the core conceptualizations that underlie them.

In considering the assessment of eating disorder symptoms and related constructs such as body image among boys and men, it is important to understand first that the historical development of the eating disorders field was characterized by a predominant conceptual and empirical focus on girls and women [2, 3]. Although historical cases of eating disorders in boys/men were noted [2], modern conceptualizations of eating disorder psychopathology that developed in the later twentieth century were mainly based on prototypical symptom presentations in young women. As such, diagnostic frameworks, assessment questionnaires, and interventions for eating disorders developed within this context, and the vast majority of the eating disorder literature has traditionally focused either primarily or exclusively on samples of girls and/or women [2, 3].

Recent years have seen progress within the eating disorders field with respect to understanding that these disorders are not in fact a rarity among boys or men, and there is now greater recognition that there may be unique attitudinal and behavioral symptom features among boys and men (e.g., related to muscularity) [2–7]. However, given that recognition, consistency, and prior experience are often strong influences in the selection of assessment measures, the historical development of the field and its predominant focus on girls/women have ongoing implications today. Notably, several measures that remain widely used within the eating disorders field were originally developed decades ago at a time in which our understanding of how disordered eating, body dissatisfaction, and related symptoms might be distinct in boys/men was extremely limited. For instance, the Eating Disorder Inventory questionnaire [8–10], originally developed in the early 1980s, and its later versions remain widely used in research and clinical settings. Although the measure has undergone updates overtime, the core eating disorder-specific scales are still reflective of traditional thinness-oriented eating disorder presentations. Similarly, the Eating Attitudes Test [11] remains in use, though it is also strongly focused on attitudes and behaviors reflective of a fear of weight gain and restrictive tendencies. Additionally, the Eating Disorder Examination [12] and its questionnaire version [13] were developed decades ago and have remain largely unchanged with respect to the core items comprising its subscales and global score. Overall, the reliance on such measures, particularly in the absence of supplemental assessments to address limitations associated with the more gendered origins of the traditional measures, may promote under-recognition of the presence and/or severity of symptoms among certain boys/men, especially for those whose symptoms do not as closely align to traditional conceptualizations of eating disorder psychopathology [2–5, 14].

Measurement Properties and Psychometrics: A Brief Primer

In the most basic sense, psychometric properties reflect the extent to which a measure is useful and meaningful with regard to its intended purpose. Core psychometric properties of a measure fall under the categories of reliability and validity, with the former addressing the consistency of a measure and the latter addressing the extent to which it actually assesses what it is purported to assess; reliability is also a necessary precondition for validity [1, 15]. It is important to recognize that even if a measure is well established and has demonstrated good psychometric properties in prior research, those properties can vary across samples and may not generalize when the measure is applied to samples that are distinctive from those used in the development and evaluation process or in previous studies [15]. This point is particularly crucial with regard to the use of eating disorder and related questionnaires with boys/men, given that many of the measures in the field were developed and evaluated using samples primarily or entirely comprised of girls/women. The following sections provide a concise, basic overview of several core measurement and psychometric properties, with an emphasis on those that are particularly relevant to understanding the use of questionnaires to assess eating disorder symptoms and related constructs in boys/men.

Reliability

The concept of measurement reliability is related to its consistency [1, 15], and there are several specific types. Two common forms that are especially important to consider when selecting a questionnaire are internal consistency reliability, which addresses the degree to which items that are posited to assess a given construct do so in a consistent way (commonly indexed by Cronbach's alpha), and test-retest reliability, which addresses the degree to which scores are consistent across time from one assessment to another (commonly indexed by a correlation coefficient or an intraclass correlation coefficient). A third type of reliability that is relevant for clinician-administered interviews (e.g., Eating Disorder Examination interview) is interrater reliability, which addresses the extent to which there is agreement across raters who are rating the same individual (commonly indexed by Cohen's kappa coefficient).

Validity

In the context of measurement, validity most generally refers to the extent to which a measure actually assesses what it is supposed to be assessing [1, 15]. As with reliability, there are several specific forms of validity. Content validity addresses the extent to which the score on a measure comprehensively reflects the breadth of the construct(s) that it is meant to represent. Convergent validity addresses the extent to which scores on a measure are associated with scores on measures of theoretically related constructs; in contrast, discriminant validity addresses whether the score on a measure is unrelated to scores on measures of constructs that are theoretically disparate (both commonly indexed by a correlation coefficient). Other forms include those addressing how scores on a measure relate to some criterion (e.g., concurrent validity, predictive validity; commonly indexed by correlation coefficients) and the extent to which a measure subjectively appears to assess what it is actually assessing (i.e., face validity).

Measurement Invariance (Equivalence)

The extent to which a measure equivalently assesses a given construct across certain specified groups is addressed by statistical tests of measurement invariance [16, 17]. Although there are alternative approaches, invariance is often categorized across three hierarchical levels, including configural (i.e., the factor structure is equivalent across groups), metric (i.e., item factor loadings are equivalent across groups), and scalar (i.e., item intercepts are equivalent across groups). Establishing measurement invariance across specific groups is especially important when using data from a measure to compare scores across those groups (e.g., across men and women) [16, 17].

Implications for Questionnaires Assessing Eating Disorder Symptoms

As described above, many of the widely used questionnaires that measure eating disorder symptoms were originally developed and validated with samples mostly or entirely comprised of girls and/or women, and as such there can be potential concerns when using traditional eating disorder measures with boys/men. For instance, if the core construct of eating disorder psychopathology or its subcomponents differ in certain ways between men and women, this could result in a traditional eating disorder measure demonstrating lower internal consistency in men, due to less consistent responding across items supposedly assessing a certain construct. One example of this concern would be for a questionnaire assessing body dissatisfaction that contains items referring to "thighs" or "hips," along with those addressing body shape more generally; in this example, men may be more likely to rate "gendered" items in a way that is inconsistent with the other items, resulting in lower internal consistency reliability for the questionnaire. Importantly, given that reliability is necessary, although not sufficient, for validity, it is therefore crucial to consider whether scores on traditional eating disorder measures exhibit adequate reliability for use in samples of boys/men.

With regard to validity, the most likely source of concern for using traditional eating disorder questionnaires among boys/men derives from the basic conceptualization that originally guided the development of the measure. For instance, certain traditional eating disorder questionnaires may have lower content validity if they are not fully capturing the breadth of the construct as it applies to samples of boys/men (e.g., absence of items addressing muscularity-oriented concerns or related behaviors). Further, if there are certain important elements of the construct that are not captured by the questionnaire, this can impact the interrelations of that questionnaire with conceptually related and unrelated measures, leading to problems with convergent and discriminant validity.

Finally, the concept of measurement invariance is particularly salient with regard to the extent to which eating disorder questionnaires are equivalently assessing a construct across men and women. For instance, it cannot be assumed that the subscales of an eating disorder measure that were developed using empirical approaches in samples of girls/women (e.g., via factor analytic methods) will also be the same in samples of boys/men (i.e., cannot assume configural invariance). In order for that questionnaire to be used for making comparisons across samples of men and women, invariance must first be evaluated to determine what degree, if any, the measure demonstrates equivalence across the groups.

Summary

In sum, when selecting a questionnaire assessing eating disorder or related symptoms for use with boys/men in either clinical or research contexts, it is important to understand the extent to which scores on that measure have demonstrated adequate psychometric properties in relevant samples. If a questionnaire has previously shown evidence of questionable psychometric properties in samples of boys/men, it might be preferable to consider using an alternative questionnaire until further studies are conducted that provide support for the use of the intended questionnaire with boys/men. Finally, even for those questionnaires that have received psychometric support in studies with relevant samples, it is also important for researchers to examine and report at least the basic psychometric properties (particularly reliability) of each measure they use in the specific sample under investigation in their study.

Overview of Assessment Questionnaires

The following section provides an overview of numerous questionnaires that assess eating disorder symptoms and related variables of conceptual relevance for boys/men that have been commonly used in research or clinical settings or that have been developed specifically for or with consideration of boys and men. This is not an exhaustive list of questionnaires, and the descriptions are primarily based on the measures as originally developed and evaluated. Further, measures specific to muscle dysmorphia are discussed in the following chapter in this section (Chap. 8) and thus are not addressed below. Finally, it is important to acknowledge the limited nature of the literature addressing the psychometric properties of many of these questionnaires in boys/men [18, 19], and much of the existing evidence derives from studies with samples of predominantly non-clinical, White, young adult, and presumably cisgender and heterosexual men (given that many studies have not assessed or reported on gender identity and/or sexual orientation). See Table 7.1 for a summary of questionnaires reviewed below.

Table 7.1 Overview of assessment questionnaires

Questionnaire	Construct	Description
Questionnaires assessing traditional eating disorder symptoms		
Eating Disorder Examination-Questionnaire (EDE-Q)	Eating disorder symptoms, broad range	28 items; 0–6 response scale with variable anchors; provides a global score and 4 subscale scores: dietary restraint, eating concern, weight concern, and shape concern; also provides separate frequency counts for various core eating disorder behaviors; time frame specified to the past 4 weeks
Eating Disorder Inventory (EDI) – Multiple versions	Eating disorder symptoms, broad range	Item total, response format, and subscale number vary across versions; 3 core subscales across versions are drive for thinness, bulimia, and body dissatisfaction; no time frame specified
Binge Eating Scale (BES)	Binge eating symptoms	16 items; multiple-choice response format with varying content and range across items; provides a total score; no time frame specified
Loss of Control Over Eating Scale (LOCES)	Loss of control eating symptoms	24 items; Likert-type response scale (1 – Never to 5 – Always); provides a total score and 3 subscale scores: behavioral, cognitive/dissociative, and positive/euphoric; time frame specified to the past 4 weeks; 7-item unidimensional abbreviated version also available and highly correlated with original
Questionnaires assessing eating disorder symptoms developed specifically for or conceptually inclusive of boys/men		
Eating Pathology Symptoms Inventory (EPSI)	Eating disorder symptoms (boys/men inclusive)	45 items; Likert-type response scale (0 – Never to 4 – Very often); provides 8 scale scores: body dissatisfaction, binge eating, cognitive restraint, purging, restricting, excessive exercise, negative attitudes toward obesity, and muscle building; time frame specified to the past 4 weeks

Table 7.1 (continued)

Questionnaire	Construct	Description
Eating Disorder Assessment for Men (EDAM)	Eating disorder symptoms (boys/men-specific)	50 items; Likert-type response scale (0 – Never to 4 – Always); provides a total score; no time frame specified
Muscularity-Oriented Eating Test (MOET)	Muscularity-oriented eating attitudes/ behaviors (boys/men inclusive)	15 items; Likert-type response scale (0 – Never true to 4 – Always true); provides a total score; time frame specified to the past 4 weeks
Eating for Muscularity Scale (EMS)	Muscularity-oriented eating attitudes/ behaviors (boys/men inclusive)	27 items; frequency-based response scale (0 – No days to 6 – Every day); provides a total score and 9 subscale scores: preoccupation, diet gain, diet loss, dietary restraint, excessive attention, functional impairment, health risk, compensatory exercise, and negative affect; time frame specified to the past 4 weeks
Questionnaires assessing body-image constructs developed specifically for or conceptually inclusive of boys/men		
Male Body Attitudes Scale (MBAS)	Body image (boys/men-specific)	24 items; Likert-type response scale (1 – Never to 6 – Always); provides a total score and 3 subscale scores: muscularity, body fat, and height; no time frame specified
Male Body Checking Questionnaire (MBCQ)	Body checking (boys/men-specific)	19 items; Likert-type response scale (1 – Never to 5 – Very often); provides a total score and 4 subscale scores: global muscle checking, chest and shoulder checking, other comparative checking, and body testing; no time frame specified
Drive for Muscularity Scale (DMS)	Muscularity-oriented attitudes/behaviors (boys/men inclusive)	15 items; Likert-type response scale (1 – Always to 6 – Never), with all items reverse scored; provides a total score and 2 subscale scores for boys/men: muscularity-related attitudes and muscle-enhancing behaviors; no time frame specified
Drive for Leanness Scale (DLS)	Leanness-oriented attitudes/behaviors (boys/men inclusive)	6 items; Likert-type response scale (1 – Never to 6 – Always); provides a total score; no time frame specified
Questionnaires assessing pathological exercise		
Compulsive Exercise Test (CET)	Compulsive exercise	24 items; Likert-type response scale (0 – Never true to 5 – Always true); provides a total score and 5 subscale scores: avoidance and rule-driven behavior, weight control exercise, mood improvement, lack of exercise enjoyment, and exercise rigidity; no time frame specified
Obligatory Exercise Questionnaire (OEQ)	Obligatory exercise	20 items; Likert-type response scale (1 – Never to 4 – Always); provides a total score; no time frame specified
Exercise Dependence Scale (EDS-21)	Exercise dependence (addiction-based conceptualization)	21 items; Likert-type response scale (1 – Never to 6 – Always); provides a total score and 7 subscale scores: tolerance, withdrawal, intention effect, lack of control, time, reductions in other activities, and continuance; time frame specified to the past 3 months

Questionnaires Assessing Traditional Eating Disorder Symptoms

The Eating Disorder Examination-Questionnaire (EDE-Q) [13], the questionnaire version of the Eating Disorder Examination interview [12], is one of the most widely used eating disorder assessments, particularly in research contexts. The 28-item questionnaire assesses a broad range of eating disorder attitudes and behaviors, providing four subscale scores (i.e., dietary restraint, eating concern, weight concern, shape concern), a global score reflecting the average of these four subscales, and frequencies of certain eating disorder behaviors (i.e., objective binge eating, self-induced vomiting, laxative use, driven/compulsive exercise). The EDE-Q has generally received qualified psychometric support, although subscale reliability has been questionable in some research with boys and men, and studies also commonly fail to replicate the original factor structure [19–23]. Core advantages of this measure in terms of use with boys and men are its broad recognition and acceptance in research and clinical contexts, the availability of published norms in various clinical and non-clinical populations of boys and men [24–26], its availability in multiple languages, and free use for non-commercial research purposes. A primary limitation of the EDE-Q with regard to eating disorder symptoms in boys and men is that it does not assess muscularity-oriented attitudes or behaviors, and the origins of the measure (i.e., traditional thinness-oriented) is evident in certain items that may have different meanings for boys/men versus girls/women [27].

The Eating Disorder Inventory, now in its third version (EDI-3) [10], is another questionnaire that has been widely used in both clinical and research contexts. The versions vary with regard to number of items, response format/scoring, and scales. Here, the description focuses on the EDI-3, which is comprised of 91 items across 12 scales that are either eating disorder-specific or general. The three core scales that comprise the Eating Disorder Risk composite are drive for thinness, bulimia, and body dissatisfaction, whereas example general scales include perfectionism, interoceptive deficits, and emotional dysregulation. Some advantages of using the EDI-3 are its wide use and recognition, general psychometric support (although reliability has been questionable in some studies of men [19]), and availability of norms for clinical samples that include boys/men [10, 24]. The measure is also available in a computerized format, with automated scoring that generates individualized reports with T-scores, percentiles, and detailed information for the scales. As with the EDE-Q, the primary limitation of the EDI-3 (and previous versions) in assessing eating disorder symptoms among boys and men is that it lacks items addressing muscularity-oriented attitudes or behaviors and certain items (particularly on the body dissatisfaction scale) are worded in a way that is more typically gendered (e.g., concern about hips and thighs being too large). Additionally, the EDI-3 (and previous versions) does not provide a frequency count for specific behaviors.

The Binge Eating Scale (BES) [28] is a 16-item questionnaire that assesses behavioral, cognitive, and affective experiences related to binge eating. Notably, the measure was originally developed in a sample of adults with obesity and provides a continuous total score that also can be used to assign a classification of no/mild binge eating, moderate binge eating, and severe binge eating. The BES has demonstrated some evidence of adequate psychometrics in mixed-gender samples of adolescents and adults [28–31]; however, there remains a need to establish the reliability and validity of the measure specifically in appropriate samples of boys and/or men. Further, the BES does not provide a frequency count for episodes of binge eating behavior.

The Loss of Control Over Eating Scale (LOCES) [32] is a 24-item questionnaire that assesses the construct of loss of control eating, irrespective of type or amount of food consumed. The measure provides a total score and three subscale scores: behavioral, cognitive/dissociative, and positive/euphoric. The LOCES, particularly the total score, has demonstrated evidence of good reliability and validity in mixed-gender college samples [32, 33] and in college men [34, 35], although the factor structure has not been consistently replicated [36]. A brief 7-item version of the scale, highly correlated with the total score of the longer version, is also available [32]. This brief LOCES has similarly demonstrated good psychometric properties in mixed-gender samples of college students [32, 36], patients with eating disorders [36], and community adolescents [37]; the brief version has also shown evidence of gender-based invariance in adult and adolescent samples [36, 37]. However, similar to the BES, neither the original nor the brief versions of the LOCES provide a frequency count for episodes of loss of control eating behavior.

Questionnaires Assessing Eating Disorder Symptoms Developed Specifically for or Conceptually Inclusive of Boys/Men

The Eating Pathology Symptoms Inventory (EPSI) [38] is a more recently developed 45-item questionnaire that assesses both traditional eating disorder symptoms and other related constructs of conceptual relevance to boys and/or men (e.g., muscularity-oriented behaviors). Items are rated in reference to the previous 4 weeks and are divided across eight scales: binge eating, purging, excessive exercise, restricting, cognitive restraint, negative attitudes toward obesity, body dissatisfaction, and muscle building. The EPSI has generally demonstrated strong psychometric properties in both men and women, including gender-based invariance, although certain scales (e.g., purging) have shown lower reliability among men in some studies [19, 34, 35, 39]. The EPSI also has been found to distinguish between those who do and do not have an eating disorder, and norms are available for both men and women [39]. Notably, a clinician-rated version of the measure also was recently developed and initially validated [40]. However, a primary limitation of the questionnaire is that it does not provide a specific frequency count for eating disorder behaviors and the body dissatisfaction scale contains items that are worded in a way that is more typically gendered (e.g., dissatisfaction with size of thighs).

The Eating Disorder Assessment for Men (EDAM) [41, 42] is another more recently developed questionnaire comprising 50 items developed specifically to assess eating disorder symptoms among men within domains including weight concerns, food issues, body image/appearance concerns, exercise issues, and disordered eating. The measure provides a total score, although initial evidence also suggests the presence of four subscales: binge eating, muscle dysmorphia, body dissatisfaction, and disordered eating [41]. Preliminary evidence also supports the psychometric properties of the measure, which has been found to distinguish between men with and without an eating disorder [41, 42]. The main advantage of the measure is that its conceptual development focused specifically on men, with the inclusion of items assessing both traditional and muscularity-oriented symptoms and concerns. However, the questionnaire has received limited use in research and clinical contexts, and further evaluation and validation of the measure is necessary.

The Muscularity-Oriented Eating Test (MOET) [43] is a recently developed 15-item unidimensional questionnaire that assesses attitudinal, affective, and behavioral components of muscularity-oriented disordered eating, such as rigid planning and control of food and macronutrient intake. A primary advantage of the measure is its unique focus on manifestations of disordered eating oriented toward pursuit of lean muscularity, as well as its relative brevity. Preliminary evidence also supports the reliability and validity of the total score among college men [43]. However, the MOET lacks items addressing other forms of disordered eating (e.g., binge eating) or other muscularity-focused behaviors (e.g., workouts), does not assess theoretically underlying attitudinal constructs (e.g., body dissatisfaction), and does not provide frequency counts for disordered eating behaviors.

The Eating for Muscularity Scale (EMS) [44] is a recently developed 27-item questionnaire that assesses an array of cognitive, behavioral, affective, and functional dimensions broadly related to the pursuit of muscularity. The measure provides a total score and nine subscale scores: preoccupation, diet gain, diet loss, dietary restraint, excessive attention, functional impairment, health risk, compensatory exercise, and negative affect. A notable advantage of the measure is the breadth of the subconstructs it assesses, and in particular, the inclusion of items assessing functional impairment related to the disordered eating behaviors. Preliminary evidence also supports reliability and validity in both men and women [44]. However, as with the MOET, the EMS does not provide frequency counts for any muscularity-oriented behaviors.

Questionnaires Assessing Body-Image Constructs Developed Specifically for or Conceptually Inclusive of Boys/Men

The Male Body Attitudes Scale (MBAS) [45] is a 24-item questionnaire developed specifically to assess body image dissatisfaction in men. The measure provides a total score and three subscale scores: muscularity, low body fat, and height. The primary advantage of this measure is its focus on body image concerns of particular salience to men, including both body fat and muscularity, consistent with the lean and muscular body ideal for boys/men. Evidence also supports the reliability and validity of the measure in men [19, 45, 46]. However, it is focused entirely on attitudinal aspects of body dissatisfaction, and thus does not capture relevant body image- or disordered eating-related behaviors. Notably, a revised and briefer 15-item version (MBAS-R) also was developed and evaluated in a sample of Irish men, with evidence supporting its reliability, validity, and a three-factor structure reflecting subconstructs similar to those in the original version (i.e., body fat, muscularity, height) [47].

The Male Body Checking Questionnaire (MBCQ) [48] is a 19-item questionnaire that assesses the frequency of various body checking behaviors specific to men, such as checking the hardness of one's biceps or taking measurements of muscle size. The questionnaire provides a total score and four subscale scores for men: global muscle checking, chest and shoulder checking, other comparative checking, and body testing. The primary advantage of this questionnaire is that its conceptual development focused on men, with items addressing body checking behaviors consistent with both muscularity and leanness, as well as body parts of particular salience for boys/men (e.g., biceps, abs). The MBCQ has demonstrated preliminary evidence of reliability and validity in college-aged men [49], although more research is needed to further evaluate and validate the measure. Further, the behavioral focus of the measure excludes other aspects of the broader experience of body image (e.g., attitudinal, affective).

The Drive for Muscularity Scale (DMS) [50, 51] is a 15-item questionnaire that assesses thoughts and behaviors related to the desire to become more muscular. The measure provides a total score and two subscale scores for boys/men: muscularity-related attitudes and muscle-enhancing behaviors. The DMS is arguably the most well-established and widely used muscularity-oriented questionnaire, and the questionnaire has demonstrated good reliability and validity in samples of boys and men [50–54]. However, the DMS does include items for assessing disordered eating behaviors, with the exception of two items that address protein intake and supplementation, and does not provide frequency counts for muscularity-oriented behaviors.

The Drive for Leanness Scale (DLS) [55] is a 6-item questionnaire that assesses the desire to have a body characterized by low body fat and toned, fit muscularity. Given the potentially greater salience of leanness over thinness for boys/men, the focus on this particular dimension is the primary strength of this questionnaire, along with its brevity. The DLS also has demonstrated evidence of good psychometric properties in college-aged men, as well as evidence supporting gender invariance [55–57]. However, contrasting with the DMS, the DLS is entirely attitudinal in nature, and does not include items assessing either disordered eating or muscularity-oriented behaviors.

Questionnaires Assessing Pathological Exercise

The Compulsive Exercise Test (CET) [58] is a 24-item questionnaire that assesses cognitive, behavioral, and affective features of compulsive exercise. The measure provides an overall score and five subscale scores: avoidance and rule-driven behavior, weight control exercise, mood improvement, lack of exercise enjoyment, and exercise rigidity. The CET has demonstrated adequate psychometric properties in a mixed-gender community sample of adolescents [59], in a community sample of sexual minority men [60], and in a clinical sample of boys/men with anorexia nervosa [61]. A primary advantage of the questionnaire is that its items and subscales are consistent with the common conceptualization of the nature of pathological exercise in eating disorders [62]. However, the factor structure of the CET has been questioned [63], and items addressing body weight/shape in relation to exercise are more consistent with traditional thinness-oriented and fear of weight gain motivations.

The Obligatory Exercise Questionnaire (OEQ) [64, 65] is a 20-item questionnaire that assesses the frequency of certain exercise-related experiences and provides an overall score. A main advantage of the OEQ, similar to the CET, is the inclusion of items addressing experiences of particular relevance to eating disorder populations (compensatory exercise, body shape motivations). The measure has demonstrated evidence of reliability and validity in mixed-gender samples of adults [64, 66] and in samples of college and community men [67, 68]. However, whereas the OEQ was originally developed as a unidimensional measure, other research in different groups (e.g., mixed-gender sample of adolescents) has suggested the utility of a briefer, multidimensional version of the measure [69].

The Exercise Dependence Scale (EDS-21) [70–72] is a 21-item questionnaire that assesses exercise dependence based on an addiction-oriented conceptualization, with items derived from the criteria for substance dependence. The measure provides an overall score and seven subscale scores: withdrawal, continuance, tolerance, lack of control, reduction in other activities, time, and intention effects. The questionnaire is also designed to classify individuals by severity, based on degree and number of symptoms endorsed. The measure has generally demonstrated evidence of adequate reliability and validity in mixed-gender samples of adults [62, 72–74] and in athletic-specific and non-athletic-specific samples of men [54, 75–77]; however, the reliability of the reduction subscale in particular has often been found to be lower [62, 73–74]. Advantages of the EDS-21 are its breadth of subconstructs and the unique addiction-oriented framework underlying the measure. However, the questionnaire is focused entirely on exercise behaviors and thus does not assess potentially salient underlying attitudes (e.g., body dissatisfaction) or other symptoms relevant to eating disorders.

Choosing Questionnaires for Assessing Boys and/or Men

General Considerations

After deciding on the particular variable of interest that one is interested in assessing, be it eating disorder symptoms broadly or a more specific construct such as binge eating or body image, one is faced with a number of choices. Ultimately the selection of a specific measure or measures will depend on a number of considerations. First, the context in which the measure will be administered is a core consideration, particularly whether the measure will be used for clinical (e.g., understanding the clinical significance of patient's symptoms at intake, tracking treatment progress over time) or research (e.g., describing symptom characteristics of a sample, examining associations of symptom severity with other constructs) purposes. For example, availability of well-established clinical norms or cut-offs for a questionnaire may be useful for clinical screening or intake assessments, as well as questionnaires that assess a wide breadth of symptomology. In contrast, within a research study, the empirical questions of interest may at times call for using questionnaires that focus on more narrowly defined constructs.

A second consideration is overall assessment burden [78], which relates particularly to the number of items on a questionnaire and the total number of questionnaires a patient or participant is asked to complete (and in the case of repeated assessments, how many times). Excessive assessment burden may result in poorer data quality and thus must be balanced with considerations of assessment depth and breadth. A third consideration is the characteristics of the individual or sample(s) one is assessing and whether the measure is appropriate for that individual or sample, as well as appropriate for comparisons across samples (e.g., evidence of invariance) if group comparison is a question of interest (e.g., men versus women). For instance, it is important to ensure that the language of a questionnaire is appropriate for the age level of the individual(s) who will be completing the assessment (particularly relevant for youth) and to confirm that a questionnaire has shown evidence of reliability and validity in samples with sociodemographic features similar to the individual or group being assessed. Finally, numerous other practical considerations may play a role in selecting a questionnaire, such as the format in which a questionnaire is administered and/or scored (e.g., computerized versus paper-and-pencil, hand-scoring versus automated scoring) and whether a questionnaire is freely available or requires purchase.

General Options

The options described below for using eating disorder and related questionnaires among boys/men should be evaluated within the context of the considerations addressed above, as well as the other general assessment and psychometric implications described earlier.

The first option involves using a traditional questionnaire, despite limitations related to the measure's original development (e.g., absence of muscularity-oriented items, presence of items that are potentially gendered). Advantages of this approach are that the traditional eating disorder questionnaires typically have a long, well-established history of use across many settings and as such are familiar to many researchers and clinicians. These measures have also had more time to undergo investigation in a variety of samples and thus may have psychometric support and norms in a wider range of specific populations. However, it is important to recognize the limitations associated with this option, including that a traditional measure in the absence of other secondary measures may not fully capture eating disorder symptom features that can be more unique to boys/men. A further limitation that is particularly relevant to assessments in clinical settings is that the use of traditional measures could promote feelings of alienation for boys/men confronted with items on a questionnaire that seem especially gendered. This could potentially lead to problems with rapport and treatment engagement, and could also inadvertently increase stigma or shame deriving from the misconception that eating disorders only affect girls or women [79, 80].

A second option involves using an existing questionnaire with modifications to certain items or content. For example, items that address thinness could be modified to address leanness or low body fat, or items that focus on dissatisfaction with body parts that may be more gendered (e.g., thighs) could be reworded to be more general (e.g., legs) or muscularity-focused (e.g., quads). One notable advantage of this approach is that it could avoid the potential for unintended alienation and stigma/shame, as described above. However, there are numerous disadvantages to this approach, and the implications must be understood and carefully considered. Namely, when modifying an existing questionnaire, prior evidence regarding psychometric support may no longer hold, and comparisons to scores from the original questionnaire, including norms and/or cut-offs, may become inaccurate or invalid. As such, it is recommended to consider an alternative approach when feasible.

The third option is to select a questionnaire that was developed conceptually and methodologically with a specific consideration for or inclusive of boys and/or men. For instance, one might choose a questionnaire that contains items assessing both traditional and muscularity-oriented eating disorder symptoms, and that included boys and/or men in the sample(s) used in the initial measure development and validation process. Examples of this include the broadly focused EPSI [38] or the more narrowly focused EMS [44], both of which were developed with consideration for eating disorder-related symptoms in men and women, or the EDAM [41, 42] or MBAS [45], which were developed specifically for men. This approach maintains the benefit of the second option (i.e., limiting alienation arising from predominantly gendered items), but also has the advantage of consistency with the original questionnaire and the associated benefits (e.g., psychometrics, facilitating comparisons to other samples and norms/cut-offs). Additionally, for questionnaires that have utility for use with both men and women, particularly if measurement invariance has been established, this approach facilitates group-based comparisons between men and women.

A final option that may have the most utility with regard to balancing depth and breadth of assessment is the use of multiple questionnaires. Each of the questionnaires included in the (non-exhaustive) list in Table 7.1 has its own unique advantages and disadvantages with regard to format, content, time frame, and psychometrics. In particular, given that eating disorder symptoms in boys and men may present traditionally, may present as more muscularity-focused, or may present with mixed features (concurrently or over time) [2, 3, 5, 81], there may be benefit in including multiple measures to capture the full spectrum of eating disorder attitudes and behaviors that boys and men may experience. This may not always be practical or feasible given the context, and as noted above, assessment burden must be considered. In addition to the rationale for the assessment (e.g., a specific research question or a general clinical assessment), understanding overlapping versus distinct content across questionnaires, as well as evidence regarding the extent to which certain questionnaires are correlated, may provide guidance in selecting which specific questionnaires to include when this approach is taken.

Conclusions

There has been much progress in recent years with regard to the assessment of eating disorder psychopathology and related constructs in boys and men, both with regard to understanding the limitations of traditional questionnaires and in terms of the development of new questionnaires that are specific to or inclusive of distinct features and symptoms relevant to boys/men (e.g., lean and muscular body ideal). Considering and selecting a questionnaire for use with boys or men in clinical or research contexts should take a number of important issues into account, including the content of the questionnaire (e.g., items addressing traditional thinness-oriented attitudes and behaviors, muscularity-oriented attitudes and behaviors, or both), the specific use of the questionnaire (e.g., understanding severity in comparison to clinical norms or cut-offs, tracking symptoms over time naturalistically or during treatment, examining in relation to another variable or construct), evidence regarding the measurement and psychometric properties of the questionnaire in samples similar to the intended respondent(s), and other issues related to practicality and feasibility (e.g., age-appropriate language and wording, assessment burden, requirement to purchase).

Despite this progress, there remain areas in need of further study. For example, given evidence that measures of certain specific symptoms may demonstrate lower reliability in men, more research on the basic nature and conceptualization of these constructs, and how they may differ in men versus women (e.g., how men recognize and perceive loss of control over eating), is warranted. Additionally, most questionnaires require further evaluation and validation in boys and men, and many require measurement and psychometric investigation in specific sub-groups that have been especially under-represented in the literature. In particular, further studies are needed in racial and ethnic minority men, sexual minority men, transgender men, and men across the lifespan (particularly children, younger adolescents, and older men), as well as in men from different countries and areas of the world (often necessitating proper language translations for questionnaires). Further, given that many of the measures were developed and evaluated in non-clinical samples, there remains a need for additional investigations of the psychometric properties of many of the measures in relevant clinical samples of boys and men.

Disclaimer The opinions and assertions expressed herein are those of the author and do not necessarily reflect the official policy or position of the Uniformed Services University or the Department of Defense.

References

1. Hinkin TR. A brief tutorial on the development of measures for use in survey questionnaires. Organ Res Methods. 1998;1:104–21.
2. Murray SB, Nagata JM, Griffiths S, Calzo JP, Brown TA, Mitchison D, Blashill AJ, Mond JM. The enigma of male eating disorders: a critical review and synthesis. Clin Psychol Rev. 2017;57:1–11.
3. Lavender JM, Brown TA, Murray SB. Men, muscles, and eating disorders: an overview of traditional and muscularity-oriented disordered eating. Curr Psychiatry Rep. 2017;19:32.
4. Strother E, Lemberg R, Chariese Stanford S, Turberville D. Eating disorders in men: underdiagnosed, undertreated, and misunderstood. Eat Disord. 2012;20:346–55.
5. Murray SB, Griffiths S, Mond JM. Evolving eating disorder psychopathology: conceptualizing muscularity-oriented disordered eating. Br J Psychiatry. 2016;208:414–5.
6. Nagata JM, Ganson KT, Murray SB. Eating disorders in adolescent boys and young men: an update. Curr Opin Pediatr. 2020;32:476–81.
7. Limbers CA, Cohen LA, Gray BA. Eating disorders in adolescent and young adult males: prevalence, diagnosis, and treatment strategies. Adolesc Health Med Ther. 2018;9:111–6.
8. Garner DM, Olmstead MP, Polivy J. Development and validation of a multidimensional eating disorder inventory for anorexia nervosa and bulimia. Int J Eat Disord. 1983;2:15–34.
9. Garner DM. Eating disorder inventory–2: professional manual. Odessa: Psychological Assessment Resources; 1991.
10. Garner DM. Eating disorder inventory–3: professional manual. Odessa/Lutz: Psychological Assessment Resources; 2004.
11. Garner DM, Garfinkel PE. The eating attitudes test: an index of the symptoms of anorexia nervosa. Psychol Med. 1979;9:273–9.
12. Fairburn CG, Cooper Z. The eating disorder examination. In: Fairburn CG, Wilson GT, editors. Binge eating: nature, assessment, and treatment. New York: Guilford Press; 1993. p. 317–60.
13. Fairburn CG, Beglin SJ. Assessment of eating disorders: interview or self-report questionnaire? Int J Eat Disord. 1994;16:363–70.
14. Darcy AM, Lin IH. Are we asking the right questions? A review of assessment of males with eating disorders. Eat Disord. 2012;20:416–26.
15. Wilkinson L. Statistical methods in psychology journals: guidelines and explanations. Am Psychol. 1999;54:594–604.
16. Putnick DL, Bornstein MH. Measurement invariance conventions and reporting: the state of the art and future directions for psychological research. Dev Rev. 2016;41:71–90.
17. Vandenberg RJ, Lance CE. A review and synthesis of the measurement invariance literature: suggestions, practices, and recommendations for organizational research. Organ Res Methods. 2000;3:4–70.
18. Burton AL, Abbott MJ, Modini M, Touyz S. Psychometric evaluation of self-report measures of binge-eating symptoms and related psychopathology: a systematic review of the literature. Int J Eat Disord. 2016;49:123–40.
19. Forbush KT, Hilderbrand LA, Bohrer BK, Chapa DAN. Test-retest reliability of common measures of eating disorder symptoms in men versus women. Assessment. 2019;26:419–31.
20. Berg KC, Peterson CB, Frazier P, Crow SJ. Psychometric evaluation of the eating disorder examination and eating disorder examination-questionnaire: a systematic review of the literature. Int J Eat Disord. 2012;45:428–38.

21. Carey M, Kupeli N, Knight R, Troop NA, Jenkinson PM, Preston C. Eating disorder examination questionnaire (EDE-Q): norms and psychometric properties in U.K. females and males. Psychol Assess. 2019;31:839–50.
22. Grilo CM, Reas DL, Hopwood CJ, Crosby RD. Factor structure and construct validity of the eating disorder examination-questionnaire in college students: further support for a modified brief version. Int J Eat Disord. 2015;48:284–9.
23. White HJ, Haycraft E, Goodwin H, Meyer C. Eating disorder examination questionnaire: factor structure for adolescent girls and boys. Int J Eat Disord. 2014;47:99–104.
24. Smith KE, Mason TB, Murray SB, Griffiths S, Leonard RC, Wetterneck CT, Smith BER, Farrell NR, Riemann BC, Lavender JM. Male clinical norms and sex differences on the eating disorder inventory (EDI) and eating disorder examination questionnaire (EDE-Q). Int J Eat Disord. 2017;50:769–75.
25. Lavender JM, De Young KP, Anderson DA. Eating disorder examination questionnaire (EDE-Q): norms for undergraduate men. Eat Behav. 2010;11:119–21.
26. Mond J, Hall A, Bentley C, Harrison C, Gratwick-Sarll K, Lewis V. Eating-disordered behavior in adolescent boys: eating disorder examination questionnaire norms. Int J Eat Disord. 2014;47:335–41.
27. Darcy AM, Doyle AC, Lock J, Peebles R, Doyle P, Le Grange D. The Eating Disorders Examination in adolescent males with anorexia nervosa: how does it compare to adolescent females? Int J Eat Disord. 2012;45:110–4.
28. Gormally J, Black S, Daston S, Rardin D. The assessment of binge eating severity among obese persons. Addict Behav. 1982;7:47–55.
29. Laghi F, Pompili S, Baumgartner E, Baiocco R. The role of sensation seeking and motivations for eating in female and male adolescents who binge eat. Eat Behav. 2015;17:119–24.
30. Celio AA, Wilfley DE, Crow SJ, Mitchell J, Walsh BT. A comparison of the binge eating scale, questionnaire for eating and weight patterns-revised, and eating disorder examination questionnaire with instructions with the eating disorder examination in the assessment of binge eating disorder and its symptoms. Int J Eat Disord. 2004;36:434–44.
31. Ricca V, Mannucci E, Moretti S, Di Bernardo M, Zucchi T, Cabras PL, Rotella CM. Screening for binge eating disorder in obese outpatients. Compr Psychiatry. 2000;41:111–5.
32. Latner JD, Mond JM, Kelly MC, Haynes SN, Hay PJ. The loss of control over eating scale: development and psychometric evaluation. Int J Eat Disord. 2014;47:647–59.
33. Stefano EC, Wagner AF, Mond JM, Cicero DC, Latner JD. Loss of control over eating scale (LOCES): validation in undergraduate men and women with and without eating disorder symptoms. Eat Behav. 2016;23:137–40.
34. Culbert KM, Shope MM, Sisk CL, Klump KL. Low testosterone is associated with dysregulated eating symptoms in young adult men. Int J Eat Disord. 2020;53:1469–79.
35. Shope MM, Prows SD, Racine SE, Culbert KM. Examining associations between emotion-based rash action and dysregulated eating symptoms in men and women. Eat Behav. 2020;37:101379.
36. Bodell LP, Forney KJ, Chavarria J, Keel PK, Wildes JE. Self-report measures of loss of control over eating: psychometric properties in clinical and non-clinical samples. Int J Eat Disord. 2018;51:1252–60.
37. Vannucci A, Ohannessian CM. Psychometric properties of the brief loss of control over eating scale (LOCES-B) in early adolescents. Int J Eat Disord. 2018;51:459–64.
38. Forbush KT, Wildes JE, Pollack LO, Dunbar D, Luo J, Patterson K, Petruzzi L, Pollpeter M, Miller H, Stone A, Bright A, Watson D. Development and validation of the eating pathology symptoms inventory (EPSI). Psychol Assess. 2013;25:859–78.
39. Forbush KT, Wildes JE, Hunt TK. Gender norms, psychometric properties, and validity for the eating pathology symptoms inventory. Int J Eat Disord. 2014;47:85–91.
40. Forbush KT, Bohrer BK, Hagan KE, Chapa DAN, Perko V, Richson B, Christian K, Christensen KA, Wildes JE. Development and initial validation of the eating pathology symptoms inventory-clinician-rated version (EPSI-CRV). Psychol Assess. 2020;32:943–55.

41. Stanford SC, Lemberg R. Measuring eating disorders in men: development of the eating disorder assessment for men (EDAM). Eat Disord. 2012;20:427–36.
42. Stanford SC, Lemberg R. A clinical comparison of men and women on the eating disorder inventory-3 (EDI-3) and the eating disorder assessment for men (EDAM). Eat Disord. 2012;20:379–94.
43. Murray SB, Brown TA, Blashill AJ, Compte EJ, Lavender JM, Mitchison D, Mond JM, Keel PK, Nagata JM. The development and validation of the muscularity-oriented eating test: a novel measure of muscularity-oriented disordered eating. Int J Eat Disord. 2019;52:1389–98.
44. Cooper M, Griffiths KM, Burns R. Getting shredded: development and validation of a measure of muscularity-oriented disordered eating. Psychol Assess. 2020;32:451–60.
45. Tylka TL, Bergeron D, Schwartz JP. Development and psychometric evaluation of the male body attitudes scale (MBAS). Body Image. 2005;2:161–75.
46. Blashill AJ, Vander Wal JS. The male body attitudes scale: a confirmatory factor analysis with a sample of gay men. Body Image. 2009;6:322–5.
47. Ryan TA, Morrison TG, Roddy S, McCutcheon J. Psychometric properties of the Revised Male Body Attitudes Scale among Irish men. Body Image. 2011;8:64–9.
48. Hildebrandt T, Walker DC, Alfano L, Delinsky S, Bannon K. Development and validation of a male specific body checking questionnaire. Int J Eat Disord. 2010;43:77–87.
49. Walker DC, Anderson DA, Hildebrandt T. Body checking behaviors in men. Body Image. 2009;6:164–70.
50. McCreary DR, Sasse DK. An exploration of the drive for muscularity in adolescent boys and girls. J Am Coll Heal. 2000;48:297–304.
51. McCreary DR. The drive for muscularity scale: description, psychometrics, and research findings. In: Thompson JK, Cafri G, editors. The muscular ideal: psychological, social, and medical perspectives. Washington, DC: American Psychological Association; 2007. p. 87–106.
52. McCreary DR, Sasse DK, Saucier DM, Dorsch KD. Measuring the drive for muscularity: factorial validity of the drive for muscularity scale in men and women. Psychol Men Masc. 2004;5:49–58.
53. McCreary DR, Karvinen K, Davis C. The relationship between the drive for muscularity and anthropometric measures of muscularity and adiposity. Body Image. 2006;3:145–52.
54. Chittester NI, Hausenblas HA. Correlates of drive for muscularity: the role of anthropometric measures and psychological factors. J Health Psychol. 2009;14:872–7.
55. Smolak L, Murnen SK. Drive for leanness: assessment and relationship to gender, gender role and objectification. Body Image. 2008;5:251–60.
56. Ryan TA, Morrison TG. Psychometric evaluation of the drive for leanness scale in a sample of Irish men. Eat Behav. 2013;14:21–15.
57. Tod D, Hall G, Edwards C. Gender invariance and correlates of the drive for leanness scale. Body Image. 2012;9:555–8.
58. Taranis L, Touyz S, Meyer C. Disordered eating and exercise: development and preliminary validation of the compulsive exercise test (CET). Eur Eat Disord Rev. 2011;19:256–68.
59. Goodwin H, Haycraft E, Taranis L, Meyer C. Psychometric evaluation of the compulsive exercise test (CET) in an adolescent population: links with eating psychopathology. Eur Eat Disord Rev. 2011;19:269–79.
60. Brewster ME, Sandil R, DeBlaere C, Breslow A, Eklund A. "Do you even lift, bro?" Objectification, minority stress, and body image concerns for sexual minority men. Psychol Men Masc. 2017;18:87–98.
61. Murray SB, Griffiths S, Rieger E, Touyz S. A comparison of compulsive exercise in male and female presentations of anorexia nervosa: what is the difference? Adv Eat Disord. 2014;2:65–70.
62. Scharmer C, Gorrell S, Schaumberg K, Anderson D. Compulsive exercise or exercise dependence? Clarifying conceptualizations of exercise in the context of eating disorder pathology. Psychol Sport Exerc. 2020;46:101586.

63. Harris A, Hay P, Touyz S. Psychometric properties of instruments assessing exercise in patients with eating disorders: a systematic review. J Eat Disord. 2020;8:45.
64. Pasman L, Thompson JK. Body image and eating disturbance in obligatory runners, obligatory weightlifters, and sedentary individuals. Int J Eat Disord. 1988;7:759–69.
65. Thompson KJ, Pasman L. The obligatory exercise questionnaire. Behav Ther. 1991;14:137.
66. Adkins EC, Keel PK. Does "excessive" or "compulsive" best describe exercise as a symptom of bulimia nervosa? Int J Eat Disord. 2005;38:24–9.
67. Pritchard ME, Beaver JL. Do exercise motives predict obligatory exercise? Eat Behav. 2012;13:139–41.
68. Coen SP, Ogles BM. Psychological characteristics of the obligatory runner: a critical examination of the anorexia analogue hypothesis. J Sport Exerc Psychol. 1993;15:338–54.
69. Steffen JJ, Brehm BJ. The dimensions of obligatory exercise. Eat Disord. 1999;7:219–26.
70. Hausenblas HA, Symons Downs D. How much is too much? The development and validation of the exercise dependence scale. Psychol Health. 2002;17:387–404.
71. Hausenblas HA, Symons Downs D. Exercise dependence scale-21 manual. Authors; 2002. http://www.personal.psu.edu/dsd11/EDS/EDS21Manual.pdf.
72. Symons Downs D, Hausenblas HA, Nigg CR. Factorial validity and psychometric examination of the exercise dependence scale-revised. Meas Phys Educ Exerc Sci. 2004;8:183–201.
73. Magee CA, Buchanan I, Barrie L. Profiles of exercise dependence symptoms in Ironman participants. Psychol Sport Exerc. 2016;24:48–55.
74. Paradis KF, Cooke LM, Martin LJ, Hall CR. Too much of a good thing? Examining the relationship between passion for exercise and exercise dependence. Psychol Sport Exerc. 2013;14:493–500.
75. Hale BD, Roth AD, DeLong RE, Briggs MS. Exercise dependence and the drive for muscularity in male bodybuilders, power lifters, and fitness lifters. Body Image. 2010;7:234–9.
76. White M, Berry R, Rodgers RF. Body image and body change behaviors associated with orthorexia symptoms in males. Body Image. 2020;34:46–50.
77. Dawson N, Hammer JH. No pain, no gains: conformity to masculine norms, body dissatisfaction, and exercise dependence. Psychol Men Masc. 2020;21:430–40.
78. Ulrich CM, Wallen GR, Feister A, Grady C. Respondent burden in clinical research: when are we asking too much of subjects? IRB. 2005;27:17–20.
79. Griffiths S, Mond JM, Li Z, Gunatilake S, Murray SB, Sheffield J, Touyz S. Self-stigma of seeking treatment and being male predict an increased likelihood of having an undiagnosed eating disorder. Int J Eat Disord. 2015;48:775–8.
80. Griffiths S, Mond JM, Murray SB, Touyz S. The prevalence and adverse associations of stigmatization in people with eating disorders. Int J Eat Disord. 2015;48:767–74.
81. Murray SB, Griffiths S, Mitchison D, Mond JM. The transition from thinness-oriented to muscularity-oriented disordered eating in adolescent males: a clinical observation. J Adolesc Health. 2017;60:353–5.

Chapter 8
Muscle Dysmorphia

William Grunewald and Aaron J. Blashill

Learning Objectives

1. Introduce Muscle dysmorphia (MD) and detail its symptoms, comorbidity, and prevalence.
2. Summarize measures for assessing MD.
3. Examine and offer suggestions for current limitations of the MD research literature.

Key Points

- MD is a disorder in which one believes they are insufficiently lean/muscular, leading to clinical distress.
- The nosology of MD is unclear due to its similarities with both eating disorders and body dysmorphic disorder.
- MD research lacks validated assessments for use with clinical populations.
- MD research lacks evidence for its theoretical models of development.
- Future MD studies must sample men diagnosed with MD in order to better inform assessment and treatment of this disorder.

W. Grunewald
Department of Psychology, San Diego State University, San Diego, CA, USA

A. J. Blashill (✉)
Department of Psychology, San Diego State University, San Diego, CA, USA

Department of Psychology, San Diego State University/University of California San Diego Joint Doctoral Program in Clinical Psychology, San Diego, CA, USA
e-mail: ajblashill@sdsu.edu

J. M. Nagata et al. (eds.), *Eating Disorders in Boys and Men*,
https://doi.org/10.1007/978-3-030-67127-3_8

What Is Muscle Dysmorphia?

Clinical Description

In the current edition of the *Diagnostic and Statistical Manual of Mental Disorders* (DSM-5), muscle dysmorphia (MD) is classified as a subtype of body dysmorphic disorder (BDD), which is defined by an excessive preoccupation with a perceived defect in one's appearance leading to marked distress [1]. Specifically, MD involves preoccupation with the thought that one is not muscular enough, coupled with a pervasive fear of muscle loss [2]. This preoccupation continues even if one is objectively muscular and may lead to withdrawal from social relationships, excessive exercise, disordered eating, and psychological distress [2]. Further symptoms of MD include persistent thoughts about muscularity, dissatisfaction with one's appearance, and functional impairment [3]. Specific behaviors associated with MD include intensive weight-lifting regimens, specialized diets meant to maximize muscle mass, compulsive mirror-checking, social comparisons, and discomfort at the presentation of one's body [4].

Prevalence

There is a paucity of data on the prevalence of clinically diagnosed MD within large community samples; however, some data exist on the prevalence of MD symptoms in the general public. Among university students taking courses in nutrition, exercise sciences, or biology, 5.9% of students showed traits of MD symptoms through the Muscle Dysmorphic Disorder Inventory (MDDI) [5]. In a sample of 472 male university students from six schools in Buenos Aires, 5.99% of participants met criteria for probable MD using the Drive for Muscularity Scale (DMS) [6]. In addition, the prevalence of MD among entry-level military personnel in the USA was 12.7% for males [7]. In a study of South-African bodybuilders (n = 28) that used structured clinical interviews to diagnosis MD, the prevalence rate for MD was estimated as 53.6% [8]. Finally, in a systematic review of studies of DSM-IV-defined BDD, it was found that approximately 2.2% of US men have been diagnosed with BDD, with 9–25% of these men fitting the subtype of MD [9]. Thus, the prevalence of MD for US men may range between 0.2% and 0.6% [9].

It is important to note that many of these studies utilized self-report instruments without validated cut scores for the diagnosis of MD and its symptoms, and that future research on MD should utilize clinician-based assessments to derive prevalence estimates. In addition, due to the narrow nature of the samples used in many existing studies (e.g., university students, military personnel, bodybuilders), more representative sampling approaches should be emphasized in future research to better capture the prevalence of MD in the general population.

Comorbidity

MD is often associated with a host of comorbid psychopathology and/or maladaptive behaviors. In a sample of 21 male patients with MD, 90% of patients endorsed lifetime use of appearance- and performance-enhancing drugs (APEDs), such as anabolic steroids, human growth hormones, laxatives, and diuretics [10]. However, due to the inclusion of laxatives and diuretics as "APEDs" in this study, these rates appear higher than in other past studies. For example, in two studies of men with MD, 10 of 23 men (44%) and 11 of 24 men (46%) reported lifetime use of anabolic-androgenic steroids [3, 11]. In a clinical comparison of men with MD vs men with BDD (no MD specifier), men with MD were shown to have significantly higher rates of anabolic steroid abuse, polysubstance abuse (inclusive of substance abuse disorders), and lifetime suicide attempts compared to men with BDD [12]. Of note, significantly higher rates of mood/anxiety disorders were found among individuals with a history of MD compared to individuals with no history of MD [3]. A study that sampled men clinically diagnosed with MD as well as men diagnosed with anorexia nervosa (AN) discovered that men with MD experience similar levels of eating pathology compared to men with AN, albeit with varied body ideals [10]. Mirroring this, in a sample of 60 natural bodybuilders, MD symptomatology was positively associated with scores on the 26-item Eating Attitudes Test, a measure of eating pathology [13]. With regard to prospective studies, data from the 2014 Growing Up Today Study (GUTS) revealed that as drive for muscularity increased, there was an increase in depressive symptoms, dieting, binge drinking, and use of muscle-building products (creatine/steroids) over time [14].

Classification Debate

There has been continued debate regarding how to classify MD. Although MD is currently classified as a subtype of BDD in the DSM-5 [1], its associations with eating pathology, anabolic steroid misuse, and strict dietary rules have cast doubt on whether this is an accurate classification [15]. In a sample of 106 male weightlifters that examined the association of certain attributes of MD with symptoms of obsessive-compulsive disorder (OCD), BDD, and eating disorders, MD symptoms were positively correlated with OCD symptoms, BDD symptoms, perfectionism, and body image dissatisfaction, but were not associated with other ED symptoms such as drive for thinness, bulimia symptoms, interoceptive awareness, etc. [16]. Furthermore, in a sample of 97 college-age men, scores on the Muscle Dysmorphia Inventory (MDI) and levels of social physique anxiety were positively correlated with obsessive-compulsive symptoms [17]. Notably, in a clinical comparison of 14 men diagnosed with MD versus 49 men diagnosed with BDD (without the MD specifier), there were no group differences on BDD severity, number of non-muscle-related areas of concern, and delusionality [12].

The positive associations between MD and OCD symptoms as well as the similarity in BDD symptomology for men with MD/BDD seem to lend support to the classification of MD as a BDD subtype. However, in a systematic review meant to aid the classification of MD, it was suggested that MD shares more similarities with eating disorders due to symptomatic overlap (perfectionism, preoccupation with diet and exercise as a means of affect regulation), comorbidity with various eating disorders, and response to similar treatment approaches such as Enhanced Cognitive Behavior Therapy (CBT-E) [15]. Further, in a clinical comparison of men with AN and men with MD, the groups showed similar levels of body image dissatisfaction, disordered eating, and compulsive exercise [10]. In contrast, it has been argued that AN, BDD, and MD should all be classified as body image disorders, in that the psychopathology associated with these disorders theoretically stems from a desire to achieve an unrealistic body image ideal [18]. Overall, the classification of MD remains unclear, and future research is needed with clinical samples in order to elucidate where MD belongs in future versions of the DSM.

Assessment of Muscle Dysmorphia

Although several measures of MD symptomatology have been published, most validation studies have lacked clinical samples of men diagnosed with MD. Specifically, only two studies have used clinically diagnosed samples of MD in empirical comparisons to other disorders [10, 12]. For this reason, it is difficult to make definitive statements regarding the psychometric properties of MD assessments in clinical MD samples. Nevertheless, a summary of different assessments commonly used in MD research is addressed below and summarized in Table 8.1.

With regard to early MD research, clinicians often used the Body Dysmorphic Disorder Modification of the Yale Brown Obsessive-Compulsive Scale (BDD-YBOCS) with modifications to some of its items to represent concerns with muscularity [26]. The BDD-YBOCS is a semi-structured clinician-based assessment that determines the number of BDD symptoms during the previous week and is comprised of two factors: preoccupations and repetitive behaviors [25]. The measure can be used in MD research to assess muscularity-oriented intrusive thoughts and behaviors, although use of the BDD-YBOCS as a semi-structured interview requires training for both assessors and raters. A further limitation is that the measure has yet to be validated in a sample of men clinically diagnosed with MD.

Several self-report measures assessing symptoms of MD are available. The Muscle Appearance Satisfaction Scale (MASS) is a 19-item self-report measure with a five-factor structure that assesses muscle checking, muscle satisfaction, substance use, injury, and bodybuilding dependence [20]. The MASS has demonstrated high internal consistency, test-retest reliability, and construct validity [20]. An alternative measure of MD symptoms is the Muscle Dysmorphia Inventory (MDI), a 27-item self-report questionnaire that consists of six subscales assessing drive for

Table 8.1 Assessments used in MD research

Measure	Construct	Description
Muscle Dysmorphic Disorder Inventory (MDDI)	MD symptoms	13-item self-report questionnaire that has shown to have strong test-retest reliability, divergent validity, and convergent validity [19]
Muscle Appearance Satisfaction Scale (MASS)	MD symptoms	19-item self-report measure with a five-factor structure: muscle checking, muscle satisfaction, substance use, injury, and bodybuilding dependence. Shown to have high internal consistency, test-retest reliability, and construct validity [20]
Muscle Dysmorphia Inventory (MDI)	MD symptoms	27-item self-report measure with six subscales: drive for size, body dissatisfaction, weight control, exercise behaviors, physique concealment, and dietary behaviors. Shown to have high internal consistency and construct/convergent validity [21]
Drive for Muscularity Scale (DMS)	Attitudes and behaviors regarding muscularity	15-item self-report measure with two subscales: attitudes toward muscularity and behaviors to increase muscularity. Found to have acceptable internal consistency and criterion-related/concurrent validity [22]
Muscularity-Oriented Eating Test (MOET)	Eating attitudes and behaviors regarding muscularity	15-item self-report measure that has shown strong internal consistency, test-retest reliability, and convergent/divergent validity [23]
Eating for Muscularity Scale (EMS)	Eating attitudes and behaviors regarding muscularity	27-item self-report measure that has shown strong internal consistency, construct validity, convergent validity, and test-retest reliability [24]
Body Dysmorphic Disorder Modification of the Yale Brown Obsessive-Compulsive Scale (BDD-YBOCS)	BDD symptoms	12-item clinician-based assessment with a two-factor structure (preoccupations and repetitive behaviors) [25]. Phillips et al. [26] demonstrated the internal consistency and convergent validity of this measure

size, body dissatisfaction, weight control, exercise behaviors, physique concealment, and dietary behaviors [21]. The MDI has demonstrated high internal consistency, construct validity, and convergent validity [21]. While these measures contain items that theoretically encompass specific aspects of MD (e.g., satisfaction with muscularity, diet/exercise behaviors), both lack validation in clinical samples of MD.

The most widely used measure of MD is the Muscle Dysmorphic Disorder Inventory (MDDI), which is a 13-item self-report questionnaire that assesses body image disturbance related to a perceived lack of muscle size/leanness [19]. The MDDI is comprised of three factors: the desire for size subscale (perceptions of being smaller/weaker than desired), the appearance intolerance subscale (anxiety regarding negative beliefs about one's body), and the functional impairment subscale (negative feelings/interference associated with body image disturbance). The total score for the MDDI as well as its three subscales has shown to demonstrate strong internal consistency, test-retest reliability, and convergent/divergent validity [19]. Notably, the MDDI focuses on muscle-related body image more than the MASS or the MDI, but has similarly not yet been validated in clinical MD samples.

Several other measures are available that address muscularity-oriented attitudes and/or behaviors more generally. The Drive for Muscularity Scale (DMS) is a 15-item self-report questionnaire that assesses participants' preoccupation with their own muscularity [22]. The measure contains two subscales, one assessing attitudes toward muscularity and one assessing behaviors meant to increase muscularity [27]. The DMS has demonstrated acceptable internal consistency, temporal stability, criterion-related validity, and concurrent validity [28]. The DMS is a methodologically sound instrument for the use of studying attitudes and behaviors related to the pursuit of muscularity more generally, but it should not be conflated with a measure specific to MD or a diagnostic instrument for MD. Additionally, two recently developed questionnaires focus on eating attitudes and behaviors associated with the pursuit of muscularity. The first of these is the 15-item single-factor Muscularity-Oriented Eating Test (MOET), which has demonstrated promising internal consistency, test-retest reliability, and convergent/divergent validity [23]. The second is the Eating for Muscularity Scale (EMS), a 27-item single-factor questionnaire that displays high construct validity, internal consistency, test-retest reliability, and concurrent validity [24].

Proposed Etiology of Muscle Dysmorphia

Theoretical models for the development of MD have been proposed, but no single model has been empirically confirmed and widely accepted. One multifaceted model states that nine interacting factors contribute to the development of MD: perfectionism, body mass, sport participation, media pressure, ideal body internalization, body dissatisfaction, low self-esteem, negative affect, and body distortion [29]. Body dissatisfaction is influenced by other factors such as ideal body internalization, low self-esteem, etc. Body dissatisfaction theoretically leads to body distortion (the inability to accurately assess one's appearance), which has a direct path to MD in the proposed model. External pressures to appear a certain way (media influence, ideal body internalization, etc.) contribute to body dissatisfaction/distortion, which can be exacerbated by traits/feelings (perfectionism and negative affect), eventually leading to the theoretical development of MD [29]. A second model for MD development based on a biopsychosocial framework includes factors such as genetics, body image consciousness, social pressures to appear a certain way, low self-esteem, and the drive for muscularity [30]. Pressures to appear a certain way, in combination with low self-esteem and other factors, can lead men to overvalue muscularity, theoretically leading to a persistent drive for muscularity that could develop into MD [30]. A third proposed model emphasizes factors including certain precipitating variables (self-esteem, body dissatisfaction), psycho-behavioral characteristics (exercise dependence, use of supplements/steroids, etc.), and negative outcomes (alienation/narcissism) [31]. In this model, MD is conceptualized as beginning with body dissatisfaction and low self-esteem, is maintained through the psycho-behavioral characteristics, and may lead to negative outcomes such as alienation or narcissism [31].

Theoretical models for the development of body image dissatisfaction/eating pathology have been applied to MD. For example, the transdiagnostic model of eating disorders [32] suggests that a dysfunction in self-evaluation (characterized by perfectionism and overvaluation of weight, shape, eating, and their control) underlies the full eating disorder spectrum, with symptoms maintained by a variety of factors such as mood intolerance, interpersonal difficulties, and low self-esteem. In a sample of 119 Australian college students, associations were found between MD symptoms and mood intolerance, perfectionism, and low self-esteem, suggesting that the transdiagnostic model of eating disorders may be applicable to MD [33]. Additionally, the tripartite model of body image [34], which states that pressures from society (media, peers, and family) may lead to body image dissatisfaction via internalization of societal body ideals, has also been investigated with regard to MD symptomology [35]. In a sample of 180 US undergraduates, internalization of the muscular ideal and the thin ideal were associated with MD symptoms. Further, the association between MD symptoms and muscular-ideal internalization was higher among those with lower thin-ideal internalization [35]. Lastly, Ricciardelli and McCabe developed a biopsychosocial model for the pursuit of muscularity in adolescent boys, which may be informative vis-à-vis the development of MD [36]. In this model, biological factors (e.g., body mass index, pubertal timing), psychological factors (e.g., body image concerns, negative affect), and sociocultural factors (e.g., pressure from parents/peers, participation in "power" sports) culminate in the pursuit of muscularity, which is theoretically associated with unsafe weight/muscle gain strategies, anabolic steroid misuse, and bodybuilding behaviors. This model was similar to a model for the development of disordered eating in adolescent boys that was posited in the same review, providing additional support for the conceptual similarity between MD and eating pathology [36]. Models of MD have utilized a biopsychosocial approach or built upon theories for the development of eating pathology/body image concerns, demonstrating the wide range of theories and lack of consensus regarding MD development.

Numerous studies have examined potential risk factors in relation to the etiology of MD symptoms. Unfortunately, there are very few studies that empirically test variables from the theoretical models outlined above [37]; however, several personality traits have been implicated in the development of MD. For example, in one study of 158 males, the association of perfectionism, sociocultural influences, and MD symptoms was investigated cross-sectionally, and perfectionism was suggested to be a mediator for the association between sociocultural influences and MD [38]. This suggests that individuals high in perfectionism may internalize sociocultural norms for how muscular one should appear, potentially leading to the development of MD symptoms. In an online study of 74 men examining self-objectification as a posited risk factor for MD, men with high levels of self-objectification also indicated a high drive for muscularity and multiple symptoms of MD [39]. In a second online study of men, self-objectification mediated the association of internalization of the mesomorphic ideal and body surveillance, with body surveillance further being associated with MD symptoms [40]. Taken together, these findings suggest that perfectionism and self-objectification might potentially be risk factors for MD; however, the cross-sectional nature of the study designs precludes the ability to make definitive statements on temporality and causality regarding their role in MD development. A summary of different models/risk factors for the development of MD is presented in Table 8.2.

One glaring limitation in the field of MD research is the lack of prospective, longitudinal studies examining potential risk factors for MD. Investigating risk factors for MD cross-sectionally certainly provides interesting insights, but the etiology of MD cannot accurately be characterized without prospective studies. Future MD research must be conducted longitudinally to evaluate theoretical risk factors for MD, such as perfectionism or self-objectification [38, 39]. Furthermore, future research must attempt to confirm the aforementioned theoretical models, as there is scant literature that tests these models empirically [37].

Prevention/Treatment

Concerning the prevention of MD, certain dissonance-based interventions (e.g., *The Body Project*) have shown to decrease internalization of body ideals, bulimic symptoms, dietary restraint, drive for muscularity, and MD symptoms, suggesting that these types of interventions should be utilized in the effort to prevent the onset of MD [41]. These reductions in bulimic and MD symptoms were mediated by a decrease in body-ideal internalization, indicating the importance of addressing internalization of body ideals in attempts at MD prevention. Further, in a mixed gender randomized control trial, delivery of dissonance-based interventions over two separate hour-long sessions was shown to reduce dissatisfaction with muscularity, body fat, and global appearance at a 2-month follow-up and dissatisfaction with body parts/body fat at a 6-month follow-up [42]. *The Body Project* has shown to be an effective program for reducing body image/muscular dissatisfaction in men, and thus shows promise with regard to the prevention of MD. See Chap. 13 for further discussion on prevention in males.

There are no known empirically supported treatments for MD, per se; however, cognitive behavioral therapy (CBT) for BDD has strong empirical support [43]. Modular-based CBT for BDD is a promising treatment which includes a module on MD; however, to date, there is no data on whether the efficacy of CBT varies as a function of MD diagnosis [44, 45]. Similarly, no known established treatments for eating disorders (e.g., CBT-E) have been tested among men with MD [46]. Given the common co-occurrence, it would also be prudent to assess for, and treat, comorbid eating pathology as necessary in individuals with MD. See Chap. 14 for further discussion on treatment in males.

Table 8.2 Theoretical models addressing MD risk factors and etiology

Manuscript	Framework	Theory/findings
Grieve (2007) [29]	Biopsychosocial	Nine factors contribute to the development of MD: perfectionism, body mass, sport participation, media pressure, ideal body internalization, body dissatisfaction, low self-esteem, negative affect, and body distortion
Olivardia (2001) [30]	Biopsychosocial	Biological factors (genetics), psychological factors (body image consciousness, low self-esteem), and sociocultural factors (societal pressures to appear a certain way) may culminate in the development of MD
Lantz, Rhea, and Mayhew (2001) [31]	Psychological	MD occurs in three stages: 1. MD arises from body dissatisfaction and low self-esteem 2. MD is maintained through psycho-behavioral characteristics (exercise dependence, steroid use, etc.) 3. MD leads to negative outcomes, such as alienation or narcissism
Murray, Rieger, Karlov, and Touyz (2013) [33]	Psychological	The transdiagnostic model of eating disorders can be applied to MD. Individuals with MD may overvalue eating, weight, and shape, as well as display mood intolerance, low self-esteem, perfectionism, and interpersonal difficulties. In an undergraduate sample, there were associations between perfectionism, mood intolerance, low self-esteem, and MD symptoms
Klimek, Murray, Brown, Gonzales IV, and Blashill (2018) [35]	Psychosocial	The tripartite influence model of body image can be applied to MD. Pressures from media, peers, and family may lead to body image dissatisfaction via internalization of societal body ideals. Muscular-ideal internalization was increasingly associated with MD symptoms as thin-ideal internalization decreased
Ricciardelli and McCabe (2004) [36]	Biopsychosocial	Biological factors (BMI, pubertal timing, etc.), psychological factors (body image concerns, negative affect, etc.), and sociocultural factors (societal pressures to appear a certain way) may culminate in the pursuit of muscularity in adolescent males
Dryer, Farr, Hiramatsu, and Quinton (2016) [38]	Psychosocial	Sociocultural norms for how to appear were associated with MD symptoms, and this association was mediated by perfectionism
Grieve and Helmick (2008) [39]	Psychological	Self-objectification was associated with drive for muscularity and MD symptoms
Heath, Tod, Kannis-Dymand, and Lovell (2016) [40]	Psychosocial	Self-objectification, internalization of the mesomorphic ideal, and body surveillance contribute to MD symptoms

Future Research

With regard to future research, there is a definitive need to isolate factors leading to thin-ideal internalization, muscular-ideal internalization, or both, in order to better understand how and why men internalize societal cues about how they "should" appear [35, 47]. Internalization of these ideals may theoretically be an important starting point for the development of the symptoms of MD, and determining why men internalize different appearance ideals may reveal further approaches for the prevention or treatment of MD. Furthermore, there is a pressing need for prospective/longitudinal designs in MD research in order to explore/confirm theoretical models for the development of MD. Existing MD research almost exclusively consists of cross-sectional designs, limiting the field's ability to make claims about the etiology of MD, as well as limiting the understanding of the course and outcomes of MD over time.

Moreover, there must be an emphasis on studies with representative sampling approaches to better understand the true prevalence of MD in the general community. As previously mentioned, there is a lack of research with clinical samples of MD, in addition to MD being compared to other clinical disorders, which limits our ability to accurately classify and tailor treatment for MD. Clinical MD research also needs to include larger sample sizes in order to increase power to detect significant effects in future research. Lastly, additional studies need to be conducted on various forms of treatments with MD, in order to illuminate which proposed therapies are efficacious in the treatment of MD and whether a distinct form of treatment for MD needs to be established.

Conclusions

MD is currently classified as a subtype of BDD defined by dissatisfaction with one's muscularity and clinical distress regarding one's appearance. MD is associated with a host of co-occurring forms of psychopathology, including various mood/anxiety disorders, eating pathology, suicidality, and substance abuse. Several risk factors/theoretical models for the development of MD have been proposed, but none have been empirically validated. Furthermore, there is no current form of treatment specific to MD, but dissonance-based interventions have shown efficacy in preventing the development of MD, and CBT for BDD shows some support as a treatment option for MD. Future research regarding MD must emphasize the use of clinical samples and longitudinal designs, as these two issues would address the most glaring limitations of the current literature on MD.

References

1. American Psychiatric Association. Diagnostic and statistical manual of mental disorders. 5th ed; 2013. https://doi.org/10.1176/appi.books.9780890425596.744053.
2. Pope HG, Gruber AJ, Choi P, Olivardia R, Phillips KA. Muscle dysmorphia: an underrecognized form of body dysmorphic disorder. Psychosomatics. 1997;38:548–57. https://doi.org/10.1016/S0033-3182(97)71400-2.
3. Cafri G, Olivardia R, Thompson KJ. Symptom characteristics and psychiatric comorbidity among males with muscle dysmorphia. Compr Psych. 2008;49:374–9. https://doi.org/10.1016/j.comppsych.2008.01.003.
4. Specter SE, Wiss DA. Muscle dysmorphia: where body image obsession, compulsive exercise, disordered eating, and substance abuse intersect in susceptible males. In: Brewerton TD, Dennis AD, editors. Eating disorders, addictions and substance use disorders: research, clinical and treatment perspectives: Springer-Verlag Publishing; 2014. p. 439–57. https://doi.org/10.1007/978-3-642-45378-6_20.
5. Bo S, Zoccali R, Ponzo V, Soldati L, De Carli L, Benso A, et al. University courses, eating problems and muscle dysmorphia: are there any associations? J Transl Med. 2014;12:1–8. https://doi.org/10.1186/s12967-014-0221-2.
6. Compte EJ, Sepulveda AR, Torrente F. A two-stage epidemiological study of eating disorders and muscle dysmorphia in male university students in Buenos Aires. Int J Eat Disord. 2015;48:1092–101. https://doi.org/10.1002/eat.22448.
7. Campagna JDA, Bowsher B. Prevalence of body dysmorphic disorder and muscle dysmorphia among entry-level military personnel. Mil Med. 2016;181:494–501. https://doi.org/10.7205/MILMED-D-15-00118.
8. Hitzeroth V, Wessels C, Zungu-Dirwayi N, Oosthuizen P, Stein DJ. Muscle dysmorphia: a South African sample. Psych & Clin Neuro. 2001;55:521–3. https://doi.org/10.1046/j.1440-1819.2001.00899.x.
9. Phillips KA, Wilhelm S, Koran LM, Didie ER, Fallon BA, Feusner J, et al. Body dysmorphic disorder: some key issues for DSM-V. Dep & Anx. 2010;27:573–91. https://doi.org/10.1002/da.20709.
10. Murray SB, Rieger E, Hildebrandt T, Karlov L, Russell J, Boon E, et al. A comparison of eating, exercise, shape, and weight related symptomatology in males with muscle dysmorphia and anorexia nervosa. Body Image. 2012;9:93–100. https://doi.org/10.1016/j.bodyim.2012.01.008.
11. Olivardia R, Pope HG, Hudson JI. Muscle dysmorphia in male weightlifters: a case-control study. Amer J Psych. 2000;157:1291–6. https://doi.org/10.1176/appi.ajp.157.8.1291.
12. Pope CG, Pope HG, Menard W, Fay C, Olivardia R, Phillips KA. Clinical features of muscle dysmorphia among males with body dysmorphic disorder. Body Image. 2005;2:395–400. https://doi.org/10.1016/j.bodyim.2005.09.001.
13. Mitchell L, Murray SB, Hoon M, Hackett D, Prvan T, et al. Correlates of muscle dysmorphia symptomatology in natural bodybuilders: distinguishing factors in the pursuit of hypermuscularity. Body Image. 2017;22:1–5. https://doi.org/10.1016/j.bodyim.2017.04.003.
14. Eik-Nes TT, Austin SB, Blashill AJ, Murray SB, Calzo JP. Prospective health associations of drive for muscularity in young adult males. Int J Eat Disord. 2018;51:1185–93. https://doi.org/10.1002/eat.22943.
15. Murray SB, Rieger E, Touyz SW, De la Garza García Y. Muscle dysmorphia and the DSM-V conundrum: where does it belong? A review paper. Int J Eat Disord. 2010;43:483–91. https://doi.org/10.1002/eat.20828.
16. Maida D, Armstrong SL. The classification of muscle dysmorphia. Int J Mens Health. 2005;4:73–91. https://doi.org/10.3149/jmh.0401.73.

17. Chandler CG, Grieve FG, Derryberry WP, Pegg PO. Are anxiety and obsessive-compulsive symptoms related to muscle dysmorphia? Int J Mens Health. 2009;8:143–54. https://doi.org/10.3149/jmh.0802.143.
18. Phillipou A, Blomeley D, Castle DJ. Muscling in on body image disorders: what is the nosological status of muscle dysmorphia? Australian & New Zealand J Psych. 2015;50:380–1. https://doi.org/10.1177/0004867415615951.
19. Hildebrandt T, Langenbucher JW, Schlundt DG. Muscularity concerns among men: development of attitudinal and perceptual measures. Body Image. 2004;1:169–81. https://doi.org/10.1016/j.bodyim.2004.01.001.
20. Mayville SB, Williamson DA, White MA, Netemeyer RG, Drab DL. Development of the muscle appearance satisfaction scale: a self-report measure for the assessment of muscle dysmorphia symptoms. Assessment. 2002;9:351–60. https://doi.org/10.1177/1073191102238156.
21. Rhea DJ, Lantz CD, Cornelius AE. Development of the muscle dysmorphia inventory (MDI). J Sports Med & Phys Fit. 2004;44:428–35.
22. McCreary DR, Sasse DK. An exploration of the drive for muscularity in adolescent boys and girls. J American Coll Health. 2000;48:297–304. https://doi.org/10.1080/07448480009596271.
23. Murray SB, Brown TA, Blashill AJ, Compte EJ, Lavender JM, Mitchison D, et al. The development and validation of the muscularity-oriented eating test: a novel measure of muscularity-oriented disordered eating. Int J Eat Disord. 2019;52:1389–98. https://doi.org/10.1002/eat.23144.
24. Cooper M, Griffiths KM, Burns R. Getting shredded: development and validation of a measure of muscularity-oriented disordered eating. Psych Assessment. 2020.;Advance online publication;32:451–60. https://doi.org/10.1037/pas0000804.
25. Phillips KA, Hart AS, Menard W. Psychometric evaluation of the Yale–Brown obsessive-compulsive scale modified for body dysmorphic disorder (BDD-YBOCS). J Obsessive-Compulsive & Rel Disord. 2014;3:205–8. https://doi.org/10.1016/j.jocrd.2014.04.004.
26. Phillips KA, Hollander E, Rasmussen SA, Aronowitz BR, DeCaria C, Goodman WK. A severity rating scale for body dysmorphic disorder: development, reliability, and validity of a modified version of the Yale-Brown Obsessive Compulsive Scale. Psychopharmacol Bull. 1997;33:17–22.
27. McCreary DR, Sasse DK, Saucier DM, Dorsch KD. Measuring the drive for muscularity: factorial validity of the drive for muscularity scale in men and women. Psych Men & Masc. 2004;5:49–58. https://doi.org/10.1037/1524-9220.5.1.49.
28. Dakanalis A, Timko A, Madeddu F, Volpato C, Clerici M, Riva G, et al. Are the male body dissatisfaction and drive for muscularity scales reliable and valid instruments? J Health Psych. 2015;20:48–59. https://doi.org/10.1177/1359105313498108.
29. Grieve FG. A conceptual model of factors contributing to the development of muscle dysmorphia. Eat Disord. 2007;15:63–80. https://doi.org/10.1080/10640260601044535.
30. Olivardia R. Mirror, mirror on the wall, who's the largest of them all? The features and phenomenology of muscle dysmorphia. Harvard Rev Psych. 2001;9:254–9. https://doi.org/10.1080/hrp.9.5.254.259.
31. Lantz CD, Rhea DJ, Mayhew JC. The drive for size: a psycho-behavioral model of muscle dysmorphia. Int Sports J. 2001;5:71–86.
32. Fairburn CG, Cooper Z, Shafran R. Cognitive behaviour therapy for eating disorders: a "transdiagnostic" theory and treatment. Beh Res & Ther. 2003;41:509–28. https://doi.org/10.1016/S0005-7967(02)00088-8.
33. Murray SB, Rieger E, Karlov L, Touyz SW. An investigation of the transdiagnostic model of eating disorders in the context of muscle dysmorphia. Euro Eat Disord Rev. 2013;21:160–4. https://doi.org/10.1002/erv.2194.
34. Cafri G, Yamamiya Y, Brannick M, Thompson JK. The influence of sociocultural factors on body image: a meta-analysis. Clin Psych: Sci Pract. 2005;12:421–33. https://doi.org/10.1093/clipsy.bpi053.

35. Klimek P, Murray SB, Brown T, Gonzales M IV, Blashill AJ. Thinness and muscularity internalization: associations with disordered eating and muscle dysmorphia in men. Int J Eat Disord. 2018;51:352–7. https://doi.org/10.1002/eat.22844.
36. Ricciardelli LA, McCabe MP. A biopsychosocial model of disordered eating and the pursuit of muscularity in adolescent boys. Psychol Bull. 2004;130(2):179–205.
37. Muller SM, Dennis DL, Schneider SR, Joyner RL. Muscle dysmorphia among selected male college athletes: an examination of the Lantz, Rhea, and Mayhew model. Int Sports J. 2004;8:119–25.
38. Dryer R, Farr M, Hiramatsu I, Quinton S. The role of sociocultural influences on symptoms of muscle dysmorphia and eating disorders in men, and the mediating effects of perfectionism. Beh Med. 2016;42:174–82. https://doi.org/10.1080/08964289.2015.1122570.
39. Grieve R, Helmick A. The influence of men's self-objectification on the drive for muscularity: self-esteem, body satisfaction and muscle dysmorphia. Int J Mens Health. 2008;7:288–98. https://doi.org/10.3149/jmh.0703.288.
40. Heath B, Tod DA, Kannis-Dymand L, Lovell GP. The relationship between objectification theory and muscle dysmorphia characteristics in men. Psych Men & Masc. 2016;17:297–308. https://doi.org/10.1037/men0000022.
41. Brown TA, Forney KJ, Pinner D, Keel PK. A randomized controlled trial of the body project: more than muscles for men with body dissatisfaction. Int J of Eat Disord. 2017;50:873–83. https://doi.org/10.1002/eat.22724.
42. Kilpela LS, Blomquist K, Verzijl C, Wilfred S, Beyl R, Becker CB. The body project 4 all: a pilot randomized controlled trial of a mixed-gender dissonance-based body image program. Int J Eat Disord. 2016;49:591–602. https://doi.org/10.1002/eat.22562.
43. Harrison A, De la Cruz L, Enander J, Radua J, Mataix-Cols D. Cognitive-behavioral therapy for body dysmorphic disorder: a systematic review and meta-analysis of randomized control trials. Clin Psych Rev. 2016;48:43–51. https://doi.org/10.1016/j.cpr.2016.05.007.
44. Wilhelm S, Phillips KA, Didie E, Buhlmann U, Greenberg JL, Fama JM, et al. Modular cognitive-behavioral therapy for body dysmorphic disorder: a randomized controlled trial. Beh Ther. 2013;45:314–27. https://doi.org/10.1016/j.beth.2013.12.007.
45. Wilhelm S, Phillips KA, Greenberg JL, O'Keefe SM, Hoeppner SS, Keshaviah A, et al. Efficacy and posttreatment effects of therapist delivered cognitive behavioral therapy vs supportive psychotherapy for adults with body dysmorphic disorder: a randomized clinical trial. JAMA Psych. 2019;76:363–73. https://doi.org/10.1001/jamapsychiatry.2018.4156.
46. Fairburn CG. Cognitive behavior therapy and eating disorders. New York: Guilford Press; 2008.
47. Murray SB, Touyz SW. Masculinity, femininity and male body image: a recipe for future research. Int J Mens Health. 2012;11:227–39. https://doi.org/10.3149/jmh.1103.227.

Part III
Medical and Substances

Chapter 9
Medical Complications of Eating Disorders in Boys and Men

Jason M. Nagata, Kyle T. Ganson, and Neville H. Golden

Learning Objectives
1. Identify cardiovascular, endocrine, skeletal, growth, gastrointestinal, neurological, and hematological complications of eating disorders in boys and men.
2. Describe gaps in evidence of medical complications of eating disorders in boys and men.

Key Points
- Eating disorders in boys and men are associated with high morbidity and high mortality rates.
- Medical complications of eating disorders in boys and men can affect nearly every organ system in the body.
- Medical complications of muscle dysmorphic disorder and muscularity-oriented disordered eating remain largely unknown.

Introduction

Eating disorders include, but are not limited to, anorexia nervosa, atypical anorexia nervosa, bulimia nervosa, binge eating disorder, and avoidant/restrictive food intake disorder, according to the *Diagnostic and Statistical Manual of Mental Disorders*,

J. M. Nagata (✉)
Division of Adolescent and Young Adult Medicine, Department of Pediatrics, University of California, San Francisco, San Francisco, CA, USA
e-mail: jason.nagata@ucsf.edu

K. T. Ganson
Factor-Inwentash Faculty of Social Work, University of Toronto, Toronto, ON, Canada

N. H. Golden
Department of Pediatrics, Stanford University School of Medicine, Stanford, CA, USA

J. M. Nagata et al. (eds.), *Eating Disorders in Boys and Men*,
https://doi.org/10.1007/978-3-030-67127-3_9

5th Edition (DSM-5) [1]. These disorders can cause significant medical complications affecting every organ system in the body [2]. Most research on medical complications of eating disorders have focused on girls and women, particularly in anorexia nervosa. However, there is a limited and growing evidence base on medical complications of eating disorders in boys and men.[1] The Minnesota Starvation Experiment conducted by Ancel Keys from 1944 to 1945 comprehensively evaluated medical consequences of starvation in young men [3]. Although these men did not necessarily experience eating disorders, many developed disordered eating through out the course of the experiment, and these findings may be applicable to young men who experience starvation from eating disorders.

The purpose of this chapter is to review the evidence on medical complications of eating disorders in boys and men. In particular, we review cardiovascular, electrolyte, refeeding syndrome, endocrine, bone density, growth and body composition, gastrointestinal and liver, neurological, and hematological consequences of eating disorders in boys and men (Table 9.1). Less is known about medical consequences of muscle dysmorphic disorder, characterized by a preoccupation with not being sufficiently muscular or lean, and muscularity-oriented disordered eating; the chapter on appearance- and performance-enhancing drugs reviews medical complications associated with use of those substances (Chap. 12).

Mortality

Eating disorders have among the highest mortality rates of any psychiatric illness. Crude mortality rates for men with eating disorders are estimated at 12.9% for anorexia nervosa, 11.1% for bulimia nervosa, and 6.4% in eating disorders not otherwise specified [4]. Standardized mortality rates in men with anorexia nervosa are six to eight times that of the male reference population [4, 5].

Cardiovascular Consequences

In a state of malnutrition, bradycardia and hypotension are cardiovascular responses due to a decreased basal metabolic rate and parasympathetic activation [6]. Among adolescent boys and young adult men evaluated for a restrictive eating disorder in an outpatient medical subspecialty clinic, 39.4% presented with bradycardia (heart rate 58.7 ± 17.5 beats/min), and 12.1% had orthostatic heart rate changes (change in heart rate 22.0 ± 21.6 beats/min) [7]. Over half (51.5%) of these patients met hospital admission criteria during their first outpatient evaluation based on vital sign instability [7]. Exercise, including team sports participation and hours of exercise per

[1] In this chapter, we use the terms males and boys/men interchangeably.

Table 9.1 Medical complications in eating disorders in boys and men

Cardiovascular	Bradycardia
	Prolonged QT interval
	Orthostatic hypotension
	Mitral valve prolapse
	Pericardial effusion
	Reduced left ventricular wall thickness and mass
	Elevated cholesterol
Electrolyte abnormalities	Refeeding syndrome
	Hypokalemia
	Hypophosphatemia
	Hypomagnesemia
	Hyponatremia
	Hypernatremic dehydration
	Hypocalcemia
Endocrine	Diminished libido
Gonadal	Low testosterone
	Low follicle-stimulating hormone (FSH)
	Low luteinizing hormone (LH) pulsatility
Thyroid	Low free triiodothyronine (fT3)
	Low free thyroxine (fT4)
Skeletal	Low bone mineral density
	Increased fracture risk
Growth	Growth stunting and retardation
Body composition	Low fat mass index
	Low lean body mass index
Gastrointestinal and liver	Impaired gastric emptying
	Superior mesenteric artery syndrome
	Elevated liver enzymes
Neurological	Cortical atrophy
	Reduced temporal and parietal volumes
	Peripheral neuropathy
	Muscle weakness
Hematological	Anemia
	Thrombocytopenia
	Leukopenia
	Neutropenia

Table adapted from Nagata and Golden, 2018 [31]

week, is associated with bradycardia in the setting of eating disorders. Bradycardia warranting hospital admission has been documented in adolescent boys with muscularity-oriented disordered eating [8]. Other cardiac complications noted in men with anorexia nervosa include supraventricular tachycardia (SVT) and cardiopulmonary arrest with subsequent tachycardic episodes and a pericardial effusion [9].

Total cholesterol abnormalities were present in 16.7–40.0% of boys and men with eating disorders [7, 10]. Abnormal triglycerides were noted in 26.1% of adolescent boys with eating disorders [10]. Cholesterol elevation in eating disorders may be related to liver dysfunction, dehydration, reduced cholesterol turnover, and delayed cholesterol metabolism, but the exact etiology is unclear [11]. Binge eating in young men is associated with incident hyperlipidemia [12].

Electrolyte Abnormalities

Eating disorders can lead to electrolyte abnormalities due to malnutrition, purging, refeeding syndrome, kidney dysfunction, or other etiologies [13]. Among a sample of 20 adolescent boys and young men presenting for eating disorder care who had available laboratory data, 25% had abnormal potassium, while 5.3% had abnormal phosphorus [7]. In the sample, three patients reported vomiting at the time of presentation. One-fifth had a creatinine level in the abnormal range [7]. In another sample of 71 male youth with eating disorders, abnormal phosphorus (23.2%), magnesium (9.1%), potassium (5.2%), chloride (4.0%), and sodium (1.7%) levels were noted [10]. In a small case series of ten adolescent boys with anorexia nervosa, one 12-year-old boy presented with hypernatremic dehydration (serum sodium 172 meq/l) [9].

Refeeding Syndrome

Refeeding syndrome is characterized by shifts in fluid and electrolyte levels from extracellular to intracellular spaces in malnourished patients who are undergoing nutritional refeeding [14]. These fluid and electrolyte shifts can have serious cardiac, respiratory, neurologic, and hematologic consequences and are associated with significant morbidity and mortality [14]. Although there is a paucity of studies examining refeeding syndrome in boys and men with eating disorders, refeeding syndrome was noted among the young men who experienced starvation and then refeeding in the Minnesota Starvation Experiment [3].

Endocrine

Malnutrition from eating disorders may suppress the hypothalamic-pituitary-gonadal axis in boys and men, leading to low luteinizing hormone (LH), follicle-stimulating hormone (FSH), and testosterone levels [10, 15]. Among male youth with eating disorders, 13.3% had abnormal testosterone levels [10]. Associated symptoms may include diminished libido. In the Minnesota Starvation Experiment, young men experiencing starvation also had decreased sperm counts and mobility [3].

Eating disorders in boys and men can also affect the hypothalamic-pituitary-thyroid axis, with dysregulation of thyroid feedback control. Among adolescent boys and young men with eating disorders, 10.5% had abnormal thyroid-stimulating hormone (TSH) levels, and 5.6% had abnormal free thyroxine (free T4) levels [7].

Bone Density

Osteoporosis and osteopenia are complications of eating disorders in boys and men [16, 17]. Adolescent boys with anorexia nervosa have significant deficits in bone mineral density [16, 17]. Bone mineral density *Z*-scores < -1 were present at the lumbar spine (48%), total hip (44%), and femoral neck (40%) among adolescent boys [18]. Atypical anorexia nervosa is associated with higher bone mineral density compared to anorexia nervosa in adolescent samples including boys [19]. In adult men, low bone mineral density *Z*-scores (<-2 at ≥ 1 site) were documented in men with anorexia nervosa (65%), atypical anorexia nervosa (33%), and avoidant/restrictive food intake disorder (18%) [20]. Weight-bearing exercise and participation in team sports may be protective of whole body bone mineral content and bone mineral density at the hip [21]. Among men older than 40 years, anorexia nervosa is associated with higher fracture risk compared to healthy controls (hazard ratio: 2.54) [22].

Growth and Body Composition

Growth stunting and retardation has been noted in adolescent boys with anorexia nervosa. In a sample of 12 boys with anorexia nervosa, 11 exhibited growth retardation as evident by a decrease in their height standard deviation score [23]. Weight restoration was associated with accelerated linear growth in all patients [23]. Complete catch-up growth was not achieved in 9 of 12 patients [23]. In terms of body composition, adolescent boys with anorexia nervosa have significant lean body mass index (mean *Z*-score $- 0.47 \pm 0.63$) and fat mass index (mean *Z*-score $- 2.41 \pm 0.96$) deficits [24]. In adolescent samples including boys, participation in team sports was associated with greater deficits in fat mass index *Z*-score, while duration of weight-bearing exercise was associated with higher lean body mass index *Z*-score [21].

Gastrointestinal and Liver

Eating disorders may affect the entire gastrointestinal tract [25]. Although most research on gastrointestinal complications has been in women with anorexia nervosa, limited research has included men with eating disorders [25]. Studies including boys and men with eating disorders have demonstrated impaired gastric emptying, but sex differences were not noted [26, 27]. Superior mesenteric artery syndrome has been documented in a 38-year-old man with a delayed diagnosis of an eating disorder [28]. Elevated liver enzymes (alanine aminotransferase ≥40 U/L) have been documented in adolescent boys with anorexia nervosa [10, 29]. Male versus female sex was associated with higher risk of elevated liver enzymes in anorexia nervosa [29].

Neurological

Brain volume may be affected in the setting of restrictive eating disorders, resulting in structural brain changes on brain imaging [2]. For instance, cortical atrophy was noted in seven of nine adolescent boys with eating disorders on computed tomography (CT) scans [9]. Another study that included an adolescent boy demonstrated reduced temporal and parietal volumes on magnetic resonance imaging (MRI) [30]. Peripheral neuropathy and muscular weakness have been noted in an adolescent boy with anorexia nervosa [9].

Hematological

Eating disorders can affect all blood lines, including red blood cells, white blood cells, and platelets [31]. In one study of adolescent boys with anorexia nervosa, seven of the ten boys had mild anemia based on normative values for their sexual development stage [9]. In another study, adolescent boys and young men with eating disorders had abnormal hemoglobin (23.8%), hematocrit (33.3%), white blood cell count (23.8%), absolute neutrophil count (10.0%), and platelet count (19.0%), presumably lower than the normal range [7].

Conclusion

This chapter summarizes the literature on medical complications of eating disorders among boys and men. See Chap. 10: Medical Management of Eating Disorders in Boys and Men: Current Clinical Guidance and Evidence Gaps for information on medical management of eating disorders. Evidence indicates that medical complications of eating disorders can affect nearly every organ system in boys and men [32]. However, there remains a need for more research on medical complications in eating disorders in boys and men, especially by diagnosis type, particularly for atypical anorexia nervosa and avoidant restrictive food intake disorder. There is a paucity of research on medical consequences of muscularity-oriented disordered eating [33], and this remains an important area of future research.

References

1. American Psychiatric Association. Diagnostic and statistical manual of mental disorders. 5th ed. Arlington: American Psychiatric Publishing; 2013.
2. Katzman DK. Medical complications in adolescents with anorexia nervosa: a review of the literature. Int J Eat Disord. 2005;37(Suppl):S52–9.
3. Keys A. The biology of human starvation. Minneapolis: University of Minnesota Press; 1950.
4. Quadflieg N, Strobel C, Naab S, Voderholzer U, Fichter MM. Mortality in males treated for an eating disorder-A large prospective study. Int J Eat Disord. 2019;52(12):1365–9.
5. Gueguen J, Godart N, Chambry J, Brun-Eberentz A, Foulon C, Divac Phd SM, et al. Severe anorexia nervosa in men: comparison with severe AN in women and analysis of mortality. Int J Eat Disord. 2012;45(4):537–45.
6. Sachs KV, Harnke B, Mehler PS, Krantz MJ. Cardiovascular complications of anorexia nervosa: a systematic review. Int J Eat Disord. 2016;49(3):238–48.
7. Vo M, Lau J, Rubinstein M. Eating disorders in adolescent and young adult males: presenting characteristics. J Adolesc Health. 2016;59(4):397–400.
8. Murray SB, Accurso EC, Griffiths S, Nagata JM. Boys, biceps, and bradycardia: the hidden dangers of muscularity-oriented disordered eating. J Adolesc Health. 2018;62(3):352–5.
9. Siegel JH, Hardoff D, Golden NH, Shenker IR. Medical complications in male adolescents with anorexia nervosa. J Adolesc Health. 1995;16(6):448–53.
10. Coelho JS, Lee T, Karnabi P, Burns A, Marshall S, Geller J, et al. Eating disorders in biological males: clinical presentation and consideration of sex differences in a pediatric sample. J Eat Disord. 2018;6:40.
11. Nakai Y, Noma S, Fukusima M, Taniguchi A, Teramukai S. Serum lipid levels in patients with eating disorders. Intern Med. 2016;55(14):1853–7.
12. Nagata JM, Garber AK, Tabler J, Murray SB, Vittinghoff E, Bibbins-Domingo K. Disordered eating behaviors and future cardiometabolic risk among young adults with overweight or obesity. Int J Eat Disord. 2018;51(8):931–41.
13. Chidiac CW. An update on the medical consequences of anorexia nervosa. Curr Opin Pediatr. 2019;31(4):448–53.
14. Fuentebella J, Kerner JA. Refeeding syndrome. Pediatr Clin N Am. 2009;56(5):1201–10.
15. Skolnick A, Schulman RC, Galindo RJ, Mechanick JI. The endocrinopathies of male anorexia nervosa: case series. AACE Clin Case Rep. 2016;2(4):e351–7.
16. Misra M, Katzman DK, Cord J, Manning SJ, Mendes N, Herzog DB, et al. Bone metabolism in adolescent boys with anorexia nervosa. J Clin Endocrinol Metab. 2008;93(8):3029–36.
17. Misra M, Katzman DK, Clarke H, Snelgrove D, Brigham K, Miller KK, et al. Hip structural analysis in adolescent boys with anorexia nervosa and controls. J Clin Endocrinol Metab. 2013;98(7):2952–8.
18. Nagata JM, Golden NH, Peebles R, Long J, Leonard MB, Carlson JL. Assessment of sex differences in bone deficits among adolescents with anorexia nervosa. Int J Eat Disord. 2017;50(4):352–8.

19. Nagata JM, Carlson JL, Golden NH, Long J, Murray SB, Peebles R. Comparisons of bone density and body composition among adolescents with anorexia nervosa and atypical anorexia nervosa. Int J Eat Disord. 2019;52(5):591–6.
20. Schorr M, Drabkin A, Rothman MS, Meenaghan E, Lashen GT, Mascolo M, et al. Bone mineral density and estimated hip strength in men with anorexia nervosa, atypical anorexia nervosa and avoidant/restrictive food intake disorder. Clin Endocrinol. 2019;90(6):789–97.
21. Nagata JM, Carlson JL, Golden NH, Murray SB, Long J, Leonard MB, et al. Associations between exercise, body composition, and bone mineral density in adolescents with anorexia nervosa. Eat Weight Disord. 2019;24(5):939–45.
22. Nagata JM, Golden NH, Leonard MB, Copelovitch L, Denburg MR. Assessment of sex differences in fracture risk among patients with anorexia nervosa: a population-based cohort study using the health improvement network. J Bone Miner Res. 2017;32(5):1082–9.
23. Modan-Moses D, Yaroslavsky A, Novikov I, Segev S, Toledano A, Miterany E, et al. Stunting of growth as a major feature of anorexia nervosa in male adolescents. Pediatrics. 2003;111(2):270–6.
24. Nagata JM, Golden NH, Peebles R, Long J, Murray SB, Leonard MB, et al. Assessment of sex differences in body composition among adolescents with anorexia nervosa. J Adolesc Health. 2017;60(4):455–9.
25. Norris ML, Harrison ME, Isserlin L, Robinson A, Feder S, Sampson M. Gastrointestinal complications associated with anorexia nervosa: a systematic review. Int J Eat Disord. 2016;49(3):216–37.
26. Robinson PH. Perceptivity and paraceptivity during measurement of gastric emptying in anorexia and bulimia nervosa. Br J Psychiatry. 1989;154:400–5.
27. Hutson WR, Wald A. Gastric emptying in patients with bulimia nervosa and anorexia nervosa. Am J Gastroenterol. 1990;85(1):41–6.
28. Recio-Barbero M, Fuertes-Soriano S, Cabezas-Garduño J, López-Atanes M, Peña-Rotella A, Sáenz-Herrero M. Delayed diagnosis of an eating disorder in a male patient with superior mesenteric artery syndrome: results from a case study. Front Psych. 2019;10:731.
29. Nagata JM, Park KT, Colditz K, Golden NH. Associations of elevated liver enzymes among hospitalized adolescents with anorexia nervosa. J Pediatr. 2015;166(2):439–43.e1.
30. Castro-Fornieles J, Bargallo N, Lazaro L, Andres S, Falcon C, Plana MT, et al. A cross-sectional and follow-up voxel-based morphometric MRI study in adolescent anorexia nervosa. J Psychiatr Res. 2009;43(3):331–40.
31. Nagata JM, Golden NH. Sex differences in eating disorders. Adolesc Med State Art Rev. 2018;29:245–59.
32. Nagata JM, Ganson KT, Murray SB. Eating disorders in adolescent boys and young men: an update. Curr Opin Pediatr. 2020;32(4):476–81.
33. Nagata JM, Ganson KT, Cunningham ML, Mitchison D, Lavender JM, Blashill AJ, Gooding HC, Murray SB. Associations between legal performance-enhancing substance use and future cardiovascular disease risk factors in young adults: A prospective cohort study. PLoS One. 2020;15(12):e0244018.

Chapter 10
Medical Management of Eating Disorders in Boys and Men: Current Clinical Guidance and Evidence Gaps

Kyle T. Ganson, Neville H. Golden, and Jason M. Nagata

Learning Objectives

1. Recognize that current clinical guidance may lack sensitivity for the unique presentations of eating disorders among boys and men.
2. Identify multiple areas, including monitoring bone health, body mass index, treatment goal weight, refeeding protocols, testosterone testing, use of performance-enhancing substances, and muscle dysmorphia, that have unique considerations for eating disorders in boys and men.
3. Identify areas for future research to address the gaps in the current clinical guidance.

Key Points

- Current clinical guidance does not disaggregate by sex, despite differences in clinical presentation of boys and men experiencing eating disorders.
- Specific areas of current clinical guidance that could be refined include monitoring bone health, body mass index, treatment goal weight, refeeding protocols, testosterone testing, use of performance-enhancing substances, and muscle dysmorphia.
- Overall, there is a need for more empirical observational and experimental medical research to develop the evidence base to inform specific clinical guidance for boys and men experiencing eating disorders.

K. T. Ganson (✉)
Factor-Inwentash Faculty of Social Work, University of Toronto, Toronto, ON, Canada
e-mail: kyle.ganson@utoronto.ca

N. H. Golden
Department of Pediatrics, Stanford University School of Medicine, Stanford, CA, USA

J. M. Nagata
Division of Adolescent and Young Adult Medicine, Department of Pediatrics, University of California, San Francisco, San Francisco, CA, USA

J. M. Nagata et al. (eds.), *Eating Disorders in Boys and Men*,
https://doi.org/10.1007/978-3-030-67127-3_10

Introduction

Guidance for the clinical treatment of eating disorders can be presented in a number of formats, including clinical practice guidelines, position papers, and review articles, among others. In this chapter, we discuss different aspects of these recommendations as they relate to boys and men[1] experiencing eating disorders. To simplify our discussion, we will refer to each of these documents more generally as clinical guidance.

Current clinical guidance lacks specificity by sex, largely due to gaps in the evidence base on eating disorders in males. Instead, guidance in the United States for adolescents [1] and adults [2] and guidelines in the United Kingdom [3] and Australia and New Zealand [4] provide direction to medical providers based on diagnosis and level of care. This guidance may not apply to boys and men given these groups experience eating disorders differently compared to girls and women. Additionally, prior to the *Diagnostic and Statistical Manual, Fifth Edition* (DSM-5), which was published in 2013, amenorrhea was a diagnostic criterion for anorexia nervosa in post-menarcheal females [5]. This criterion did not apply to males and may have led to inaccurate diagnosis for boys and men that presented with the remaining criteria of anorexia nervosa. Ultimately, current clinical guidance does not provide adequate direction on how medical professionals can provide effective assessment and treatment for boys and men. In the age of precision medicine [6, 7], developing specific clinical guidance for the treatment of boys and men experiencing eating disorders is imperative [8]. This chapter will focus on additions and updates needed to current clinical guidance in order to effectively include boys and men.

While eating disorders treatment often requires an interdisciplinary team, the role of the medical professional is critical and multifaceted. Medical professionals may be the first point of contact for boys and men who are experiencing an eating disorder. Therefore, it is crucial that medical professionals are knowledgeable and skilled at screening for eating disorders among these populations [9]. Medical professionals are the primary member of the treatment team who assess medical stability, which will ultimately inform the treatment provided by psychiatrists, dietitians, and psychotherapists. Subsequently, assessment of medical stability will inform the appropriate level of care (i.e., inpatient versus outpatient management) necessary for the individual to receive optimal clinical intervention. It is clear that the role of the medical professional is critical to providing effective eating disorders treatment, as is guidance used to provide appropriate medical care.

[1] In this chapter, we use the terms "males" and "boys/men," as well as "females" and "girls/women," interchangeably.

Summary of Current Medical Treatment Guidance

Medical treatment guidelines have been published by the American Psychiatric Association (APA) [2], the National Institute for Health and Care Excellence (NICE) [3], and the Royal Australian and New Zealand College of Psychiatrists (RANZCP) [4]. Further, the Society for Adolescent Health and Medicine (SAHM) has published a position paper [1] with an accompanying review article to update the medical management of restrictive eating disorders in adolescents [9]. See Table 10.1 for the characteristics of these publications. While there are many components of these recommendations that apply to both sexes (i.e., the role of the medical provider and standardization of terminology), the clinical guidance is not disaggregated by sex. This may inhibit males from receiving appropriate care.

Overall, major components of the current clinical guidance that do not account for the unique differences in the presentation of eating disorders in boys and men may negatively impact these individuals. These recommendations include guidance for monitoring bone health, body mass index (BMI), target weight goals, refeeding protocols, testosterone testing, use of performance-enhancing substances, and muscle dysmorphia. The remainder of this chapter will discuss each of these problems as it relates to the treatment of boys and men. It is important to note that the lack of specific clinical guidance for boys and men is due to the overall lack of evidence to support specific recommendations. Therefore, we provide potential solutions and areas of needed research aimed at remedying these problems and building the evidence base to develop clear medical treatment guidelines.

Table 10.1 Clinical guidance referred to in this chapter

	Year published	Country published	Population
Clinical practice guidelines			
American Psychiatric Association (APA)	2006	United States	Adolescents and adults
National Institute for Health and Care Excellence (NICE)	2017	United Kingdom	Adolescents and adults
Royal Australian and New Zealand College of Psychiatrists (RANZCP)	2014	Australia and New Zealand	Adolescents and adults
Position paper			
Society for Adolescent Health and Medicine (SAHM)	2015	United States	Adolescents
Review paper			
Society for Adolescent Health and Medicine (SAHM) "Update"	2015	United States	Adolescents

Monitoring Bone Health

Clinical guidance outlined in the SAHM review article indicates that dual-energy X-ray absorptiometry (DXA) scans should be conducted to monitor bone health when there has been a loss of menses for 6 or more months in adolescent girls [9]. This does not provide adequate guidance on how to monitor the bone health of adolescent boys, despite boys experiencing similar bone deficits compared to adolescent girls [10]. The APA guidelines also indicate that amenorrhea should be used as a marker for monitoring bone health in adult patients [2]. The NICE [3] and RANZCP [4] guidelines recommend that the monitoring of bone health via DXA scans should be based on duration of illness. This improved language is more inclusive and appropriate for boys and men who may be at risk for reduced bone mineral density (BMD) for age or osteoporosis. Additionally, medical professionals should consider the degree of weight-bearing exercise boys and men engage in when assessing and monitoring bone health. Boys and men may engage in excessive exercise behaviors, which may be protective of BMD at the hip and whole-body bone mineral content (BMC) [11].

Further studies examining the progression of BMD and fractures through the time course and duration of illness could help guide when to obtain a DXA. In particular, understanding how BMI, duration of illness, specific eating disorder diagnosis, age, and other factors may affect BMD and fracture risk in males could inform future clinical practice guidelines.

Body Mass Index

The use of BMI as a measure of health or severity of illness presents a significant issue for boys and men experiencing eating disorders. As noted by the SAHM position paper, BMI is used in conjunction with other measures to assess the degree of malnutrition [1]. Ultimately, this assessment of malnutrition guides treatment goals for weight gain and refeeding and meal planning.

The SAHM review article indicates that the degree of malnutrition is based on percent median BMI, Z-scores, and percent weight loss [9]. Adolescent boys and young adult men may present higher percent median BMI and have a higher mean weight loss [12]. This updated definition of the degree of malnutrition recognizes that an individual can be severely malnourished even at a normal or high weight if he or she has lost a great deal of weight (>20% in 1 year or > 10% in 6 months). However, medical professionals who strictly use BMI as a measure of malnutrition may miss boys and men experiencing eating disorders who are more likely to be at a normal weight or are overweight based on their BMI [12]. Low BMI is indicated in the NICE guidelines as a primary eating disorder assessment measure, as well as a marker of recovery [3]. Similarly, the RANZCP guidelines recommend that BMI be used as a primary measure to differentiate between a psychiatric and medical admission criteria in adults [4]. BMI may not effectively differentiate between fat mass and muscle mass. Therefore, BMI will not be able to effectively identify boys and men who are attempting to gain muscle mass and may have deficits in body fat. BMI is also used in the APA guidelines; however, it is noted that both degree of muscularity and body frame size may decrease the validity of the BMI as a marker of medical condition in adult patients [2]. Therefore, medical professionals should consider using multiple measures, such as the patient's growth charts, percent weight loss, BMI, and pubertal stage to accurately measure body composition in boys and men.

Future research could characterize to what extent BMI is associated with medical instability in specific eating disorder diagnoses in males, especially atypical anorexia nervosa, avoidant/restrictive food intake disorder, and muscle dysmorphia. Furthermore, alternative markers such as weight suppression, weight loss, or body composition could be explored as alternative predictors of medical instability.

Determining Treatment Goal Weight

The SAHM position paper proposes a two-step process to calculate treatment goal weight: (1) determination of degree of malnutrition and (2) determination of a healthy weight range for that particular individual. For the determination of degree of malnutrition, as discussed above, percent median BMI, BMI Z-score, and amount and rate of weight loss may have limitations in males who may seek to gain weight or muscularity [1]. In particular, evaluating for weight loss may miss boys who are seeking a larger body size and muscularity given that these boys may not experience weight loss [13]. The APA guidelines for the treatment of anorexia nervosa indicate that a goal weight is reached when normal testicular functioning is resumed [2]. The APA guidance indicates that atypical anorexia nervosa, which may be more prevalent among males, poses challenges for identifying a treatment goal weight. The RANZCP guidelines emphasize that BMI percentiles can be used as a marker for determining weight goals in children and adolescents with eating disorders [4]. The current NICE guidelines do not have specific recommendations for treatment goal weight [3].

Ideally, future randomized controlled trials could compare different treatment goal weight methods in males for markers of remission, including medical stability, psychological stability, and others. Additionally, studies should investigate the optimal (if any) treatment goal weights (or alternative goal markers) for boys and men experiencing atypical anorexia nervosa and muscle dysmorphia. This may include comparisons of treatment outcomes for different treatment goal weight needs and methods.

Refeeding Protocols

In conjunction with treatment goal weight, the measurement of refeeding protocols may not provide effective guidance for the treatment of boys and men despite early research on refeeding protocols focusing solely on young adult men [14]. The review article on medical management of eating disorders in adolescents indicates that for inpatient treatment, initial caloric intake should be between 1400 and 2000 calories per day [9]. The APA guidelines indicate that caloric intake should be measured from 30 to 40 calories per kilogram of weight per day (approximately 1000–1600 calories per day) [2]. The APA guidelines appropriately note that caloric intake may need to be higher (upward of 4500 calories per day) for male patients with anorexia nervosa as men may have higher lean body mass and lower fat mass compared to women [2]. Additionally, men have generally larger body frames compared to women, which may require greater weight gain to return to a normal weight [2]. The current NICE guidelines for refeeding indicate starting with 5–10 calories per kilogram of weight for severely underweight patients, eventually increasing caloric intake to 20 calories per kilogram of weight within the first 2 days of inpatient treatment [15]. Lastly, the RANZCP guidelines recommend starting at roughly 1400 calories per day and increasing by roughly 500 calories per day every 2–3 days until the individual's weight goal has been achieved [4].

The current SAHM, APA, NICE, and RANZCP recommendations all neglect to discuss specific refeeding protocols for boys and men who are engaging in muscularity-oriented disordered eating (see Chap. 3 on Muscularity-Oriented Disordered Eating). These boys and men often engage in behaviors that include increasing exercise (i.e., exercising for the sole purpose of gaining muscle), changing dietary intake (i.e., increasing protein intake and decreasing fat and carbohydrate intake or cycling between bulking and cutting eating), and even using muscle-enhancing supplements (i.e., creatine, whey protein, etc.) and steroids in order to gain muscle mass [16]. These are unique behaviors that will require targeted nutrition protocols for effective treatment.

Future research could design randomized controlled trials using various refeeding protocols in males to determine short- and long-term treatment outcomes, such as refeeding syndrome (short-term) and clinical remission (long-term). Different refeeding protocols, such as weight-based and fixed calories (i.e., starting at 2000 calories and advancing by 200 calories per day), could be compared using multiple study sites to increase sample sizes.

Testosterone Testing

Chronic dieting or excessive exercise in patients with eating disorders leads to hypothalamic suppression as an adaptive response to an energy deficit. Impaired pulsatility of gonadotropin-releasing hormones suppresses the secretion of gonadotropins. In females, this manifests as primary or secondary amenorrhea with low luteinizing hormone (LH), follicle-stimulating hormone (FSH), and estradiol levels and regression of the ovaries and uterus to prepubertal size. Duration of amenorrhea is directly correlated with low BMD [17, 18], providing an evidence base to recommend prolonged duration of amenorrhea (>6 months) as a reason to order a DXA in females with eating disorders [9, 19–21]. Resumption of menses in females is one indicator of restoration of hypothalamic-pituitary-gonadal function, and an estradiol level > 30 pg/mL has been shown to be predictive of resumption of menses within 3–6 months in adolescent females with eating disorders [22]. Serial estradiol levels have been used by some to help set treatment goal weights in females [23, 24]. Others have used serial pelvic ultrasound [25–28].

In males, hypothalamic suppression leads to low LH, FSH, and testosterone levels [29–33], accompanied by the symptoms of diminished libido and loss of early morning erections. Testosterone has both an anabolic and antiresorptive effect on bony structures, and low testosterone levels may contribute to reduced bone mineral density and increased fracture risk in males with anorexia nervosa. Testosterone levels improve with weight restoration [34, 35]. However, data are lacking on specific testosterone cutoffs to guide clinical decision-making, such as when to order a DXA or how to determine treatment goal weight. Future research could determine clinically significant testosterone levels and associations with DXA, medical stability, and treatment goal weight.

Muscle Dysmorphia and Performance-Enhancing Substances

As already noted in this chapter, boys and men commonly engage in muscularity-oriented disordered eating [16, 36, 37] and are often more concerned with muscularity and leanness rather than thinness [13]. These characteristics are emblematic of muscle dysmorphia. Currently, the DSM-5 does not classify muscle dysmorphia as an eating disorder, but instead classifies this disorder as a subtype of body dysmorphic disorder under the obsessive-compulsive disorders [5]. Given the similarities between the characteristics of eating disorders among boys and men and muscle dysmorphia, it may be important to reclassify muscle dysmorphia as an eating disorder and, therefore, develop specific medical treatment recommendations for this disorder.

An additional concern for boys and men experiencing eating disorders is the use of performance-enhancing substances (PES). PES are legal (i.e., creatine) and illegal (i.e., anabolic-androgenic steroids) substances that are used to improve athletic performance and increase muscularity [38, 39]. These substances are widely used by adolescent boys [36] and men [37] and are often used in conjunction with other disordered eating behaviors [40, 41]. It is crucial for medical professionals to be screening for PES use among boys and men who present for treatment for an eating disorder or who are engaging in muscularity-oriented behaviors. Additionally, there is a need to develop treatment recommendations on how medical professionals can assist patients in safely tapering off the use of PES.

Future research could design randomized controlled trials to investigate tapering protocols based on type of PES, frequency of use, and dosage. Future research is also needed to investigate the longitudinal health outcomes of legal PES use specifically related to physiological (i.e., cardiovascular, endocrine, and circulatory systems), psychological (i.e., mental health diagnoses and substance use), and social (i.e., relational, violence, and criminal justice) health outcomes. These data will assist in developing effective treatment protocols related to these domains.

Conclusion

This chapter outlines areas of the current adolescent and adult eating disorder medical treatment guidance from SAHM, APA, NICE, and RANZCP that do not effectively consider the unique presentation of eating disorders among boys and men, largely due to gaps in the evidence base among males with eating disorders. We provide some suggestions to address the knowledge gap; however, there remains a need for the development of a more robust research base in order to develop more inclusive medical treatment guidelines specific to the needs of boys and men.

References

1. Golden NH, Katzman DK, Sawyer SM, Ornstein R. Position paper of the society for adolescent health and medicine: medical management of restrictive eating disorders in adolescents and young adults references. J Adolesc Health. 2015;56(1):121–5.
2. Yager J, Devlin MJ, Halmi KA, Herzog DB, Mitchell JE, Powers P, et al. Practice guidelines for the treatment of patients with eating disorders. Am J Psychiatry. 2006:1–128.
3. Eating disorders: recognition and treatment [Internet]. National Institute for Health and Care Excellence. 2017. Available from: https://www.nice.org.uk/guidance/ng69/resources/eating-disorders-recognition-and-treatment-pdf-1837582159813.
4. Hay PJ, Chinn D, Forbes D, Madden S, Newton R, Sugenor L, et al. Royal Australian and New Zealand College of Psychiatrists clinical practice guidelines for the treatment of eating disorders. Aust N Z J Psychiatry. 2014;48(11):1–62.
5. American Psychiatric Association. Diagnostic and statistical manual of mental disorders: diagnostic and statistical manual of mental disorders. 5th ed: American Psychiatric Association; 2013.
6. Legato MJ, Johnson PA, Manson JE. Consideration of sex differences in medicine to improve health care and patient outcomes. JAMA. 2016;316(18):1865–6.
7. Miller VM, Rocca WA, Faubion SS. Sex differences research, precision medicine, and the future of women's health. J Women's Health. 2015;24(12):969–71.
8. Ganson KT, Murray SB, Nagata JM. Last word: a call to develop specific medical treatment guidelines for adolescent males with eating disorders. Eat Disord. 2019;17:1–7.
9. Golden NH, Katzman DK, Sawyer SM, Ornstein RM, Rome ES, Garber AK, et al. Update on the medical management of eating disorders in adolescents. J Adolesc Heal [Internet]. 2015;56(4):370–5. Available from:. https://doi.org/10.1016/j.jadohealth.2014.11.020.

10. Nagata JM, Golden NH, Peebles R, Long J, Leonard MB, Carlson JL. Assessment of sex differences in bone deficits among adolescents with anorexia nervosa. Int J Eat Disord. 2017;50(4):352–8.
11. Nagata JM, Carlson JL, Golden NH, Murray SB, Long J, Leonard MB, et al. Associations between exercise, body composition, and bone mineral density in adolescents with anorexia nervosa. Eat Weight Disord. 2019;24(5):939–45.
12. Vo M, Lau J, Rubinstein M. Eating disorders in adolescent and young adult males: presenting characteristics. J Adolesc Health. 2016;59(4):397–400.
13. Murray SB, Nagata JM, Griffiths S, Calzo JP, Brown TA, Mitchison D, Blashill AJ, Mond JM. The enigma of male eating disorders: a critical review and synthesis. Clin Psychol Rev. 2017;57:1–1.
14. Keys A. The biology of human starvation. Minneapolis: University of Minnesota Press; 1950.
15. College of Psychiatrists. MARSIPAN: management of really sick patients with anorexia nervosa (2nd edn) (college report CR189): Royal College of Psychiatrists; 2014.
16. Murray SB, Griffiths S, Mond JM. Evolving eating disorder psychopathology: conceptualising muscularity-oriented disordered eating. Br J Psychiatry. 2016;208(5):414–5.
17. Castro J, Lazaro L, Pons F, Halperin I, Toro J. Predictors of bone mineral density reduction in adolescents with anorexia nervosa. J Am Acad Child Adolesc Psychiatry. 2000;39(11):1365–70.
18. Maïmoun L, Guillaume S, Lefebvre P, Philibert P, Bertet H, Picot MC, Gaspari L, Paris F, Courtet P, Thomas E, Mariano-Goulart D. Role of sclerostin and dickkopf-1 in the dramatic alteration in bone mass acquisition in adolescents and young women with recent anorexia nervosa. J Clin Endocrinol Metabol. 2014;99(4):E582–90.
19. Gordon CM, Ackerman KE, Berga SL, Kaplan JR, Mastorakos G, Misra M, Murad MH, Santoro NF, Warren MP. Functional hypothalamic amenorrhea: an endocrine society clinical practice guideline. J Clin Endocrinol Metabol. 2017;102(5):1413–39.
20. Golden NH, Abrams SA. Optimizing bone health in children and adolescents. Pediatrics. 2014;134(4):e1229–43.
21. Bachrach LK, Gordon CM. Bone densitometry in children and adolescents. Pediatrics. 2016;138(4):e20162398.
22. Golden NH, Jacobson MS, Schebendach J, Solanto MV, Hertz SM, Shenker IR. Resumption of menses in anorexia nervosa. Arch Pediatr Adolesc Med. 1997;151(1):16–21.
23. Golden NH, Jacobson MS, Sterling WM, Hertz S. Treatment goal weight in adolescents with anorexia nervosa: use of BMI percentiles. Int J Eat Disord. 2008;41(4):301–6.
24. Pitts S, Blood E, Divasta A, Gordon CM. Percentage body fat by dual-energy X-ray absorptiometry is associated with menstrual recovery in adolescents with anorexia nervosa. J Adolesc Health. 2014;54(6):739–41.
25. Lai KY, De Bruyn R, Lask B, Bryant-Waugh R, Hankins M. Use of pelvic ultrasound to monitor ovarian and uterine maturity in childhood onset anorexia nervosa. Arch Dis Child. 1994;71(3):228–31.
26. Sobanski E, Hiltmann WD, Blanz B. Pelvic ultrasound scanning of the ovaries in adolescent anorectic patients at low weight and after weight recovery. Eur Child Adolesc Psychiatry. 1997;6(4):207–11.
27. Key A, Mason H, Allan R, Lask B. Restoration of ovarian and uterine maturity in adolescents with anorexia nervosa. Int J Eat Disord. 2002;32(3):319–25.
28. Allan R, Sharma R, Sangani B, Hugo P, Frampton I, Mason H, Lask B. Predicting the weight gain required for recovery from anorexia nervosa with pelvic ultrasonography: an evidence-based approach. Eur Eating Disord Rev: Prof J Eating Disord Assoc. 2010;18(1):43–8.
29. Misra M, Katzman DK, Cord J, Manning SJ, Mendes N, Herzog DB, Miller KK, Klibanski A. Bone metabolism in adolescent boys with anorexia nervosa. J Clin Endocrinol Metabol. 2008;93(8):3029–36.
30. Coelho JS, Lee T, Karnabi P, Burns A, Marshall S, Geller J, Lam PY. Eating disorders in biological males: clinical presentation and consideration of sex differences in a pediatric sample. J Eat Disord. 2018;6(1):40.

31. Mehler PS, Sabel AL, Watson T, Andersen AE. High risk of osteoporosis in male patients with eating disorders. Int J Eat Disord. 2008;41(7):666–72.
32. Skolnick A, Schulman RC, Galindo RJ, Mechanick JI. The endocrinopathies of male anorexia nervosa: case series. AACE Clin Case Rep. 2016;2(4):e351–7.
33. Galusca B, Leca V, Germain N, Frere D, Khalfallah Y, Lang F, Estour B. Normal inhibin B levels suggest partial preservation of gonadal function in adult male patients with anorexia nervosa. J Sex Med. 2012;9(5):1442–7.
34. Wheeler MJ, Crisp AH, Hsu LK, Chen CN. Reproductive hormone changes during weight gain in male anorectics. Clin Endocrinol. 1983;18(4):423–9.
35. Wabitsch M, Ballauff A, Holl R, Blum WF, Heinze E, Remschmidt H, Hebebrand J. Serum leptin, gonadotropin, and testosterone concentrations in male patients with anorexia nervosa during weight gain. J Clin Endocrinol Metabol. 2001;86(7):2982–8.
36. Eisenberg ME, Wall M, Neumark-Sztainer D. Muscle-enhancing behaviors among adolescent girls and boys. Pediatrics. 2012;130(6):1019–26.
37. Nagata JM, Murray SB, Bibbins-Domingo K, Garber AK, Mitchison D, Griffiths S. Predictors of muscularity-oriented disordered eating behaviors in U.S. young adults: a prospective cohort study. Int J Eat Disord. 2019;(February):1–9.
38. LaBotz M, Griesemer BA. Use of performance-enhancing substances. Pediatrics. 2016;138(1):e20161300.
39. Pope HG, Wood RI, Rogol A, Nyberg F, Bowers L, Bhasin S. Adverse health consequences of performance-enhancing drugs: an endocrine society scientific statement. Endocr Rev. 2014;35(3):341–75.
40. Murray SB, Accurso EC, Griffiths S, Nagata JM. Boys, biceps, and bradycardia: the hidden dangers of muscularity-oriented disordered eating. J Adolesc Health. 2018;62(3):352–5.
41. Nagata JM, Brown TA, Lavender JM, Murray SB. Emerging trends in eating disorders among adolescent boys: muscles, macronutrients, and biohacking. Lancet Child Adolesc Health. 2019;4642(19):19–20.

Chapter 11
Nutritional Considerations for Boys and Men with Eating Disorders

Melissa Whitelaw and Jason M. Nagata

Learning Objectives

1. Recognize that energy requirements for boys and men with eating disorders may differ compared to girls and women with eating disorders due to sex, weight, age, and energy expenditure.
2. Identify refeeding syndrome in the nutritional management of eating disorders.
3. Describe unique nutritional considerations for males with eating disorders with regard to macronutrients, micronutrients, and diagnosis.

Key Points

- Energy requirements for boys and men with eating disorders may differ compared to girls and women with eating disorders due to sex, weight, age, and energy expenditure.
- Refeeding syndrome can occur with the commencement of refeeding following prolonged dietary restriction and starvation.
- A dietician with experience in nutritional counselling for eating disorders is an important member of the interdisciplinary team caring for boys and men with eating disorders.

M. Whitelaw (✉)
Department of Adolescent Medicine, Department of Nutrition and Food Services, The Royal Children's Hospital, Melbourne, VIC, Australia
e-mail: melissa.whitelaw@rch.org.au

J. M. Nagata
Division of Adolescent and Young Adult Medicine, Department of Pediatrics, University of California, San Francisco, San Francisco, CA, USA

J. M. Nagata et al. (eds.), *Eating Disorders in Boys and Men*,
https://doi.org/10.1007/978-3-030-67127-3_11

Introduction

The lower prevalence of eating disorders in males[1] compared to females has resulted in the under-representation of males in eating disorder research [1, 2]. This under-representation is not surprising as males are underdiagnosed and undertreated [3]. Males are more susceptible to the stigma associated with mental health [4], the perception that eating disorders are a "female condition" [5], and they are less likely to seek treatment and experience longer duration of eating disorder pathology before seeking treatment [2, 4]. Further, eating disorder diagnostic criteria are skewed to the female pursuit of thinness and therefore less reflective of males who frequently strive for leanness and increased muscle mass [4, 6–8].

The absence of specific guidelines for treatment of males and the unique nutritional requirements for boys and men diagnosed with eating disorders is problematic. Evidence-based protocols for refeeding and nutritional support in males are currently based on research that has been undertaken predominantly in females. This chapter describes the limited published recommendations to guide nutritional support in boys and men diagnosed with eating disorders. The chapter focuses predominantly on eating disorders that involve dietary restriction leading to weight loss and the state of starvation. These are the eating disorders that require dietetic expertise to prescribe nutrition to reduce the risk of refeeding syndrome, to support weight gain to reverse the complications of malnutrition, and, finally, for weight restoration with normalized eating. Nutrition is discussed in the following eating disorders: anorexia nervosa, atypical anorexia nervosa, and bulimia nervosa.

Energy Considerations for Eating Disorders in Males

Calculating energy requirements in eating disorders is complex. In healthy populations, energy calculations may differ among males and females based on age, sex, body weight, and physical activity [9–11]. Daily energy expenditure includes the energy requirement for basal metabolic rate that accounts for approximately 60–70% of the expenditure. Diet-induced thermogenesis from the effect of food consumption requires approximately 10% of additional energy expenditure. The most variable component of energy expenditure is physical activity that can be 10% in a sedentary person and up to 70% of the total daily expenditure in an athlete [12].

In general, males may have greater estimated energy requirements than females from adolescence to adulthood. Males with eating disorders may present at a later age (due to delayed diagnosis), have a higher body weight, and have more engagement in excessive or compulsive exercise compared to females with eating disorders [1], which may contribute to greater energy requirements. For example, boys with eating disorders self-reported over 8 hours of exercise per week on average in the

[1] In this chapter, we use the terms males and boys/men interchangeably.

prior month, with approximately half participating in team sports [13]. Further, male athletes, who may have high energy expenditures due to physical activity, may be at a particularly high risk for eating disorder symptoms [14].

The landmark Minnesota Starvation Experiment undertaken by Ancel Keys in the 1940s among 36 men aged 22–33 years provided the first scientific evidence for the multisystem physiological and psychological complications that can arise from refeeding in starvation [15]. After a 12-week control period when participants ate normally, they subsequently underwent a 24-week period of semi-starvation when the average daily energy intake was reduced to 1570 kcal/day. Participants were then refed on a strictly controlled diet during this refeeding phase; the young men required approximately 4000 kcal/day in order to promote weight gain. In clinical samples of participants diagnosed with eating disorders, two studies undertaken in women [16, 17] and one study in girls diagnosed with anorexia nervosa [18] demonstrated that refeeding was associated with an increased resting energy expenditure that was not explained by an increased body mass index. The metabolic adaptive response to semi-starvation was found to lower energy requirements, and this lowered rate was subsequently reversed with refeeding [19]. This response to refeeding suggests that monitoring of individual nutritional intake and change in weight is recommended in anorexia nervosa, rather than a reliance on calculations of energy requirements [16, 17]. The research gaps highlight the need for large, prospective studies in males to explore refeeding and the association with resting energy expenditure and weight gain.

The position statement of the American Dietetic Association [20] recommends that treatment for all eating disorders be undertaken by an interdisciplinary team that includes a dietitian with expertise in eating disorders in collaboration with clinicians from mental health and medicine. The dietitian has a role in eating disorder prevention, assessment, and nutrition support for recovery. Dietitians working in the eating disorders field require an understanding of the nutritional requirements for different ages in order to provide nutritional rehabilitation to restore weight and assist to normalize eating. The important role of the dietitian in eating disorders is also supported by the American Academy of Pediatrics [21], the American Psychiatric Association [22], and the Academy for Eating Disorders [23].

The American Academy of Dietetics and the American Psychiatric Association have published recommendations for refeeding. However, there is little consensus for nutritional provision as reflected in the wide variations in clinical practice [20, 22]. Recent studies have challenged the historical recommendations for conservative refeeding with new evidence to support the efficacy in mildly and moderately malnourished patients with more aggressive refeeding. To date, these studies have been undertaken in hospital specialist eating disorder services which provide rigorous medical supervision for inpatients [24–29].

The recommendations for refeeding are based on studies undertaken predominantly in females with a few studies that have included small numbers of male participants. In 2019, Reber et al. summarized 12 published guidelines and reviews for the management of refeeding. The recommendations for initial energy prescription

Table 11.1 Summary of refeeding recommendations for males with anorexia nervosa

	Boys	Men
Energy prescriptions		
Initiation of refeeding energy (kcal/day)	1400–2000 [26]	1000–1200 [20, 21]
Daily increments in energy (kcal/day) [29]	Incremental advancement 100–300	Incremental advancement 100–300
Energy for weight gain (kcal/day) [29]	2400–3000	3000
Electrolyte monitoring and use of supplements [31]	No guidelines	No guidelines
Macronutrients (percentage of total energy input) [9–11]		
Carbohydrate (normal guidelines)	50–60%	50–60%
Fat (normal guidelines)	25–35%	25–35%
Protein (normal guidelines)	15–20%	15–20%
Micronutrients [32]		
Calcium (mg/day)	1200–1500	1200–1500
Vitamin D (IU/day)	400–800	400–800

ranged from 10 kcal/kg (42 kJ/kg) to 20 kcal/kg (84 kJ/kg), with high-risk cases recommended to commence at 5 kcal/kg (21 kJ/kg). Macronutrient provision was recommended at 50–60% of carbohydrate and 15–40% fat [30]. Notably, these studies were predominantly undertaken in females, with no specific recommendations for males. A summary is provided of refeeding recommendations used in boys and men who have been diagnosed with anorexia nervosa (Table 11.1).

Refeeding Syndrome

Refeeding syndrome and death can occur as the sequelae following prolonged dietary restriction and starvation in eating disorders with the commencement of refeeding. This can occur in both inpatient and outpatient settings. The multisystem cardiopulmonary and neurological complications that can arise from refeeding in starvation are attributable to the severe electrolyte and fluid shifts from the extracellular to intracellular space due to insulin surges following the re-introduction of nutrition. Hypophosphatemia is considered the hallmark of refeeding syndrome, a condition that can result in respiratory, cardiac, neurologic, renal, and hematologic complications [33–35].

Historically, the fear of refeeding syndrome led to conservative approaches in refeeding with delays in weight gain, prolonged hospital admissions, and long-term outcomes [36]. More recently the conservative approaches in refeeding have been challenged, with increasing evidence that higher calorie refeeding can result in faster weight gain and shorter length of hospital admissions. More aggressive approaches to refeeding have been safely used in hospitalized patients provided with appropriate monitoring [24, 25, 29]. An update of medical management of eating disorders in adolescents suggests that there is now sufficient evidence to support initiating refeeding in moderately malnourished hospitalized patients with more aggressive refeeding at 1400–2000 kcals/day, provided there is close medical and biochemical monitoring [28, 29].

Wide variations in practice are evident for the commencement of refeeding, with no consensus in monitoring electrolytes or for the use of electrolyte supplementation as prophylaxis or for correction of electrolyte imbalances [30]. Although the earliest data were from young men [15], these findings have not been replicated, and subsequent studies in clinical eating disorder samples undergoing refeeding have included entirely or predominantly female samples.

In the absence of studies in males, there is concern about more aggressive refeeding in boys and men due to the frequent delays in diagnosis and treatment, which may confer a higher risk of the development of refeeding syndrome [2, 4]. As the safety of higher calorie initiation of refeeding is yet to be established in males, close monitoring in clinical contexts is required, and further research is recommended.

Macronutrients

The assessment for an eating disorder requires a food history to be undertaken by a dietitian to assess the consumption of energy, macronutrients, micronutrients, and patterns of disordered eating [20]. Differences in macronutrient consumption in boys and men diagnosed with eating disorders compared to girls and women have been described. Protein consumption is frequently increased as males strive for leanness and muscularity, with intakes of up to 5 gm of protein per kilogram of weight, evident in some males [37]. This intake is well above the recommended dietary intake of 0.8 gm/kg among boys 14–18 years and 0.85 gm/kg among men aged over 19 years [38] or 40–60 gm/day in boys and 64 gm/day in men up to 70 years [10]. For some males this may involve the consumption of a high-protein diet as well as the use of protein supplements.

One of the concerns of high-protein diets is the corresponding low intake of carbohydrates and fats [37, 39]. Adequate carbohydrate consumption is important for provision of energy, to avoid ketoacidosis, and for fiber. Dietary fats are the most concentrated form of energy for the body and are important for absorption of the fat soluble vitamins, A, D, E and K, and for provision of essential fatty acids. An additional concern is that high-protein diets have been found to produce a sustained decrease in ad libitum kilojoule intake due to the anorexic effect of protein [40]. Within the context of refeeding, this intake pattern does not promote a return to responding to hunger and satiety cues [41]. A further disadvantage is the higher diet-induced thermic effect of protein that increases the difficulty in achieving weight gain [42]. Given that protein supplement use in male university students has also been found to be associated with higher eating disorder symptoms [43], these collective findings highlight the importance of assessing intake of fat, carbohydrate, and protein, including protein supplements, among males with eating disorders.

In a systematic review undertaken by Garber et al. [29], six studies examined meal-based refeeding to determine if there was any effect of macronutrient content on refeeding outcomes. Five studies were undertaken in adolescents [24–27, 44], and one study was undertaken in adults [45]. In all studies, the macronutrient distributions were consistent with the current guidelines for normal eating: 25–35% calories from fat, 15–20% from protein, and 50–60% from carbohydrates [9–11]. It is unknown if a variation in the recommendations for macronutrient distribution would provide a benefit in refeeding males. Future research is needed to determine if the normal macronutrient dietary guidelines should be recommended for refeeding boys and men diagnosed with eating disorders.

Micronutrients

Calcium is one particularly important micronutrient consideration in males and females diagnosed with eating disorders. For adolescents, during the period of growth and bone accretion, and also in adults, there is the potential for long-term complications that can affect bone health. Osteoporosis is the increased bone turnover and bone fragility from progressive bone loss that has been well documented in females with anorexia nervosa [46]. However, less is known about males. In a retrospective chart review of 33 boys diagnosed with an eating disorder, ten percent were found to have abnormal serum calcium levels [47]. However, there is an overall lower prevalence of osteoporosis among males in general [48], which is usually associated with bone loss in aging. Notably, males have several protective factors that include the greater accumulation of skeletal bone mass during adolescence, larger bone size, shorter lifespan, and not experiencing menopause [49].

Males with anorexia nervosa have lower bone mineral density compared to healthy controls [50], and men over 40 years with anorexia nervosa have higher fracture risk compared to healthy controls [51]. Further, males with anorexia nervosa have equally severe deficits in bone mineral density as females with anorexia nervosa [52]. Dual-energy X-ray absorptiometry (DXA) scans are recommended to be undertaken yearly when amenorrhea has been experienced for 6 or more months [28], which does not apply to males, and when disease duration has been longer than 6–12 months [53]. The best predictor for improved bone mineral density is weight gain, with nutritional recommendations for calcium intake (1200–1500 mg/day) [32] and vitamin D (400–800 IU/day) [32] being considered helpful in bone restoration [54]. Future research is needed with randomized controlled trials focused on bone health and the contribution of weight regain and the role of calcium and vitamin D in bone health in boys and men.

Few studies have explored micronutrients and eating disorders. However, one retrospective, non-randomized study in severely malnourished adults diagnosed with anorexia nervosa compared a low-sodium diet (1600–2000 mg) to a normal-sodium diet (4000–4800 mg). In the normal-sodium diet, weight gain and peripheral edema were greater, suggesting that, in malnourished adults (<15 kg/m^2), a low-sodium diet may assist in managing fluid shifts [55].

Electrolyte derangements in response to refeeding have been well documented. Hypophosphatemia is considered the hallmark of refeeding syndrome and occurs in response to the sudden increase in carbohydrates [34]. Hypomagnesemia occurs in response to refeeding and also from gastrointestinal losses due to vomiting and diarrhea (including laxative and diuretic abuse) [56]. Hypokalemia occurs from refeeding, vomiting, and medication misuse [56]. There is no consensus in electrolyte monitoring and supplementation, with evidence of wide variation in practice [31]. With a lack of recommendations about micronutrients in eating disorders, further studies are needed to support the study about sodium and other micronutrients in eating disorders.

Considerations for Other Specific Diagnoses

The final two diagnoses to be considered are atypical anorexia nervosa and bulimia nervosa. There is limited evidence about the nutritional management in both of these eating disorders; atypical anorexia nervosa is a relatively new diagnosis, and bulimia nervosa is a more secretive eating disorder that also has nutritional implications in boys and men.

Atypical Anorexia Nervosa

Atypical anorexia nervosa is diagnosed in patients who meet all diagnostic criteria for anorexia nervosa but are not sufficiently underweight to meet the low weight criterion. The increasing identification of atypical anorexia nervosa as a serious disorder highlights the importance of identifying early signs of starvation and malnutrition regardless of body size, particularly in males who frequently experience delays in diagnosis and treatment [2, 4, 57]. This is especially important given evidence that a large proportion of males with eating disorders have a history of overweight or obesity [47].

Patients diagnosed with atypical anorexia nervosa have been found to have similar clinical complications as anorexia nervosa. These include bradycardia, orthostatic changes in pulse rate or blood pressure, incidence of hypophosphatemia, hypomagnesemia, hypokalemia, and lower nadirs of phosphate, magnesium potassium, and amenorrhea [57, 58]. Further, compared to anorexia nervosa, adolescents with atypical anorexia nervosa report higher rates of premorbid obesity (71% compared to 12%) and greater losses of weight (17.6 kg compared to 11.0 kg) over a longer period of time (13.3 months compared to 10.2 months) [58].

Atypical anorexia nervosa challenges the concept of severity of underweight as a primary marker of the degree of malnutrition. Future research is needed to assist clinicians in determining expected weight ranges and guidelines in refeeding. It is currently unknown in atypical anorexia nervosa if weight stabilization is sufficient for resolution of clinical and psychological complications or if weight gain is required. Finally, future studies should clarify the nutritional needs of boys and men diagnosed with atypical anorexia nervosa.

Bulimia Nervosa

Bulimia nervosa is characterized by recurrent episodes of binge eating, with associated compensatory behaviors of a purging or non-purging nature. The presentation of bulimia nervosa in males can present differently compared to females. Males are more likely to undertake extreme exercise compared to females who are more likely to compensate by purging [59, 60], which may have implications for energy requirements. Further, females are described as having a preference for consumption of sweet foods during binge episodes, versus males who may prefer high-protein and high-fat foods [61]. Further, males may seek to pursue the muscular and lean body ideal through cyclical eating patterns characterized by low-carbohydrate, high-protein meals interspersed with "cheat meals" that can include consumption of a large number of calories and more energy-dense foods [62, 63].

Conclusion

This chapter highlights the importance of nutritional considerations in boys and men with eating disorders, including in the detection and treatment of these serious conditions. Greater clinician and public awareness is needed to appreciate the differences in how eating disorders may present and respond to intervention among males versus females. Furthermore, a dietician with experience in nutritional counseling for eating disorders is an important member of the interdisciplinary team caring for males with eating disorders [64]. Delays in diagnosis and treatment seeking for eating disorders in males have been associated with greater severity of complications and prolonged length of illness attributed to these delays. The current dietary recommendations for eating disorders are based on studies of predominantly females and therefore are not evidence based for males. Greater scientific attention and research is needed to be undertaken to explore the specific nutritional requirements of boys and men [64]. In particular, randomized controlled trials in males are needed to establish appropriate refeeding guidelines for energy requirements and macronutrient and micronutrient needs in boys and men diagnosed with eating disorders.

References

1. Murray SB, Nagata JM, Griffiths S, Calzo JP, Brown TA, Mitchison D, et al. The enigma of male eating disorders: a critical review and synthesis. Clin Psych Rev. 2017;57:1–11.
2. Limbers CA, Cohen LA, Gray BA. Eating disorders in adolescent and young males: prevalence, diagnosis and treatment strategies. Adolesc Health Med Ther. 2018;9:111–6.
3. Ganson KT, Murray SB, Nagata JM. Last word: a call to develop specific medical treatment guidelines for adolescent males with eating disorders. Eat Disord. 2019;17:1–7.
4. Griffiths S, Mond JM, Li Z, Gunatilake S, Murray SB, Sheffield J, Touz S. Self-stigma of seeking help and being male predicts an increased likelihood of having an undiagnosed eating disorder. Int J Eat Disord. 2015;48(6):775–8.
5. Griffiths S, Mond JM, Murray SB, Touz S. Young peoples's stigmatizing attitudes and beliefs about anorexia nervosa and muscle dysmorphia. Int J Eat Disord. 2014;47:189–95.
6. Strober M, Freeman R, Lampert C, Diamond J, Teplinsky C, DeAntonio M. Are there gender differences in core symptoms, temperament and short-term prospective outcome in anorexia nervosa? Int J Eat Disord. 2006;39:570–5.
7. Darcy AM, Doyle AC, Lock J, Peebles R, Doyle P, Le Grange D. The eating disorders examination in adolescent males with anorexia nervosa: how does it compare to adolescent females? Int J Eat Disord. 2012;45:110–4.
8. Murray SB, Griffiths S, Mond JM. Evolving eating disorder psychopathology: conceptualizing muscularity-oriented disordered eating. Br J Psychiatry. 2016;208:414–5.
9. US Department of Agriculture and Us Department of Health and Human Services. Dietary guidelines for Americans, 2010. 7th ed. Washington, DC: US Government Printing Office; 2010.
10. National Health and Medical Research Council (Australia), Commonwealth Department of Health and Ageing (Australia), Ministry of Health (New Zealand). Nutrient and reference values for Australia and New Zealand including recommended dietary intakes. Canberra: Commonwealth of Australia and New Zealand Government; 2006.
11. Department of Health. Dietary Reference Values for Food and Energy and Nutrients for the United Kingdom. Report of the Panel on Dietary reference values of the committee on Medical Aspects of Food Policy. Report on Health and Social Subjects 41. HSMO: London; 1991.
12. Schebendach J. The use of indirect calorimetry in the clinical management of adolescents with nutritional disorders. Adolescent Medicine: State of the Art Reviews. 14, 1, 2003. Philadelphia, Hanley & Belfus, Inc.
13. Nagata JM, Carlson JL, Kao JM, Golden NH, Murray SB, Peebles R. Characterization and correlates of exercise among adolescents with anorexia nervosa and bulimia nervosa. Int J Eat Disord. 2017;50(12):1394–403.
14. Gorrell S, Nagata JM, Hill KB, Carlson JL, Shain AF, Wilson J, Alix Timko C, Hardy KK, Lock J, Peebles R. Eating behavior and reasons for exercise among competitive collegiate male athletes. Eat Weight Disord. 2019:1–9.
15. Keys A. The biology of human starvation. Minneapolis: University of Minnesota Press; 1950.
16. Krahn DD, Rock C, Dechert RE, Narin KK, Hasse SA. Changes in resting energy expenditure and body composition in anorexia nervosa patients during refeeding. J Am Diet Assoc. 1993;93(4):434–8.
17. Obarzanek E, Lesem MD, Jimerson DC. Resting metabolic rate of anorexia nervosa patients during weight gain. Am J Clin Nutr. 1994;60:666–75.
18. Cuerda C, Ruiz A, Velasco C, Breton I, Camblor M, Garcia-Peris P. How accurate are predictive formulas calculating energy expenditure in adolescent patients with anorexia nervosa? Clin Nutr. 2007;26:100–6.
19. Schebendach JE, Golden NH, Jacobson MS, Hertz S, Schenker IR. The metabolic responses to starvation and refeeding in adolescents with anorexia nervosa. Ann N Y Acad Sci. 1997;817:110–9.

20. Position of the American Dietetic Association. Nutrition intervention in the treatment of eating disorders. J Am Diet Assoc. 2011;111:1236–41.
21. Rosen DS. American Academy of Pediatrics Committee on Adolescence. Identification and management of eating disorders in children and adolescents. Pediatrics. 2010;126:1240–53.
22. American Psychiatric Association. Treatment of patients with eating disorders, third edition. Am J Psychiatry. 2006;163(7 Suppl):4–54.
23. Klump KL, Bulik CM, Kaye WH, Treasure J, Tyson E. Academy of eating disorders position paper: eating disorders are serious mental illnesses. Int J Eat Disord. 2009;42:97–103.
24. Whitelaw M, Gilbertson H, Lam PY, Sawyer SM. Does aggressive refeeding in hospitalized adolescents with anorexia nervosa result in increased hypophosphatemia? J Adolesc Health. 2010;46:577–82.
25. Garber AK, Michihata N, Hetnal K, Schafer MA, Moscicki AB. A prospective examination of weight gain in hospitalized adolescents with anorexia nervosa on a recommended refeeding protocol. J Adolesc Health. 2012;50:24–9.
26. Garber AK, Mauldin K, Michihata N, Bucklew SM, Shafer MA, Moscicki AB. Higher calorie diets increase rate of weight gain and shorten hospital stay in hospitalized adolescents with anorexia nervosa. J Adolesc Health. 2013;53:579–84.
27. Golden NH, Keane-Miller C, Sainani KL, Kapphahn CJ. Higher caloric intake in hospitalized adolescents with anorexia nervosa is associated with reduced length of stay and no increased rate of refeeding syndrome. J Adolesce Health. 2013;53:573–8.
28. Golden NH, Katzman DK, Sawyer SM, Ornstein RM, Rome ES, Garber AK, Kohn M, Kreipe RE. Update on the medical management of eating disorders in adolescents. J Adolesc Health. 2015;56:370–5.
29. Garber AK, Sawyer SM, Golden NH, Guarda AS, Katzman DK, Kohn MR, Le Grange D, Madden S, Whitelaw M, Redgrave GW. A systematic review of approaches to refeeding in patients with anorexia nervosa. Int J Eat Disord. 2016;49(3):293–310.
30. Reber E, Friedli N, Vasiloglou MF, Schuetz P, Stanga Z. Management of refeeding syndrome in medical patients. http://www.mdpi.com/journal/jcm. Accessed 18 Dec 2019.
31. Schwartz BI, Mansbach JM, Marion JG, Katzman DK, Forman SF. Variations in admission practices for adolescents with anorexia nervosa: a North American sample. J Adolesc Health. 2008;43:425–31.
32. Position of the American Dietetic Association. Nutrition intervention in the treatment of anorexia nervosa, bulimia nervosa, and other eating disorders. J Am Diet Assoc. 2006;106:2073–82.
33. Solomon SM, Kirby DF. The refeeding syndrome. A review. J Parenter Enteral Nutr. 1990;14:90–7.
34. Ornstein RM, Golden NH, Jacobson MS, Shenker IR. Hypophosphatemia during rehabilitation in anorexia nervosa: implications for refeeding and monitoring. J Adolesc Health. 2003;32:83–8.
35. Marinella MA. The refeeding syndrome and hypophosphatemia. Nutr Rev. 2003;61:320–3.
36. Lund BC, Hernandez ER, Yates WR, Mitchell JR, McKee PA, Johnson CL. Rate of inpatient weight restoration predicts outcome in anorexia nervosa. Int J Eat Disord. 2009;42:301–5.
37. Mosley PE. Bigorexia: bodybuilding and body dysmorphia. Eur Eat Disord Rev. 2009;17:191–8.
38. Institute of Medicine. Dietary reference intakes for energy, carbohydrate, fiber, fat, fatty acids, cholesterol, protein, and amino acids. Washington, DC: The National Academies Press; 2005.
39. Murray SB, Rieger E, Hildebrand T, Karlov L, Russell J, Boon E, Dawson RT, Touz SW. A comparison of eating, exercise, shape, and weight related symptomatology in males with muscle dysmorphia and anorexia nervosa. Body Image. 2012;9:193–200.
40. Weigle DS, Breen PA, Matthys CC, Callahan HS, Meeuws KE, Burden KE, Burden VR, Purnell JQ. A high-protein diet induces reductions in appetite, ad libitum caloric intake, and body weight despite compensatory changes in diurnal plasma leptin and ghrelin concentrations. Am J Clin Nutr. 2005;82:41–8.
41. Griffiths S, Murray SB, Touz S. Disordered eating and the muscular ideal. J Eat Disord. 2013;1:15.

42. Westerterp KR, Wilson SAJ, Rolland. Diet induced thermogenesis measured over 24h in a respiration chamber: effect of diet composition. Int J Obes Metab Disord. 1999;23:287–92.
43. Nagata JM, Peebles R, Bell Hill K, Gorrell S, Carlson JL. Associations between ergogenic supplement use and eating behaviors among university students. Eat Disord. 2020. In Press.
44. Leclerc A, Turrini T, Sherwood K, Katzman DK. Evaluation of a nutrition rehabilitation protocol in hospitalized adolescents with restrictive eating disorders. J Adolesc Health. 2013;53:585–9.
45. El Goch M, Milanese C, Calugi S, Pelligrini M, Battistini NC, Dalle GR. Body composition, eating disorder psychopathology, and psychological distress in in anorexia nervosa. A longitudinal study. Am J Clin Nutr. 2014;99:771–8.
46. Misra M, Golden NH, Katzman DK. State of the art systematic review of bone disease in anorexia nervosa. Int J Eat Disord. 2016;49(3):276–92.
47. Vo M, Lau J, Rubinstein M. Eating disorders in adolescent and young adult males: presenting characteristics. J Adolesc Health. 2016;59(4):397–400.
48. Khosla S, Amin S, Orwoll E. Osteoporosis in men. Endoc Rev. 2008;29(4):441–64.
49. Mehler PS, Sabel AL, Watson T, Anderson AE. High risk of osteoporosis in male patients with eating disorders. Int J Eat Disord. 2008;41:666–72.
50. Misra M, Katzman DK, Cord J, Manning SJ, Mendes N, Herzog DB, Miller KK, Klibanski A. Bone metabolism in adolescent boys with anorexia nervosa. J Clin Endocrinol Metab. 2008;93(8):3029–36.
51. Nagata JM, Golden NH, Leonard MB, Copelovitch L, Denburg MR. Assessment of sex differences in fracture risk among patients with anorexia nervosa: a population-based cohort study using the health improvement network. J Bone Miner Res. 2017;32(5):1082–9.
52. Nagata JM, Golden NH, Peebles R, Long J, Leonard MB, Chang AO, Carlson JL. Assessment of sex differences in bone deficits among adolescents with anorexia nervosa. Int J Eat Disord. 2017;50(4):352–8.
53. Mészáros S, Tóth E, Ferencz V, Csupor E, Hosszú É, Horváth C. Calcaneous quantitative ultrasound measurements predicts vertebral fractures in idiopathic male osteoporosis. Joint Bone Spine. 2007;74(1):79–84.
54. Grinspoon S, Thomas L, Miller K, Herzog D, Klibanski A. Effects of recombinant human IGF-1 and oral contraceptive administration on bone density in anorexia nervosa. J Clin Endocrinol Metab. 2002;87:2883–91.
55. Rigaud D, Boulier A, Tallonneau I, Brindisi MC, Rozen R. Body fluid retention and body weight change in anorexia nervosa patients during refeeding. Clin Nutr. 2010;29:749–55.
56. Stheneur C, Bergeron S, Lapeyraque AL. Renal complications in anorexia nervosa. Eat Weight Disord. 2014;19:455–60.
57. Whitelaw M, Gilbertson H, Lee KJ, Sawyer SM. Restrictive eating disorders among adolescent inpatients. Pediatrics. 2014;134:e758–64.
58. Sawyer SM, Whitelaw M, Le Grange D, Yeo M, Hughes EK. Physical and psychological morbidity in adolescents with atypical anorexia nervosa. Pediatrics. 2016;137:e20154080.
59. Striegel-Moore RH, Rosselli F, Perrin N, DeBar L, Wilson GT, May A, Kraemer HC. Gender difference in the prevalence of eating disorder symptoms. Int J Eat Disord. 2009;42(5):471–4.
60. Lavender JM, De Young KP, Anderson DA. Eating disorder examination questionnaire (EDE-Q): norms for undergraduate men. Eat Behav. 2010;11(2):119–21.
61. Wansink B, Cheney MM, Chan N. Exploring comfort food preferences across age and gender. Physiol Behav. 2003;79(4–5):739–47.
62. Murray SB, Griffiths S, Hazery L, Shen T, Wooldridge T, Mond JM. Go big or go home: a thematic content analysis of pro-muscularity websites. Body Image. 2016;16:17–20.
63. Pila E, Mond JM, Griffiths S, Mitchison D, Murray SB. A thematic content analysis of# cheat meal images on social media: characterizing an emerging dietary trend. Int J Eat Disord. 2017;50(6):698–706.
64. McMaster CM, Wade T, Franklin J, Hart S. A review of treatment manuals for adults with an eating disorder: nutrition content and consistency with current dietetic evidence. Eat Weight Disord. 2020; https://doi.org/10.1007/s40519-020-00850-6. [Epub ahead of print].

Chapter 12
Appearance- and Performance-Enhancing Substances Including Anabolic-Androgenic Steroids Among Boys and Men

Mitchell L. Cunningham and Scott Griffiths

Learning Outcomes

1. To gain an appreciation of various classes of APESs one may use to improve weight, shape, and/or performance
2. To better understand the physical and psychological health complications connected to the use of anabolic-androgenic steroids (AASs)
3. To better understand the link between male body image psychopathology and AAS use
4. To better understand some of the complexities inherent in addressing AAS use and important recommendations to facilitate the treatment of this psychopathology

Key Points

- Men may seek out and use appearance- and performance-enhancing substances (APESs) to facilitate the growth of lean muscle mass.
- Arguably the most widely recognized and studied class of illicit APESs are anabolic-androgenic steroids (AASs), which are associated with significant physical and psychological health complications.
- Problematic body image, namely that related to muscularity, is likely to be an crucial risk factor for engagement in AASs among boys and men.
- While our understanding of best-practice approaches to addressing AAS use is limited, there are important considerations and recommendations to help support health professionals deal with this complex psychopathology.

M. L. Cunningham (✉)
School of Psychology, The University of Sydney, Sydney, NSW, Australia
e-mail: Mitchell.cunningham@sydney.edu.au

S. Griffiths
School of Psychological Sciences, The University of Melbourne, Melbourne, VIC, Australia

J. M. Nagata et al. (eds.), *Eating Disorders in Boys and Men*,
https://doi.org/10.1007/978-3-030-67127-3_12

Introduction

Body dissatisfaction continues to be a common issue among boys and men.[1] Many are motivated to attain a physique characterized by overt muscularity, perhaps unsurprisingly, as this represents the ideal male appearance widely portrayed and promoted in Western media and society [1, 2]. Concerningly, this male muscular ideal appears to be permeated to the extent that boys as young as 6 years of age may acquire and report a preference for them [3]. This hyper-muscular body ideal is extraordinarily difficult, if not impossible, for most boys and men to attain. Consequently, it is easy to conceive how appearance- and performance-enhancing substances (APESs) may acquire their allure. APESs, including anabolic-androgenic steroids, prohormones, and clenbuterol, can be used to influence one's physical appearance (e.g., boost muscle mass, reduce body adiposity) and/or enhance one's performance in a variety of areas (e.g., sports, sexual interactions) [4]. Narrowing in on the attainment of overt muscularity, certain APESs can lead to gains in lean muscle mass that often exceedingly surpass that achievable through natural means such as exercise alone [5]. However, while such substance use may serve to enhance appearance or performance in the short term, such "gains" may be accompanied by a multitude of physical and psychological health issues in the longer term.

This chapter describes APESs in the context of male body image and appearance-related psychopathology (e.g., eating disorders, muscle dysmorphia). We focus on one class of APESs in particular, anabolic-androgenic steroids (AASs), which are not only one of the most widely and illegally used APESs, but are also associated with a constellation of potentially serious physical and psychological health issues [6–9]. To provide the reader with a sense of what APESs are available, in this chapter we first highlight a variety of classes of APESs and their associated functions. Second, we focus on the serious, and potentially life-threatening, physical and psychological health concerns linked to AAS use. Third, we underscore the relationship between problematic male body image, conceptualized through both eating disorder and muscle dysmorphia psychopathology, and AAS use. Lastly, we synthesize available literature to offer important (albeit preliminary) considerations, guidance, and recommendations for clinicians who may be faced with assisting individuals who use AASs.

Classes of APESs

Anabolic-Androgenic Steroids

A summary of several classes of APESs is contained in Table 12.1. AASs represent a class of pharmacological substances that include the male hormone testosterone and substances which share its chemical structure [7] and are believed to account for the largest proportion of illicit APES use [9]. As the name implies, the uses of these

[1] In this chapter, we use the terms males and boys/men interchangeably.

substances are associated with both *anabolic* and *androgenic* effects that an individual may wish to procure. The anabolic effects of these substances are well recognized – they expedite the growth of lean muscle mass at a rate surpassing that typically possible via more conventional or natural means [5, 10]. On the other hand, the androgenic impact of these substances involves the promotion of the masculinization of secondary sexual characteristics (e.g., deepened voice, beard growth, baldness) [7]. While certain AASs can be taken orally, most are administered via intramuscular injection [9].

Pope and colleagues [9] note that, despite AAS use being prevalent across several Western regions, the United States is home to the highest absolute number of users of the substance. In their study, Pope and colleagues [11] analyzed four large national youth datasets and developed equations to estimate the lifetime prevalence of AAS use in the US general population. The study estimated that among Americans aged 13–50 years, approximately 2.9–4.0 million have engaged in AAS use. Further, the authors reason that since approximately 30% of AAS users experience AAS dependence (i.e., using AASs despite significant physical and/or psychological consequences), they estimate that around 1 million users have experienced AAS dependence in their lifetime. The study also highlights that while a large sex discrepancy exists among AAS users (i.e., men make up around 98.2% of users, a male/female ratio of approximately 50 to 1), there does not appear to be evidence for substantial differences in the prevalence of AAS use across racial/ethnic groups. On a global scale, epidemiological estimates of the lifetime prevalence of AAS use among men are around 6.4% [12].

Prohormones

Prohormones are substances that can be utilized by the body's own metabolic processes to produce anabolic hormones (i.e., serve as a precursor to testosterone) [13, 14]. This is in contrast to AASs, which involve testosterone (or testosterone analogues) that can readily used by the body upon administration. Although sometimes described as *legal steroids* and marketed to produce similar effects as AAS use (e.g., enhanced performance), we do not yet have a comprehensive understanding of their efficacy and safety for human use [13]. In fact, many studies do not support such marketed claims [14]. Concerningly, as these substances are precursors to anabolic hormones, they may be associated with aversive health implications akin to those observed with AAS use [14].

Clenbuterol

Clenbuterol hydrochloride (clenbuterol for short) is a synthetic β2-adrenergic agonist that typically serves as a prescribed bronchodilator for both humans and animals [15, 16]. However, the drug has been exploited for its accelerated fat-burning properties by both professional and amateur bodybuilders, as well as fitness enthusiasts more generally [15, 16]. Having been dubbed colorful (informal) names such as the *size zero pill* or *weight-loss wonder drug* in the media, clenbuterol has been shown to expedite lipolysis, which understandably may attract misuse from both those wishing to be overtly thin or to enhance muscular leanness (e.g., to become increasingly "cut") [15, 16]. Non-prescribed use of the drug has been linked to serious medical complications and high rates of hospitalization, particularly for tachycardia, gastrointestinal disturbances, tremors, and anxiety/agitation [15, 16].

Testosterone Boosters

Testosterone boosters are legal supplementary substances often used with the intention of naturally increasing testosterone levels in the blood [17, 18]. These substances typically lack a standardized composition and can consist of a variety of ingredients and/or compounds (e.g., herbal, nutrients) [17]. Ostensibly by virtue of increasing testosterone in the body, these products tend to be heavily marketed as having the potential to improve lean muscle mass and enhance one's sex drive (among other purported benefits) [18]. However, available published evidence supporting these marketed claims is very limited [17, 18].

Nutritional and Dietary Supplements

Nutritional and dietary supplements can include a number of substances that are often easily accessible and legally available from supermarkets, pharmacies, and specialty fitness stores. The specific functions of these substances vary across supplements, but of most relevance to this chapter, many are designed to enhance aspects of muscle development or recovery. Examples of such substances include dietary protein powder (supplementary protein to support muscle growth) [19], creatine monohydrate (i.e., a nutritional ergogenic supplement which may be used to enhance exercise performance and/or recovery) [20], and other substances such as L-carnitine, another popular ergogenic aid [21].

Health and Medical Risks Associated with AAS Use

Given AASs are believed to be one of the most widely used illicit APESs, and that this class of substance has garnered empirical and clinical attention which surpasses that devoted to most other APESs (e.g., testosterone boosters or prohormones), we have devoted this section to discussing the physical and psychological health concerns associated with AAS use. Recent reviews have previously discussed these risks in detail and have typically categorized them into several broad groups that warrant particular attention: cardiovascular toxicity, psychiatric effects, AAS-withdrawal hypogonadism, and neurotoxicity [7, 9, 22]. While we focus on the potential negative health impacts of AAS use here, we acknowledge that, in certain contexts and for certain populations, exogenous testosterone may bear some positive health benefits (e.g., significant weight loss and reduced cardiovascular issues for overweight and hypogonadal men) [23].

Cardiovascular Toxicity

There is wide consensus that supraphysiological doses (i.e., amounts greater than that normally found in the body) of AASs can negatively affect numerous aspects of cardiovascular health. Anecdotally, there is a growing number of cardiac-related deaths among AAS user athletes (or believed to be using) at a young age, namely, being in their 20s or 30s (see for review [24]). Although the prevalence and mechanisms underpinning the effects of AAS use on cardiovascular systems are not yet well understood, chronic use has been linked to myocardial pathology and coronary atherosclerosis [25, 26]. Goldman and colleagues [7] note that these complications likely exacerbate the likelihood of heart attacks, strokes, and in extreme cases death. Indeed, a nationwide population study in Sweden found that AAS users exhibited a cardiovascular morbidity and mortality rate which was around double that of non-users [27].

Psychiatric Effects

Long-term AAS use may also have deleterious effects on one's psychological health, with research indicating associations between AAS use and a range of psychiatric symptoms [9, 22]. For instance, AAS use has been linked to major mood syndromes (e.g., hypo/mania) [28], although argued to be for only a minority of users [22]. Moreover, several case reports describes uncharacteristic episodes of aggression and violence among individuals who had never exhibited such behaviors before AAS use (e.g., [29]), as well as links between AAS use and violent behaviors more broadly [30]. Research also suggests that users can exhibit depressive symptoms, occasionally accompanied with suicidal ideation, upon the discontinuation of use [9, 31, 32].

AAS-Withdrawal Hypogonadism

Exogenous testosterone through the administration of AASs suppresses the body's natural production of the hormone, and as a result, especially after long-term use, one can become hypogonadal (i.e., fail to naturally produce testosterone through the testes) [9, 33, 34]. Hypogonadism can have both physical (e.g., erectile/sexual dysfunction) and psychological symptoms (e.g., major depressive episodes), which typically become most salient after discontinuation of use [34]. Given the distressing nature of some of these symptoms, some men may be driven to recommence AAS use in an attempt to self-medicate, consequently precipitating a cycle of AAS dependence [9, 22]. We discuss AAS-withdrawal hypogonadism further under *Clinical Considerations, Guidance, and Recommendations* in this chapter.

Neurotoxicity

Supraphysiological doses of AASs may also negatively impact neurochemical and other brain structures. For instance, evidence hints at the possibility that chronic AAS use may heighten the risk for neuropathologies such as early-onset dementia [35]. Indeed, AAS use is associated with several similar cognitive, structural, and neurochemical abnormalities to those exhibited by individuals diagnosed with or at risk of dementia (see for review [35]). Other brain abnormalities have also been associated with long-term AAS use. For example, neuroimaging research has shown that AAS users may exhibit reduced overall cortical, grey matter, and putamen volume, the degree to which may correlate with the duration of AAS use (i.e., be more likely after prolonged use) [36]. Such findings add to the concern that AAS use is linked to the degeneration of certain brain structures, and this may be particularly salient among longer-term users [36].

The 1980s mark the period in which illicit AAS use became particularly widespread, and consequently, the cohorts who used (and could still use) during this time are only now in their middle ages and reaching older age [8, 24]. As such, worryingly, it is believed that certain neurotoxicity (and other deleterious) effects of long-term use may not yet have had the opportunity to fully develop and be evident within these groups [8].

AAS Use and Male Body Image

The serious and potentially life-threatening adverse impacts of AAS use beg the question of why men are driven to use these substances. Indeed, when men are asked about what motivates them to use AASs, common themes emerge. For example, among 500 AAS users, the primary motivations for use were to attain greater muscular development, enhance physical appearance, and improve strength [37]. This is compared to other motivations for use such as peer acceptance, pressure to perform, and improving sexual drive/function, all of which were endorsed less in the study. Similarly, among 1955 users in the United States, enhanced muscle mass, strength, and attractiveness were the top rated motivations for use [38]. Interestingly, the lowest ranked reasons for use were largely concerned with professional and recreational sports and bodybuilding. Recent research by Murray and colleagues [39] builds on this literature, delineating the motivation to use AAS *initially* versus *current* use. Among their 122 AAS users, the study found that 50.4% were initially motivated to use by improving appearance exclusively, followed by enhancing performance exclusively (30.6%), and lastly to improve appearance in conjunction with performance (19.0%). However, a distinct pattern was observed for *current* motivations for AAS use, with appearance (only) remaining the primary motivator (41.3%), followed by both appearance and performance (33.1%), and then performance only (25.6%) [39], suggesting performance may be a stronger motivator driving initial AAS use rather than maintaining it. However, together, this body of research provides clear evidence that AAS users want to look better and that motivations for use associated with appearance appear to be more salient than those related to performance.

Given many use AASs with the intention of improving appearance, it is unsurprising that problematic body image may represent a key risk factor for AAS use among men. In Western nations, many men report a preference for, and drive to acquire, an overtly muscular physique [1, 2]. Specifically, this muscular appearance ideal is often characterized by a well-developed upper-body and minimal body fat to ensure one's muscles are readily visible and look defined [40, 41]. Indeed, research suggests that around 90% of university men in the United States want higher levels of muscularity [42] and preferences for enhanced muscularity have even been observed in boys from a very young age (e.g., 6 years old) [3]. Recent analyses of epidemiological data suggest that significant proportions of boys and young men across the United States strive to gain weight or "bulk up" and indeed engage in efforts to do so, indicative of the widespread muscularity dissatisfaction, and concomitant body change efforts, among these male populations [43–45].

This lean muscular body ideal is extraordinarily difficult, if not impossible, for many boys and men to attain through natural ways. Consequently, men who negatively appraise their bodies, and firmly believe they are insufficiently muscular, may be at risk of using AASs to facilitate the attainment of big muscles. Indeed, empirical research supports this theoretical position. Pope et al. [46] found that concerns with one's physical attractiveness, body, and preoccupation with muscularity among weightlifters were relatively strong risk factors for AAS use. Moreover, among AAS users ($n = 74$), appearance concerns (conceptualized through social physique anxiety) were associated with increasingly severe symptoms of AAS dependence, the said relationship exhibiting a large effect size [47]. Recent qualitative research among male weightlifters further supports the importance of problematic body image, implicating poor self-esteem and body dissatisfaction, namely, tied to the perception one was too small, as key motivators for both the initiation and ongoing use of AASs [48]. While a dearth of research has been devoted to uncovering the temporal relationships between indicators of poor body image and AAS use, preliminary earlier longitudinal research found that, among adolescent boys, the desire for a larger body size/weight (i.e., a proxy indicator of muscularity dissatisfaction) predicted AAS use 5 years later [49]. Together, the literature converges in underscoring the importance of poor muscularity-oriented body image in potentially precipitating illicit AAS use, even to the extent that problematic body image is argued to be a primary mechanism (one of three; see below) for AAS initiation and ongoing use [22, 50].

Eating Disorders and AAS Use

Limited published research has examined AAS use in the context of eating disorders (EDs). Among the research that exists, findings appear to be mixed. Some studies have found no relationship between AAS and ED pathology, with AAS users no more likely meet diagnostic criteria for a comorbid eating disorder than non-users [28, 37]. However, others have found a link. For instance, research has shown that AAS users exhibit significantly greater (albeit modest) ED pathology than non-using controls as indexed through psychometrically validated self-report measures (e.g., [51]). A recent study of 2733 sexual minority men across Australia and New Zealand found that ED pathology distinguished users from non-users and was a relatively strong predictor of participants' frequency of thoughts about using AASs [52]. Importantly, Murray et al. [39] demonstrated that AAS users motivated exclusively to improve appearance, compared to motivations related to performance, may be particularly susceptible to experiencing ED pathology. These empirical associations between ED pathology and AAS use are consistent with the lean muscular physique revered by many men. That is, it may be the case that AAS users are in part driven to enhance muscularity using "traditional" thinness-oriented pathology (e.g., rigid dietary restriction, fasting) with the intention of minimizing body fat so one's musculature is increasingly prominent (i.e., to look "cut") [53].

Muscle Dysmorphia

In contrast to EDs, the psychiatric condition which has arguably received the greatest public and empirical attention in the context of AAS use is muscle dysmorphia (MD). MD is a form of body dysmorphic disorder (BDD) characterized by a severe preoccupation with the notion that one is insufficiently muscular [54, 55]. Formerly named "reverse anorexia" [56], MD is hallmarked by a pathological extreme drive to attain overt muscularity despite, in many cases, the afflicted individual already presenting with hypertrophic muscles. The condition is characterized through a multitude of symptoms that often cause significant distress and/or impairments in psychosocial functioning. These can include chronic obsessions about one's muscularity and getting bigger (in some cases for 5+ hours per day), repeated body scrutiny and checking in the mirror (in some cases more than 13 times per day), and frequent camouflaging or avoidance behaviors in relation to one's body (e.g., wearing heavy sweatshirts in summer) [57, 58]. Importantly, MD is also earmarked by rigid diet and exercise regimes aimed at expediting musculature development (e.g., large and frequent intakes of protein, excessive rule-driven weight lifting activities) [32, 59]. As such, the nosology of MD has been previously questioned, with an active discussion continuing as to whether MD may be more appropriately classified as a form of ED [41, 60].

MD is closely associated to AAS use, with afflicted individuals driven to use AASs to address severe muscularity concerns [22]. The drive to use, and the actual use of, such substances among those with MD is so widely acknowledged that it is argued to be a part of the diagnostic criteria for the condition [55]. Indeed, AAS use can distinguish men with pathological (i.e., MD) from non-pathological pursuits of muscularity. For instance, Olivardia and colleagues [58] found that 46% of their MD sample used AASs compared to only 7% of weightlifting controls. Similarly, Pope and colleagues [61] found that 21.4% of their sample of men with a history of MD reported having experienced AAS abuse/dependence in their lifetime, a strikingly larger prevalence than that found among men with a non-muscle form of BDD (0%). These findings align with Cafri et al. [57] in that 44% of men with a history of MD reported AAS use, which was greater than three times that among weightlifting men with no history of MD (i.e., 14%). While showing few differences between AAS users and matched non-using controls on several other psychological variables (e.g., self-esteem), Kanayama and colleagues [51] demonstrated that the groups could be distinguished by the severity of MD symptoms experienced, with AAS users being 5.5 times more likely to report being preoccupied with being too small (and becoming more muscular) than non-users. This finding was particularly salient among heavier AAS users (lifetime use for 6–150 months), highlighting the importance of the duration of use in the context of muscularity-oriented psychopathology that may be experienced. Furthermore, the study found that users were over four times likely to report always covering their body with clothes (to hide percieved inadequacies in muscularity) than non-users. This early seminal work is supported by more recent evidence with Kanayama and team [62] suggesting that, through the use of a directed acyclic graph analysis, MD symptoms may contribute to the development of AAS use.

Regrettably, since the discontinuation of AAS use may be met with the prospect of (or actual) loss of lean muscle mass, it is easy to fathom how significant distress may be experienced by individuals with a pronounced preoccupation with their muscularity as a result [22, 32]. Consequently, this may spur a swift resumption of AAS use and exacerbate the risk of AAS dependence [9, 22].

Clinical Considerations, Guidance, and Recommendations

Knowledge of effective strategies to address AAS use remains limited [22]. However, here we synthesize the available literature to provide preliminary guidance and recommendations to clinicians and health-care practitioners in helping address AAS use.

A key issue is that AAS users may not, or be extremely reluctant to, seek treatment in the first place. This is for several potential reasons. First, AAS use attracts considerable stigma, likely serving as a conduit for its secrecy among users and impede help-seeking behaviors [63]. Second, users may also hold egosyntonic beliefs about AAS use, lacking insight into its potential physical and/or psychological harms or just not caring about them, or believe it can be integrated into a healthy lifestyle [32, 64]. As such, some men may simply not want to stop using AASs. Given the lack of help-seeking behaviors among AAS users, many clinicians may not have been exposed to and fully understand the complexity of problems associated with AAS use and consequently be rendered ill-prepared to assist these individuals in the best way possible.

Once (and if) this initial help-seeking hurdle is overcome, the therapeutic relationship and dialogue between the AAS user and clinician are critical. Dunn et al. [65] note that, from the outset, there may be an incongruence in the type of care AAS users seek from clinicians and that which clinicians are inclined to provide. Specifically, while users may want to continue use in a *health-conscious* way under the guardianship of a clinician, the clinician could instead exhibit a proclivity toward preventing use altogether and an unwillingness to help [65]. As such, once a dialogue is established and when users open up about their AAS use, it is critical that clinicians maintain an inclusive and supportive environment, with special care to not react in a negative way, be judgmental, shame, or unnecessarily counsel users [65]. Kanayama et al. [22] note that "persuading an AAS user to stop using the drugs and potentially lose muscle is often as difficult as persuading patients with anorexia nervosa that they need to gain weight" (p. 69), therefore necessitating a level of sensitivity and understanding from clinicians for the appearance-related concerns of AAS users. However, while oppositional reactions may be used as a therapeutic strategy, this can further deter the user from providing key information about their use and health, possibly portending a poor therapeutic alliance and clinical outcomes [10, 65].

Another important consideration in the development of a therapeutic relationship is the perceived or actual lack of knowledge of AASs among clinicians. It is vital that clinicians be well versed in AAS use and associated complications, as users may be particularly reluctant to enter into a meaningful dialogue with and trust clinicians as a reliable source of information if they are viewed as being uneducated in this area [65, 66]. Indeed, there is seemingly a systemic lack of trust among AAS users toward clinicians, with earlier research finding that 56% never discussed their use with a primary health carer and trusting their advice no more than that available from friends or on the web [66].

One such key piece of information in helping clinicians address and treat AAS use for a particular individual is an understanding of the underlying mechanism(s) that may be driving its use [22, 50]. The mechanism of most relevance to this chapter is the *body image mechanism* [22, 50]; that is, AAS use is driven by a preoccupation with, and obssession of, the idea that one is inadequately muscular or too scrawny, the concomitant desire to enhance muscularity and, in achieving this, improve one's appearance. This mechanism of AAS use is exemplified among individuals afflicted with MD as discussed earlier. One could reason, therefore, that addressing body image concerns among those with MD would then ameliorate their desire and propensity to use AASs. However, the relationship between appearance concerns and AAS is not that simple, with concerns likely to have a reciprocal relationship with AAS use [50]. Further research utilizing prospective designs will be crucial in helping us disentangle the temporal relationships between problematic body image and AAS use.

Regrettably, a scarcity of research has specifically examined the treatment efficacy and outcomes of men with severe preoccupations with muscularity (i.e., afflicted with MD). However, a recent review highlights several treatment approaches that have been assessed through the lens of related disorders, BDD and EDs, which may also bear clinical utility in the context of MD [67].

Clinicians should also be informed of other potential mechanisms driving AAS use. For example, the *androgenic* or *neuroendocrine mechanism* [22, 50] focuses on AAS-induced hypogonadism, and a reduction in endogenous production of testosterone, as a result of prolonged use. Hypogonadism can have critical flow-on dysphoric effects, which may be pronounced upon discontinuation of long-term AAS use (and the body is no longer receiving exogenous testosterone). These can include deflation of muscle mass and increased body fat, reduction in libido, symptoms of major depressive disorder, and in rare cases suicide [34, 50]. However, as poignantly alluded to earlier, these symptoms can be extremely distressing for the individual, precipitating a strong motivation to resume AAS as self-medication, and potentially lead to dependence [9, 22]. As such, to deter relapse after discontinuation, it may be crucial that clinicians aggressively treat such withdrawal-type symptoms when presented [22, 50]. If hypogonadal symptoms are persistent and severe, an endocrinologist may need to be engaged to help treat and expedite the restoration of endogenous testosterone [22, 68]; however, unfortunately, endocrinologists who are well-versed in AAS-withdrawal symptoms may be particularly difficult to find [22].

Clinicians should also be cognizant of the *hedonic mechanism* of AAS use [22, 50]. AAS use is not typically described as having intoxicating effects or producing a "high" in the classical sense in humans; however, it may nevertheless create other pleasurable/reinforcing experiences (e.g., feelings of enhanced self-confidence and self-esteem, social praise or recognition) [48, 50, 69]. The potential hedonic effects of AASs have been further extrapolated from findings of laboratory rodent studies, which describe not only the establishment of conditioned place preferences to testosterone but also through the repeated self-administration of testosterone solutions, even to the extent that results in death (see for review [22, 50]). Research even suggests that the rewarding effects of AAS may be similar to that of opioid use and that AAS use may be in part underpinned by opioidergic mechanisms (see for review [9]). As such, although there exists a lack of treatment research pertaining to problematic AAS use per se, it may be in some cases useful to approach AAS use with therapies and/or medication that have demonstrable efficacy for other types of drug dependence [22, 50].

Conclusion

Particularly in Westernized nations, societal pressures are likely playing a key role in motivating men to attain a (for most) unattainable appearance characterized by overt muscularity and minimal body fat. Such pressures are exemplified by the prevalence of body and muscularity dissatisfaction we find among boys and men in these nations. It is then no surprise that certain APESs may be sought and used to facilitate the attainment of this lean muscular body ideal. As highlighted in this chapter, a myriad of both legal and illicit APESs exist which individuals may use for different functions (e.g., muscle growth, fat loss, recovering). For some of these substances (e.g., testosterone boosters, prohormones), we do not yet have a comprehensive and empirical understanding of their prevalence of use, efficacy, and safety. However, the class of illicit APES which has perhaps received the greatest empirical and clinical attention are AASs. While AASs may be used to rapidly achieve a degree of muscularity that is essentially impossible through diet and exercise alone, our chapter presents medical research to underscore the serious physical and psychological health harms linked to its use.

The motivations men report in relation to using AASs showcase the close relationship between problematic body image and AAS use. Questioning the stereotype that AAS use is predominantly confined to athletes who want to enhance performance, the research findings presented here converge in highlighting that appearance-related motivations are a critical driver of use. And while links have been found among AAS use and ED psychopathology, ostensibly deriving from the motivation to minimize body adiposity and enhance the visibility of one's musculature, AAS use has been researched perhaps most extensively within the context of MD. Those who are preoccupied with being too small or puny, and who are driven to attain an increasingly muscular stature, are at a high risk of using AASs.

Despite the emerging research indicating the prevalence of AAS use, its poor health correlates, and close-knit relationship with body image psychopathology, we currently have a limited understanding of evidence-based strategies to address it. However, our chapter synthesizes available literature to provide an overview of important (but preliminary) considerations, guidance, and recommendations that may help support clinicians in dealing with the complexities of AAS use. For example, given the significant stigma associated with AAS use, we believe it is critical for clinicians to respond to users in a non-judgmental way to facilitate a therapeutic dialogue. Moreover, it is important that clinicians are knowledgeable in terms of what the drug is and its associated effects, therefore making it more likely users perceive the clinician as a reliable source of information. Finally, having a comprehensive understanding of the distinct mechanism(s) which are theorized to drive AAS use, and how these might apply to different users, will likely inform the most appropriate route of treatment.

Table 12.1 Summary descriptions of APESs

APES	Examples	Typical form of intake	Sought-after function
Anabolic-androgenic steroids [70]	Anadrol (oxymetholone) Anavar (oxandrolone) Dianabol (methandienone) Winstrol (stanozolol) Restandol (testosterone undecanoate) Deca-Durabolin (nandrolone decanoate) Durabolin (nandrolone phenpropionate)	Intramuscular injection, oral	Increase lean muscularity and/or strength
Prohormones [71]	Dehydroepiandrosterone (DHT) Androstenedione Androstenediol Norandrostenedione Norandrostenediol	Oral	Convert to testosterone to provide similar anabolic functions as AAS – increase lean muscularity and/or strength
Beta-2 androgenic agonist	Clenbuterol	Oral	Rapid reduction in body adiposity
Testosterone boosters [18]	Ingredients will vary from product to product. Commonly included ingredients include: Zinc Fenugreek Tribulus terrestris Vitamin B6	Oral	Naturally increase blood testosterone concentrations
Protein supplements	Available in a variety of powders, shakes and drinks, and other snacks	Oral	Provide macronutrients (i.e., protein) to support muscle growth
Creatine monohydrate supplements	Available in powder form	Oral	Enhance energy provision to muscles to facilitate exercise
Amino acids [72]	Available in individual or compound forms: Arginine Glutamine Leucine Isoleucine Valine	Oral	Varies depending on amino acid or compound. May be sought after to support fat loss and muscle growth and/or facilitate exercise

References

1. Leit R, Gray J, Pope H. The media's representation of the ideal male body: a cause for muscle dysmorphia? Int J Eat Disord. 2002;31(3):334–8.
2. Pope H, Phillips K, Olivardia R. The Adonis complex: the secret crisis of male body obsession. New York: Free Press; 2000.
3. McLean S, Wertheim E, Paxton S. Preferences for being muscular and thin in 6-year-old boys. Body Image. 2018;26:98–102.
4. Hildebrandt T, Lai J, Langenbucher J, Schneider M, Yehuda R, Pfaff D. The diagnostic dilemma of pathological appearance and performance enhancing drug use. Drug Alcohol Depend. 2011;114(1):1–11.
5. Bhasin S, Storer T, Berman N, Callegari C, Clevenger B, Phillips J, et al. The effects of supraphysiologic doses of testosterone on muscle size and strength in normal men. N Engl J Med. 1996;335(1):1–7.
6. Begley E, Mcveigh J, Hope VD. Image and performance enhancing drugs: 2016 National survey results survey. Public Health Institute, Liverpool John Moores.
7. Goldman A, Pope H, Bhasin S. The health threat posed by the hidden epidemic of anabolic steroid use and body image disorders among young men. J Clin Endocrinol Metab. 2019;104(4):1069–74.
8. Kanayama G, Hudson J, Pope H. Illicit anabolic–androgenic steroid use. Horm Behav. 2010;58(1):111–21.
9. Pope H, Wood R, Rogol A, Nyberg F, Bowers L, Bhasin S. Adverse health consequences of performance-enhancing drugs: an endocrine society scientific statement. Endocr Rev. 2014;35(3):341–75.
10. Griffiths S, Murray S, Mitchison D, Mond J. Anabolic steroids: lots of muscle in the short-term, potentially devastating health consequences in the long-term. Drug Alcohol Rev. 2016;35(4):375–6.
11. Pope H, Kanayama G, Athey A, Ryan E, Hudson J, Baggish A. The lifetime prevalence of anabolic-androgenic steroid use and dependence in Americans: current best estimates. Am J Addict. 2014;23(4):371–7.
12. Sagoe D, Molde H, Andreassen C, Torsheim T, Pallesen S. The global epidemiology of anabolic-androgenic steroid use: a meta-analysis and meta-regression analysis. Ann Epidemiol. 2014;24(5):383–98.
13. Brown G, Vukovich M, King D. Testosterone prohormone supplements. Med Sci Sports Exerc. 2006;38(8):1451–61.
14. Van Thuyne W, Van Eenoo P, Delbeke F. Nutritional supplements: prevalence of use and contamination with doping agents. Nutr Res Rev. 2006;19(1):147–58.
15. Brett J, Dawson A, Brown J. Clenbuterol toxicity: a NSW Poisons Information Centre experience. Med J Aust. 2014;200(4):219–21.
16. Spiller H, James K, Scholzen S, Borys D. A descriptive study of adverse events from clenbuterol misuse and abuse for weight loss and bodybuilding. Subst Abus. 2013;34(3):306–12.
17. Balasubramanian A, Thirumavalavan N, Srivatsav A, Lipshultz L, Pastuszak A. 126 testosterone imposters: an analysis of popular online testosterone boosting supplements. J Sex Med. 2019;16(4):S65.
18. Clemesha C, Thaker H, Samplaski M. 'Testosterone boosting' supplements composition and claims are not supported by the academic literature. World J Mens Health. 2020;38(1):115.
19. Morton R, Murphy K, McKellar S, Schoenfeld B, Henselmans M, Helms E, et al. A systematic review, meta-analysis and meta-regression of the effect of protein supplementation on resistance training-induced gains in muscle mass and strength in healthy adults. Br J Sports Med. 2018;52(6):376–84.
20. Kreider RB, Kalman DS, Antonio J, Ziegenfuss T, Wildman R, Collins R, et al. International Society of Sports Nutrition position stand: safety and efficacy of creatine supplementation in exercise, sport and medicine. J Int Soc Sports Nutr. 2017;14:18.

21. Karlic H, Lohninger A. Supplementation of l-carnitine in athletes: does it make sense? Nutrition. 2004;20(7–8):709–15.
22. Kanayama G, Hudson J, Pope H Jr. Anabolic-androgenic steroid use and body image in men: a growing concern for clinicians. Psychother Psychosom. 2020;89(2):65–73.
23. Saad F, Doros G, Haider K, Haider A. Differential effects of 11 years of long-term injectable testosterone undecanoate therapy on anthropometric and metabolic parameters in hypogonadal men with normal weight, overweight and obesity in comparison with untreated controls: real-world data from a controlled registry study. Int J Obes (Lond). 2020;44(6):1264–78.
24. Kanayama G, Hudson J, Pope HG. Long-term psychiatric and medical consequences of anabolic–androgenic steroid abuse: a looming public health concern? Drug Alcohol Depend. 2008;98(1–2):1–12.
25. Baggish A, Weiner R, Kanayama G, Hudson J, Lu M, Hoffmann U, et al. Cardiovascular toxicity of illicit anabolic-androgenic steroid use. Circulation. 2017;135(21):1991–2002.
26. D'Andrea A, Caso P, Salerno G, Scarafile R, De Corato G, Mita C, et al. Left ventricular early myocardial dysfunction after chronic misuse of anabolic androgenic steroids: a Doppler myocardial and strain imaging analysis. Br J Sports Med. 2007;41(3):149–55.
27. Thiblin I, Garmo H, Garle M, Holmberg L, Byberg L, Michaëlsson K, et al. Anabolic steroids and cardiovascular risk: a national population-based cohort study. Drug Alcohol Depend. 2015;152:87–92.
28. Pope HG. Psychiatric and medical effects of anabolic-androgenic steroid use. Arch Gen Psychiatry. 1994;51(5):375.
29. Pope HG, Kouri EM, Powell KF, Campbell C, Katz DL. Anabolic-androgenic steroid use among 133 prisoners. Comprehensive Psychiatry. 1996;37:322–27.
30. Beaver K, Vaughn M, DeLisi M, Wright J. Anabolic-androgenic steroid use and involvement in violent behavior in a nationally representative sample of young adult males in the United States. Am J Public Health. 2008;98(12):2185–7.
31. Griffiths S, Henshaw R, McKay F, Dunn M. Post-cycle therapy for performance and image enhancing drug users: a qualitative investigation. Perform Enhanc Health. 2017;5(3):103–7.
32. Mosley P. Bigorexia: bodybuilding and muscle dysmorphia. Eur Eat Disord Rev. 2009;17(3):191–8.
33. Coward R, Rajanahally S, Kovac J, Smith R, Pastuszak A, Lipshultz L. Anabolic steroid induced hypogonadism in young men. J Urol. 2013;190(6):2200–5.
34. Kanayama G, Hudson J, DeLuca J, Isaacs S, Baggish A, Weiner R, et al. Prolonged hypogonadism in males following withdrawal from anabolic-androgenic steroids: an under-recognized problem. Addiction. 2015;110(5):823–31.
35. Kaufman M, Kanayama G, Hudson J, Pope H. Supraphysiologic-dose anabolic–androgenic steroid use: a risk factor for dementia? Neurosci Biobehav Rev. 2019;100:180–207.
36. Bjørnebekk A, Walhovd K, Jørstad M, Due-Tønnessen P, Hullstein I, Fjell A. Structural brain imaging of long-term anabolic-androgenic steroid users and nonusing weightlifters. Biol Psychiatry. 2017;82(4):294–302.
37. Ip E, Barnett M, Tenerowicz M, Perry P. The anabolic 500 survey: characteristics of male users versus nonusers of anabolic-androgenic steroids for strength training. Pharmacotherapy. 2011;31(8):757–66.
38. Cohen J, Collins R, Darkes J, Gwartney D. A league of their own: demographics, motivations and patterns of use of 1,955 male adult non-medical anabolic steroid users in the United States. J Int Soc Sports Nutr. 2007;4(1):12.
39. Murray S, Griffiths S, Mond J, Kean J, Blashill A. Anabolic steroid use and body image psychopathology in men: delineating between appearance- versus performance-driven motivations. Drug Alcohol Depend. 2016;165:198–202.
40. Ridgeway R, Tylka T. College men's perceptions of ideal body composition and shape. Psychol Men Masculinity. 2005;6(3):209–20.
41. Murray S, Nagata J, Griffiths S, Calzo J, Brown T, Mitchison D, et al. The enigma of male eating disorders: a critical review and synthesis. Clin Psychol Rev. 2017;57:1–11.

42. Frederick D, Buchanan G, Sadehgi-Azar L, Peplau L, Haselton M, Berezovskaya A, et al. Desiring the muscular ideal: men's body satisfaction in the United States, Ukraine, and Ghana. Psychol Men Masculinity. 2007;8(2):103–17.
43. Nagata J, Bibbins-Domingo K, Garber A, Griffiths S, Vittinghoff E, Murray S. Boys, bulk, and body ideals: sex differences in weight-gain attempts among adolescents in the United States. J Adolesc Health. 2019;64(4):450–3.
44. Nagata J, Murray S, Bibbins-Domingo K, Garber A, Mitchison D, Griffiths S. Predictors of muscularity-oriented disordered eating behaviors in U.S. young adults: a prospective cohort study. Int J Eat Disord. 2019;52(12):1380–8.
45. Nagata J, Ganson K, Griffiths S, Mitchison D, Garber A, Vittinghoff E, et al. Prevalence and correlates of muscle-enhancing behaviors among adolescents and young adults in the United States. Int J Adolesc Med Health. 2020.
46. Pope H, Kanayama G, Hudson J. Risk factors for illicit anabolic-androgenic steroid use in male weightlifters: a cross-sectional cohort study. Biol Psychiatry. 2012;71(3):254–61.
47. Griffiths S, Jacka B, Degenhardt L, Murray S, Larance B. Physical appearance concerns are uniquely associated with the severity of steroid dependence and depression in anabolic-androgenic steroid users. Drug Alcohol Rev. 2018;37(5):664–70.
48. Greenway C, Price C. A qualitative study of the motivations for anabolic-androgenic steroid use: the role of muscle dysmorphia and self-esteem in long-term users. Perform Enhanc Health. 2018;6(1):12–20.
49. vandenBerg P, Neumark-Sztainer D, Cafri G, Wall M. Steroid use among adolescents: longitudinal findings from project EAT. Pediatrics. 2007;119(3):476–86.
50. Kanayama G, Brower K, Wood R, Hudson J, Pope H Jr. Treatment of anabolic–androgenic steroid dependence: emerging evidence and its implications. Drug Alcohol Depend. 2010;109(1–3):6–13.
51. Kanayama G, Barry S, Hudson J, Pope H. Body image and attitudes toward male roles in anabolic-androgenic steroid users. Am J Psychiatry. 2006;163(4):697–703.
52. Griffiths S, Murray S, Dunn M, Blashill A. Anabolic steroid use among gay and bisexual men living in Australia and New Zealand: associations with demographics, body dissatisfaction, eating disorder psychopathology, and quality of life. Drug Alcohol Depend. 2017;181:170–6.
53. Lavender J, Brown T, Murray S. Men, muscles, and eating disorders: an overview of traditional and muscularity-oriented disordered eating. Curr Psychiatry Rep. 2017;19(6):32.
54. Diagnostic and statistical manual of mental disorders. Arlington: American Psychiatric Publishing; 2013.
55. Pope H, Gruber A, Choi P, Olivardia R, Phillips K. Muscle dysmorphia: an underrecognized form of body dysmorphic disorder. Psychosomatics. 1997;38(6):548–57.
56. Pope H, Katz D, Hudson J. Anorexia nervosa and "reverse anorexia" among 108 male bodybuilders. Compr Psychiatry. 1993;34(6):406–9.
57. Cafri G, Olivardia R, Thompson J. Symptom characteristics and psychiatric comorbidity among males with muscle dysmorphia. Compr Psychiatry. 2008;49(4):374–9.
58. Olivardia R, Pope H, Hudson J. Muscle dysmorphia in male weightlifters: a case-control study. Am J Psychiatry. 2000;157(8):1291–6.
59. Murray S, Rieger E, Touyz S. Muscle dysmorphia symptomatology during a period of religious fasting: a case report. Eur Eat Disord Rev. 2011;19(2):162–8.
60. Murray S, Rieger E, Touyz S, De la Garza García Lic Y. Muscle dysmorphia and the DSM-V conundrum: where does it belong? A review paper. Int J Eat Disord. 2010;43(6):483–91.
61. Pope C, Pope H, Menard W, Fay C, Olivardia R, Phillips K. Clinical features of muscle dysmorphia among males with body dysmorphic disorder. Body Image. 2005;2(4):395–400.
62. Kanayama G, Pope H, Hudson J. Associations of anabolic-androgenic steroid use with other behavioral disorders: an analysis using directed acyclic graphs. Psychol Med. 2018;48(15):2601–8.
63. Griffiths S, Murray S, Mond J. The stigma of anabolic steroid use. J Drug Issues. 2016;46(4):446–56.

64. Kimergård A. A qualitative study of anabolic steroid use amongst gym users in the United Kingdom: motives, beliefs and experiences. J Subst Abus. 2014;20(4):288–94.
65. Dunn M, Henshaw R, McKay F. Do performance and image enhancing drug users in regional Queensland experience difficulty accessing health services? Drug Alcohol Rev. 2016;35(4):377–82.
66. Pope H, Kanayama G, Ionescu-Pioggia M, Hudson J. Anabolic steroid users' attitudes towards physicians. Addiction. 2004;99(9):1189–94.
67. Cunningham M, Griffiths S, Mitchison D, Mond J, Castle D, Murray S. Muscle dysmorphia: an overview of clinical features and treatment options. J Cogn Psychother. 2017;31(4):255–71.
68. Brower K. Anabolic steroid abuse and dependence in clinical practice. Phys Sportsmed. 2009;37(4):131–40.
69. Vassallo M, Olrich T. Confidence by injection: male users of anabolic steroids speak of increases in perceived confidence through anabolic steroid use. Int J Sport Exerc Psychol. 2010;8(1):70–80.
70. https://www.drugabuse.gov/publications/research-reports/steroids-other-appearance-performance-enhancing-drugs-apeds/how-are-anabolic-steroids-used.
71. https://en.wikipedia.org/wiki/Androgen_prohormone.
72. https://en.wikipedia.org/wiki/Essential_amino_acid.

Part IV
Prevention and Treatment

Chapter 13
Prevention of Eating Disorders in Boys and Men

Marie Nebel-Schwalm and Tiffany A. Brown

Learning Objectives

1. Describe the efficacy of school-based eating disorder prevention and intervention programs for boys.
2. Describe the efficacy of cognitive-behavioral in-person eating disorder prevention in young adult men.
3. Describe the efficacy of Internet-based prevention programs for men.
4. Describe the efficacy of dual eating and weight prevention programs for boys and men.

Key Points

- School-based interventions feature universal mixed-gender programs for elementary and middle school students and have not demonstrated efficacy in relation to eating pathology.
- Regarding in-person cognitive-behavioral programs for young adults, mixed-gender programs generally fail to report results separately for men and are less effective than male-specific programs; however, few programs exist for men only. Dissonance-based interventions specific to men appear promising to reduce eating pathology.
- Internet-based prevention programs for boys and men remain in their infancy, and it is unknown whether they demonstrate efficacy.
- Dual-focused prevention programs targeting eating and weight show potentially promising results.

M. Nebel-Schwalm
Illinois Wesleyan University, Department of Psychology, Bloomington, IL, USA

T. A. Brown (✉)
Department of Psychiatry, University of California, San Diego, San Diego, CA, USA

San Diego State University Research Foundation, San Diego, CA, USA
e-mail: tiffanybrown@ucsd.edu

J. M. Nagata et al. (eds.), *Eating Disorders in Boys and Men*,
https://doi.org/10.1007/978-3-030-67127-3_13

- Despite growing awareness, current programs remain hampered by inappropriate measurement and extension of existing programs for girls and women, rather than bottom-up program development for boys and men. More evidence-based efforts for this population are needed.

Introduction

Although often overlooked, eating disorders (EDs) in boys and men represent a serious and deadly public health problem, which will affect up to seven million men in the United States in their lifetime [1, 2]. Despite the impairment and distress associated with these conditions [3–6], men are less likely to seek treatment than women, in part due to stigma [7, 8]. Unfortunately, even for those men who do seek help, existing treatments are targeted mostly toward women, rarely address male-specific risk factors, and are ineffective for a substantial proportion of patients [9, 10]. This disparity highlights the need for greater clarity and focused effort regarding intervention development for boys and men. In particular, well-accepted, disseminable prevention programs that target male-specific ED risk factors *prior* to disorder onset are critical to reduce the public health burden and disparities associated with boys and men with EDs. Importantly, these unique factors for men include muscularity-oriented body image and eating and related body change behaviors that correspond with these concerns (e.g., steroid use, excessive protein intake, binge eating, and unhealthy exercise).

Though still a burgeoning area of research in men, an increasing number of programs aimed at prevention of EDs, muscle dysmorphia, and their associated features have been developed and evaluated. As such, the primary purpose of this chapter is to provide an overview of the ED prevention research in men and provide directions for future research.

Across disciplines, there are several frameworks for classifying different levels of prevention programs. The Institute of Medicine (IOM) classifications are perhaps one of the most prominent, differentiating between universal, selected, and indicated interventions [11]. *Universal prevention* refers to programs that target the general population and are not directed at any particular risk group (e.g., a program is provided to all boys and girls in a school). *Selected prevention* refers to programs targeted toward individuals with probable increased risk for a given disorder (e.g., individuals who report body image concerns). Finally, *indicated prevention* refers to programs targeted to those with known risk, symptoms, or subclinical presentations of a given disorder (e.g., individuals who do not meet criteria for an ED but exhibit binge eating or purging symptoms). Throughout the chapter, we will use these terms, as relevant, to help provide greater context on the types of programs that have been developed or adapted for boys and men.

It is important to note that, to date, few studies in boys and men have examined true ED "prevention," that is, demonstrating that a program reduces the onset of an ED compared to a control condition. Thus, most of the preventative intervention efforts described in this chapter are more accurately described as efforts to reduce risk factors for EDs. The present chapter summarizes research on (1) school-based prevention programs for boys, (2) in-person prevention programs for young men, (3) Internet-based prevention programs for boys and men, and (4) dual prevention programs targeting weight and eating for boys and men.

School-Based Prevention Programs (See Table 13.1)

For youth, school-based settings provide an ideal environment to disseminate ED prevention programs [12]. School-based programs for boys have largely been implemented universally in elementary and middle schools with both boys and girls simultaneously. The use of mixed-gender samples is likely due to the higher prevalence of EDs in women [13] and the ease of including both genders in intervention groups.

Elementary and Middle School ED Prevention Programs

Several universal school-based programs have been developed for elementary [14–16] and middle school students [17–22]. All of these programs with the exception of one [19] included both boys and girls in the same program. However, none of these programs have demonstrated significant improvements in eating pathology or disordered eating behavior compared to class as usual. This may be due to the lack of focus on male-specific content and muscularity in larger school-based programs [20], the use of female-validated measures [20], and the floor effects for traditional measures of eating pathology in boys at baseline assessments [18, 20].

While none of these programs have reduced eating pathology per se, programs have demonstrated behavioral improvements in self-reported dieting [22] and obligatory or compulsive exercise [20]. Many school-based programs have actively targeted and demonstrated improvements in ED knowledge [15] and body image attitudes including body dissatisfaction, weight and shape concerns [14, 17, 20–22], appearance comparisons [16, 20], and body-ideal internalization [16, 21]. Some programs have also found evidence for reducing risk factors that affect EDs beyond body image including perfectionism [20, 21], self-esteem [19], and mood or negative affect [19].

Most school-based prevention programs have included at least some elements of media literacy programming. Media literacy prevention programs aim to reduce disordered eating through promoting education and activism around ED risk factors of pressures to be attractive and fulfill gender-specific body ideals as communicated by the media. Students are educated about gender stereotypes that are promoted through media, how these contribute to western body ideals, and techniques used to create media images (i.e., airbrushing and digital manipulation). One of the most

Table 13.1 School-based ED prevention programs for boys

Authors	Program (no. of sessions)	Control condition	Age	N (% male)	Program type	Assessments	Result summary for boys
Elementary and middle school-based ED prevention programs							
Smolak et al. [15]	Eating Smart, Eating for Me [10]	Class as usual	5th grade	222 (45.9%)	Universal Mixed gender	• Body esteem (BES) • Exercise frequency • Beliefs about body fat and fat people • Weight-related teasing • Fruit/vegetable consumption	• Boys increased vegetable consumption and overall sample decreased negative beliefs about fat people • No changes in physical activity, body esteem, and weight-related teasing
Kater et al. [14]	Healthy Body Image: Teaching Kids to Eat and Love Their Bodies Too! [10]	n/a	4th and 6th grade	222 (unknown)	Universal Mixed gender	• Questionnaire developed by authors to assess attitudes and behavioral intentions regarding body image and dieting	• In the mixed-gender sample at post-intervention: improvements in responses regarding their own body development, attitudes about body sizes, factors influencing body size/shape, attitudes toward dieting, body image, and critical thinking regarding media image • Results were not analyzed separately by gender
O'Dea and Abraham [17]	Everybody's Different [9]	Class as usual	11–14 years	470 (37%)	Universal Mixed gender (examined high and low risk)	• Eating pathology (EDI) • Self-perception • Depression (Depression Inventory) • Anxiety (STAI) • Body image questionnaires	• Post-intervention across boys and girls: improvements in body dissatisfaction, drive for thinness, physical appearance ratings, and less importance of social acceptance and physical appearance, with most effects maintained at 12-month follow-up • High-risk boys and girls also improved in drive for thinness and physical appearance ratings at post-intervention and body dissatisfaction through 12-month follow-up

Varnado-Sullivan et al. [18]	Body Logic (universal, 3; selected, 4)	n/a	10–13 years	287 (45.3%)	Universal (stage 1) Selected (stage 2) Mixed gender	• Eating pathology (ChEAT, MAEDS) • Depression (CDI) • Body image (BIA) • Self-esteem (RSES)	• No significant improvements for boys across assessments • Data for boys in selected program were too small to analyze ($n = 9$)
Stanford and McCabe [19]	Adolescent male program [2]	Class as usual	12–13 years	121 (100%)	Universal Males only	• Body Satisfaction and Body Change Inventory • Exercise (EES) • Eating pathology (EDI-2) • Depression, anxiety, stress (DASS)	• Improvements in satisfaction with muscles, self-esteem, and negative affect • No differences in overall body satisfaction, body image importance, or the use of steroids/food supplements, excessive exercise, or eating pathology
Wilksch and Wade [22]	Media Smart [8]	Class as usual	8th grade	540 (49.4%)	Universal Mixed gender	• Shape and weight concerns (EDE-Q) • Dieting (DEBQ) • Body dissatisfaction (EDI) • Media internalization (SATAQ) • Perceived pressure (PSPS) • Depression (CDI) • Self-esteem (RSES)	• Boys demonstrated greater reductions in dieting, body dissatisfaction, and weight/shape concerns at post-intervention and 6-month follow-up compared to class as usual

(continued)

Table 13.1 (continued)

Authors	Program (no. of sessions)	Control condition	Age	N (% male)	Program type	Assessments	Result summary for boys
Bird et al. [16]	Happy Being Me [3]	Class as usual	10–11 years	88 (52.3%)	Universal Mixed gender	• Body Satisfaction Visual Analogue Scale • Appearance internalization (SATAQ) • Appearance-related teasing, conversations, and comparisons • Restrained, emotional eating (TFEQ) • Self-esteem	• Boys post-intervention: improvements in body-ideal internalization and appearance comparison • Boys at 3-month follow-up: no significant effects
Wilksch et al. [21]	Media Smart [8]	LifeSmart (ED + obesity prevention) HELPP (ED prevention) Class as usual	7th–8th grade	1316 (36.2%)	Universal Mixed gender	• Shape, weight, eating concerns (EDE-Q) • Dieting (DEBQ) • Body dissatisfaction (EDI) • Media internalization (SATAQ) • Perceived pressure (PSPS) • Depression (CDI) • Weight-related teasing (McKnight Risk Factor Survey) • Perfectionism (MPS) • Regular eating • Screen time • Physical activity	*Media Smart* • Boys post-program: improvements in body dissatisfaction, media internalization, weight-related teasing, perfectionism • Boys at 6- and 12-month follow-up: improvements in media internalization and depression *LifeSmart* • Boys post-program: improvements for body dissatisfaction, while media internalization increased • Boys at 6- and 12-month follow-up: increases in media internalization (6-month) and depression (6- and 12-month) *HELPP* • Boys post-program: improvements in media internalization. Higher levels of being a victim of weight-related peer teasing than Media Smart • Boys at 6- and 12-month follow-up: improvements in media internalization, depression

Warschburger and Zitzmann [20]	POPS program [9]	Class as usual	10–16 years	568 (48%)	Universal Mixed gender	• Eating pathology (EDI-2, EAT-26) • Body dissatisfaction (EDI-2, CDRS) • Appearance internalization (SATAQ) • Exercise (OEQ) • Social comparison (PACS) • Teasing (POTS)	• In the combined sample of boys and girls: At 3-month follow-up: greater improvements in body dissatisfaction, perceived media pressures, obligatory exercise, social comparison, and perfectionism compared to class as usual
High school-based ED prevention programs							
Goldberg et al. [26]	ATLAS [7]	Educational (pamphlet) control	15 years (average)	1506 (100%)	Selected Boys only	• AAS and other drug use • Knowledge of drug effects • Attitudes toward and behavioral intent to use AAS • Nutrition and exercise knowledge • Belief in media messages • Body image • Drug refusal skills	• Improvements in intent to use AAS, greater knowledge of AAS and their effects, more negative attitudes about AAS users, improved feeling of athletic abilities, higher self-esteem, more competent drug refusal skills, less belief in media messages, and improved nutrition and exercise behaviors through 9–12-month follow-up • No change in body image
Buddeberg-Fischer et al. [24]	Swiss high school [3]	Class as usual	14–19 years	314 (34.7%)	Universal	• Eating pathology (EAT-26) • Overall distress (GSCL-C) • Psychological impairment (SCL-90-R)	• No differences between intervention and control post-intervention, although both groups improved in eating pathology, overall distress, and general psychiatric symptoms • Data for high-risk boys were too small to analyze

(continued)

Table 13.1 (continued)

Authors	Program (no. of sessions)	Control condition	Age	N (% male)	Program type	Assessments	Result summary for boys
Gumz et al. [25]	Germany [3]	Class as usual	14 and 17 years (8th and 11th grade)	1452 (44.4%)	Universal Mixed gender	• Eating pathology (ChEDE) • ED knowledge • Internalization of appearance ideals (SATAQ) • (Body-related) self-concept (MCSC) • Depression (PHQ-9) • Anxiety (GAD-7)	• For 8th grade boys, eating pathology decreased post-intervention and remained stable at follow-up • For 11th graders, both boys and girls in the intervention group exhibited lower ED pathology than the control group at follow-up • ED knowledge increased for the intervention group through 6-month follow-up
Yager et al. [29]	ATLAS [10]	Waitlist	10th grade	211 (100%)	Universal Boys only	• Body esteem (BES) • Drive for muscularity (DMS) • Body appearance rating • Body satisfaction (Embodied Image Scale) • Knowledge, attitudes, intentions to use, and use of substances and steroids	• ATLAS participants had greater improvements (small effect sizes) in functional and aesthetic body image and attitudes towards APEDs compared to WL post-intervention and 3-month follow-up; however, after adjustment for multiple comparisons, effects were no longer significant • No significant effects were found for body esteem, drive for muscularity, or use of APEDS/steroids

Note. *AAS* anabolic-androgenic steroids, *BIA* Body Image Assessment for Children and Adolescents, *BES* Body Esteem Scale, *CDI* Children's Depression Inventory, *CDRS* Contour Drawing Rating Scale, *ChEDE* Child Eating Disorder Examination, *DASS* Depression Anxiety Stress Scales, *DEBQ* Dutch Eating Behavior Questionnaire, *EAT-26* Eating Attitudes Test, *EDI* Eating Disorder Inventory, *EES* Excessive Exercise Scale, *GAD-7* Generalized Anxiety Disorder 7-Item Scale, *GSCL-C* Giessen Physical Complaint List for Children and Adolescents, *MAEDS* Multiaxial Assessment of Eating Disorder Symptoms, *MSCS* Multidimensional Self-Concept Scale, *MPS* Multidimensional Perfectionism Scale, *OEQ* Obligatory Exercise Questionnaire, *PACS* Physical Appearance Comparison Scale, *PHQ-9* Patient Health Questionnaire, *POTS* Perception of Teasing Scale, *PSPS* Perceived Sociocultural Pressures Scale, *RSES* Rosenberg Self-Esteem Scale, *SATAQ* Sociocultural Attitudes Towards Appearance Scale, *SCL-90-R* Self-Report Symptom Checklist, *STAI* State Trait Anxiety Inventory, *TFEQ* Three-Factor Eating Questionnaire successful and empirically supported media literacy programs to date has been *Media Smart* [22], an 8-week program for 7th–8th grade boys and girls. Across two trials, boys in *Media Smart* demonstrated reductions in weight-related peer teasing, perfectionism, and body dissatisfaction at post-intervention [21]; dieting, body dissatisfaction, and weight/shape concerns at post-intervention and 6-month follow-up [22]; and depression and media internalization at 6-month and 12-month follow-up [21], compared to class as usual. While the program has traditionally been delivered by professional (graduate-level) facilitators, recent research has supported similar effects when the program is delivered in school by teachers as well [21], which may make this program more easily disseminable to a wider audience.

As noted above, the lack of significant effects on eating pathology for boys in school-based programs may be due, in part, to the lack of muscularity-oriented program content and muscularity-oriented body image assessments. Research supports that adolescent boys with EDs report lower scores on traditional assessments of eating pathology compared to girls with equally as severe EDs [23]. Thus, use of appropriate measures to assess male-specific concerns is critical. Further, while mixed-gender groups may be easier to implement in practice, there may be advantages to separating boys and girls to allow for more candid and honest conversations among peers. In a small trial, Stanford and McCabe [19] evaluated a two-session, male-only program focusing on self-esteem and body acceptance for 12–13-year-old boys. Participants in the program showed increased muscle satisfaction and self-esteem, as well as decreased negative affect, relative to those in class as usual. Importantly, while the program found significant effects for muscularity satisfaction, a significant effect was not found for overall body dissatisfaction, highlighting that intervention effects for boys may be obscured when using assessments that are not specific to body image concerns in boys.

High School ED Prevention Programs

Fewer ED prevention programs have been implemented for high school-age boys [24, 25]. One program examined the effects of a universal ED prevention program in Swiss high school students [24], but did not find any significant differences between the intervention and class as usual in a mixed-gender sample. More recently, a large-scale universal prevention trial in Germany [25] implemented with 8th and 11th grade students found no significant differences in ED pathology between the intervention and control group at 6-month follow-up. However, gender and grade moderated the intervention effects, such that 11th graders (both girls and boys) in the intervention group exhibited lower ED pathology than the control group at follow-up, whereas for 8th graders, boys experienced decreased eating pathology directly after the intervention that remained stable through follow-up, but girls exhibited increased ED pathology. Thus, in at least one case, a universal high school-based prevention program may show some promise for reducing ED risk in boys.

While few school-based programs have focused on ED prevention exclusively in boys, programs have targeted athletes' use of appearance- and performance-enhancing drugs (APEDs). Specifically, the Athletes Training and Learning to Avoid Steroids (*ATLAS*) program, which focuses on preventing steroid and food supplement abuse, has been well researched among boys and men. Originally developed as a selective prevention program with high school athletes [26–28], it uses a multifactorial approach to change group norms, increase skills, and promote media literacy. The program has been successful in reducing both the intention to use steroids and use of APEDs in male athletes [27, 28], with research demonstrating that effects are mediated by changes in team norms around steroid use and knowledge and perceived severity of anabolic steroids [28]. Further, recent research has supported the utility of *ATLAS* in improving functional and aesthetic body satisfaction and attitudes toward supplement use in non-athlete boy high school students compared to waitlist control [29]. Results support that programs focused on targeting relevant risk factors for appearance-based concerns in boys can be efficacious in improving body image and attitudes and, potentially, the use of unhealthy substances.

In-Person Cognitive-Behavioral Programs in Adults (See Table 13.2)

In meta-analyses of cognitive-behavioral ED prevention programs prior to 2007, programs that were associated with greater efficacy were interactive (versus didactic), were selected (versus universal), involved multiple sessions (versus a single session), and included cognitive dissonance-based content [30, 31]. Further, prevention programs targeting women as opposed to mixed-gender programs had better effects; however, none of the programs included in these meta-analyses were specific programs for men only.

Cognitive Dissonance-Based Programs

The *Body Project* is a cognitive dissonance-based program that was originally developed to target and reduce thin-ideal internalization in young women through a series of verbal, written, and behavioral exercises aimed at exploring the negative effects of pursuing the thin ideal of beauty. These exercises generate cognitive dissonance, or psychological discomfort, which prompts participants to reduce their pursuit of this unrealistic ideal, as people are motivated to align their attitudes with their public behaviors [32]. Consistent with the dual pathway model of eating pathology in women [33], reducing internalization of the thin ideal has demonstrated significant reductions in body dissatisfaction, disordered eating symptoms,

Table 13.2 In-person cognitive-behavioral programs in men

	Program (no. of sessions)	Control condition	Age (SD)	N (% male)	Program type	Assessments	Result summary for men
Dissonance-based programs							
Kilpela et al. [38]	Body Project 4 All (2 sessions, 120 minutes)	WL	19.9 (1.2)	185 (38%)	Universal Mixed gender	• Negative affect (PANAS) • Appearance-ideal internalization (SATAQ) • Body satisfaction (BPSSR) • Eating pathology (EDEQ) • Male body attitudes (MBAS)	• Men had improved body satisfaction at post, 2-month, and 6-month follow-up • Men did not show improvements in eating pathology or internalization • Improved negative affect scores at post only • Improved muscularity dissatisfaction through 2-month but not 6-month follow-up
Brown et al. [36]	Body Project: More than Muscles (2 sessions, 120 minutes)	Assessment only	20.4 (2.4)	93 (100%)	Selected: body or muscle dissatisfaction Men only Peer-led	• Body-ideal internalization (SATAQ) • Dietary restraint (EDEQ) • Bulimic symptoms (EDEQ) • Muscularity and body fat dissatisfaction (MBAS) • Drive for muscularity (DMS) • Muscle dysmorphia (MDDI)	• Decreases in body-ideal internalization, dietary restraint, bulimic symptoms, muscle dysmorphia symptoms, and drive for muscularity, and at post and 1-month follow-up • Improvements in body fat and muscularity dissatisfaction at follow-up

(continued)

Table 13.2 (continued)

	Program (no. of sessions)	Control condition	Age (SD)	N (% male)	Program type	Assessments	Result summary for men
Jankowski et al. [37]	Body Project M (2 sessions, 90 minutes)	Assessment only	20.8 (4.5)	108 (100%)	Universal Men only Clinician-led	• Body fat dissatisfaction (MBAS-R) • Drive for muscularity (DMS) • Body appreciation (BAS) • Bulimic pathology (EDEQ) • Appearance comparison (PACS) • Body-ideal internalization (SATAQ)	• Improvements on body-ideal internalization and muscularity dissatisfaction at post (nonsignificant at 3-month follow-up) • Results favored men who reported higher body-ideal internalization at BL • No improvements on eating pathology
Unikel-Santoncini et al. [39]	Body Project: Mexican University Students (5 sessions, 120 mins)	n/a	22.4 (3.5)	133 (21%)	Universal Mixed gender	• Disordered eating behaviors • Internalization of thin ideal (IATI) • Depressive symptoms (CES-R)	• Did not examine gender as a potential moderator of treatment • Large improvements in disordered eating behaviors at 1-year follow-up (based on completer analysis; 44% attrition)

Cognitive-behavioral programs							
Sepulveda et al. [40]	Healthy Eating Workshops (16 weeks, 90 minutes)	Low-risk comparison group	18.2 (0.5)	135 (31.4%)	Universal (intended as indicated EDI >=40) Mixed gender	• Eating pathology (EDI-2) • Body dissatisfaction (BSQ) • Self-esteem (RSES) • Exercise frequency • Knowledge of treatment-seeking	• No benefits for men regarding eating pathology or body dissatisfaction • Dieting rates significantly higher in comparison group • Marginal evidence of worsening of drive for thinness and body satisfaction in intervention group • Treatment-seeking knowledge significantly higher in comparison group
Cognitive-behavioral programs for sexual minority males							
Brown and Keel [35]	PRIDE Body Project (2 sessions, 120 minutes)	Assessment only	21.48 (2.5)	87 (100%)	Selected: sexual minority Men only	• Body dissatisfaction (BSQ) • Drive for muscularity (DMS) • Body-ideal internalization (SATAQ) • Restraint, bulimic symptoms (EDEQ) • Self- and partner objectification (SOQ)	• Decreases in body dissatisfaction, drive for muscularity, self-objectification, partner objectification, dietary restraint, and bulimic symptoms at post and 1-month follow-up • Body-ideal internalization was lower at post but not at follow-up

(continued)

Table 13.2 (continued)

	Program (no. of sessions)	Control condition	Age (SD)	N (% male)	Program type	Assessments	Result summary for men
Blashill et al. [44]	CBT-Body Image and Self-Care (12 sessions, 50 minutes)	Enhanced treatment as usual	Not reported	44 (100%)	Indicated (HIV+) Men only	• Body image disturbance (BDD-YBOCS) • Medication adherence • Depressive symptoms (MADRS) • Global functioning (GAF)	• Body image significantly improved through 6-month follow-up • Depressive symptoms and global functioning improved through 6-month follow-up • Medication adherence improved through follow-up

Note. *AUDIT*-C Alcohol Use Disorders Identification Test-Consumption, *BAS* Body Appreciation Scale, *BDD-YBOCS* Body Dysmorphic Disorder-Yale-Brown Obsessive-Compulsive Scale, *BFQ* Body Figure Questionnaire, *BPSSR* Body Parts Satisfaction Scale-Revised, *BSQ* Body Shape Questionnaire, *CDI* Child Depression Inventory, *CESR* Center for Epidemiologic Studies Revised Depression Scale, *DASS* Depression Anxiety Stress Scales, *DMS* Drive for Muscularity Scale, *EDE*-Q Eating Diagnostic Examination Questionnaire, *FFQ* Food Frequency Questionnaire, *GAF* Global Assessment of Functioning, *IES-2* Intuitive Eating Scale-2, *MADRS* Montgomery-Asberg Depression Rating Scale, *MBAS* Male Body Attitudes Scale, *MBICS* Male Body Image Concerns Scale, *MDDI* Muscle Dysmorphic Disorder Inventory, *PACS* Physical Appearance Comparison Scale, *PANAS* Positive and Negative Affect Schedule, *PAQ* Paffenbarger Activity Questionnaire, *SATAQ* Sociocultural Attitudes Towards Appearance Questionnaire, *SCL-90-R* Self-Report Symptom Checklist, *SOQ* Self-Objectification Questionnaire, *WCS* Weight Concerns Scale, *WL* waitlist and the likelihood of developing an ED in young women through a 3-year follow-up (see Becker and Stice [34] for review).

Despite the relevance of targeting internalization of the increasingly lean and muscular ideal for men in western culture, men were not included in dissonance-based interventions until recently. To ensure relevance for men (including the differences between internalization concerns), the *Body Project* was modified for use with men-only and mixed-gender samples. These *Body Project* variants designed specifically for men include the *PRIDE Body Project* [35] (to be discussed in the next section), the *Body Project: More Than Muscles* (*MTM*; [36]), and the *Body Project M* (*BPM*; [37]). Of the latter two, *MTM* is a selected prevention program, whereas *BPM* is a universal prevention program. Despite *MTM* and *BPM* being created for men only, results varied between these two programs. *MTM* found significant and large improvements in eating pathology and muscle dysmorphia symptoms post-intervention and at 1-month follow-up [36]. *BPM* reported significant differences at post-intervention for muscularity dissatisfaction and internalization of appearance ideals; however, these were not significant at 3-month follow-up. The divergent results observed here are consistent with the selected program (*MTM*) outperforming the universal program (*BPM*). It is not clear if the different program lengths (4 hours *MTM* versus 3 hours *BPM*), group size (4–10 *MTM* versus 2–6 *BPM*), facilitator features (one female graduate clinician with male peer facilitators *MTM* versus one graduate male clinician *BPM*), or randomization status (yes *MTM* versus no *BPM*) further contributed to differential effects. However, these findings converge with previous reviews regarding effective elements of ED prevention programs [30, 31].

Variants of the *Body Project* have also included mixed-gender groups, with lesser effects found for men. In the *Body Project 4 All* [38], men experienced general body image improvement at post-intervention and 2- and 6-month follow-up; however, body-ideal internalization and ED psychopathology did not show improvement. Men also demonstrated improvements in muscularity dissatisfaction at post-intervention and 2-month, but not 6-month, follow-up. Another mixed-gender group, an expanded 10-hour *Body Project* program delivered in Mexico, did not analyze men separately and lacked a comparison group [39]; thus results for men are unknown.

ED Prevention Interventions Without Dissonance-Based Elements

Consistent with results in women supporting increased efficacy when using dissonance-based content in ED prevention programs, few cognitive-behavioral programs exist for adult men that do not primarily feature cognitive dissonance-based activities and strategies. One such program is the *Healthy Eating Workshop* (*HEW*; [40]), a mixed-gender program implemented as a college course. Disseminated across 16 weeks, this program featured guest speakers, role-play, drama, games, videos, and media literacy aimed at improving body image and eating pathology for men and women. It included non-ED-related topics as well (e.g., self-esteem, relaxation, and coping skills). Due to low base rates, small samples, and high attrition, the final sample used for analyses failed to retain any men with high risk for eating pathology. The resulting comparisons for men reflect a universal design, which did not yield any significant benefits.

Cognitive-Behavioral Programs for Sexual Minority Males

The increased prevalence rates of EDs among sexual minority men (gay, bisexual+) highlight the need for effective interventions among this population [41]. Despite this increased risk, existing interventions for this population were almost non-existent until recently. Using a sociocultural perspective, the *PRIDE Body Project* [35] uses the cognitive dissonance-based approach to address risk factors relevant to sexual minority men. Results from a randomized control trial showed that *PRIDE Body Project* program was associated with significantly greater decreases in bulimic symptoms, body dissatisfaction, drive for muscularity, self-objectification, partner-objectification, body-ideal internalization, and dietary restraint compared to assessment-only control from pre- to post-intervention. Improvements were maintained at 4-week follow-up, with the exception of body-ideal internalization. Additional analyses demonstrated that the intervention's effects on bulimic symptoms were mediated by reductions in body-ideal internalization, supporting models of ED risk in sexual minority men [35].

Increased risk for body image concerns and EDs among sexual minority men can be compounded for those diagnosed with human immunodeficiency virus (HIV), particularly when viewed in light of the premium placed on appearance concerns [42]. It is not uncommon for HIV and antiretroviral therapy (ART) treatments to result in undesirable bodily changes, spawning a potentially cyclical risk for increased body image disturbances, depressive symptoms, and poor ART adherence. Thus, recent programs have targeted body image concerns and their link to ART adherence for sexual minority men diagnosed with HIV. A group intervention targeting body image and healthy eating [43] aimed to improve immune system health and reduce the risk of poor ART adherence using cognitive dissonance-based activities, media literacy, nutrition education, and awareness-building. The program was well-accepted; however, the authors did not evaluate intervention efficacy. Another more recent program, *Cognitive Behavioral Treatment for Body Image and Self-Care* (*CBT-BISC*; [44]) was created to improve body image and quality of life for sexual minority men with HIV. Importantly, *CBT-BISC* led to significant and large effects on body image disturbance at post, 3-month, and 6-month follow-up, and for depression at 6-month follow-up, compared to enhanced treatment as usual. Finally, ART adherence was high, but results varied based on the methodology used to measure adherence, and unusually high baseline rates signify a potential ceiling effect for this sample.

Internet-Based Programs

Recently, ED prevention programs have also been delivered in online formats. Internet-based prevention programs can help minimize barriers to treatment, reduce in-person clinical demands, increase access to services, and reduce costs compared to in-person delivery methods. For boys and men, Internet-based programs may be especially helpful to address barriers to in-person programs around body image, such as stigma. Currently no Internet-based programs have been developed specifically for men; thus, in this section, we review screening and Internet-based intervention programs currently available for mixed-gender groups.

Screening Programs

The rise of mental health concerns on college campuses, and ED symptomatology in particular, has spawned interest in effective screening measures to improve prevention efforts and identify individuals in need of services. Using a five-item ED screener, Eisenberg and colleagues [45] found positive screens for 9–13% of women and 3–4% of men. This 3:1 women-to-men ratio was in contrast to the lifetime ED diagnostic rate of 20:1 women-to-men and the commonly quoted 10:1 rate for ED prevalence, providing a clear rationale for including both men and women in such efforts.

Although a variety of screeners and Internet-based programs exist, evidence remains underdeveloped regarding the efficacy of Internet-based interventions [46]. However, a recent meta-analysis supported that Internet-based programs as a whole are successful at reducing ED risk, with small but significant effects on reducing symptoms, albeit primarily in women [47]. Programs for mixed-gender population screening include *ProYouth*, a European-based program [48, 49], and the *Healthy Body Study* (a population-level survey [50]). Designed to prevent EDs and enhance treatment utilization for men and women, the efficacy of *ProYouth* is currently unknown. The *Healthy Body Study*, however, is part of a network designed to provide referrals and Internet-based interventions based on risk level and uses one of the most studied Internet-based prevention programs for women – *Student Bodies*. The *Student Bodies* program utilizes traditional cognitive-behavioral prevention techniques to improve knowledge of ED risk factors, body image, unhealthy weight regulation behaviors, and ED behaviors [51]. Results from the *Healthy Body Study* are used to refer individuals to appropriate Internet-based interventions from a group of programs referred to collectively as *Healthy Body Image* [52]. Those with low risk for ED and/or obesity are referred to *Staying Fit* [53], individuals with high-risk for ED are referred to *Student Bodies*, and those with subclinical or clinical symptoms are recommended for more intense interventions including clinician referrals [54]. The potential benefits of using online screeners among populations such as college students are compelling, but the challenge to successfully connect individuals with effective interventions, Internet-based or otherwise, remains. Currently, more work is needed to reach men with these efforts.

Dual-Focused Behavior Modification Programs Targeting Both Weight and ED Symptoms (See Table 13.3)

Given concerns regarding the increasing prevalence and health consequences of obesity, programs have been developed to target dual concerns of both weight and disordered eating behaviors in adolescents and young adults in mixed-gender samples. Further, overweight and/or obesity is associated with body image concerns, greater frequency of weight change behaviors, and binge eating symptoms [55, 56]. Although potential ethical concerns have been raised that obesity interventions could place participants at risk for EDs, especially children and adolescents [57], only two of the studies reviewed in this chapter found some evidence for potential iatrogenic effects (i.e., a small temporary increase in dietary restraint [64] and moderate temporary increase in depression and media internalization [21]).

School-Based Programs Targeting Weight and ED Symptoms

One school-based program targeting eating and weight is *Healthy Buddies* [58], a peer-based program in which 4th–7th grade girls and boys are paired with a student in K–3rd grade to promote a healthy body image, physical activity, and eating healthy foods. Compared with students in school as usual, both older and younger students in *Healthy Buddies* showed an increase in healthy living knowledge, behavior, and attitude scores. Compared to control, weight increased less in the students participating in *Healthy Buddies* in 4th through 7th grade, and height increased more in the *Healthy Buddies* condition for kindergarten through 3rd grade. Notably, body image and eating pathology were not significantly improved by the intervention, and the authors did not examine gender as a potential moderator of outcomes. Wilksch and colleagues [21] developed and evaluated *LifeSmart*, a universal program targeting risk factors shared between both EDs and obesity, and compared this program to (i) Media Smart; (ii) Helping, Encouraging, Listening, and Protecting Peers (HELPP, a more focused ED prevention program); and (iii) class as usual. *LifeSmart* resulted in improvements in body satisfaction compared to class as usual but did not result in greater improvements in physical activity, mood, body mass index, or eating pathology. Further, the program was associated with increases in depression and internalization of appearance ideals from media through follow-up. Thus, while programs have aimed to target both risk factors for EDs and obesity, there is little evidence that these programs have been successful thus far at achieving both aims for boys.

Table 13.3 Dual-focused behavior modification programs targeting both weight and ED symptoms for boys and men

Authors	Program (no. of sessions)	Control condition	Age	N (% male)	Program type	Assessments	Result summary for boys and men
School-based behavior modification-based programs targeting weight and eating							
Stock et al. [58]	Healthy Buddies (21 weeks)	Class as usual	K–3rd and 4th–7th grade	382 (41.8%)	Universal Mixed gender	• Healthy living questionnaire • Self-competence (Perceived Self-Competence Scale) • Body image (Figure Rating Scale) • Eating pathology (ChEAT)	• All students improved in healthy living knowledge, behavior, and attitudes • Weight increased less in the 4th–7th graders in Healthy Buddies • Height increased more in the K–3rd graders in Healthy Buddies • Body image and eating pathology were not significantly improved • Did not examine gender as a potential moderator of treatment
Programs targeting weight and ED symptoms in adult men							
Stice et al. [60]	Healthy Weight (6 sessions, 60 minutes)	Obesity prevention and obesity education video control	19.3 (1.2)	148 (28%)	Selected: weight, diet, and exercise concerns Mixed gender	• BMI • Eating pathology (EDDI) • Dietary intake (BFFQ)	• Did not examine gender as a potential moderator of treatment • HW had improved ED symptoms than obesity prevention and video control groups • BMI was maintained with HW and increased in obesity prevention at post and 6-month follow-up • HW had lower BMI v. video control (NS compared to obesity prevention)

(continued)

Table 13.3 (continued)

Authors	Program (no. of sessions)	Control condition	Age	N (% male)	Program type	Assessments	Result summary for boys and men
Stice et al. [61]	Project Health (6 sessions, 60 minutes)	Healthy Weight and video control	19.1 (1.2)	364 (28%)	Selected: weight, diet, and exercise concerns Mixed gender	• Obesity onset (BMI) • Eating pathology (EDDI) • ED onset (EDDI)	• Did not examine gender as a potential moderator of treatment • HW and PH had lower ED symptoms than controls (small effect) post and through 2-year follow-up • PH smaller increases in BMI through 2-year follow-up than controls and HW (small effect) • PH had lower overweight and obesity onset than HW and controls (41% reduction in onset vs HW and 43% reduction vs controls) • HW and PH had a trend towards lower onset of ED than controls (62% reduction for both)
Rohde et al. [63]	Project Health (6 sessions, 60 minutes)	Same as above	Same as above		Same as above	• Obesity onset (BMI) • Eating pathology (EDDI) • ED onset (EDDI) • Body dissatisfaction (BES) • Negative affect (PANAS) • Physical activity (PAQ) • Dietary intake (BFFQ)	• Did not examine gender as a potential moderator of treatment • PH and HW had reduced body dissatisfaction and negative affect vs control

Castillo et al. [62]	OBEyTA, Mexican University (8 sessions, 90 minutes)	Study skills control and assess-ment-only control	19.8 (2.1)	388 (32%)	Universal Mixed gender	• Media internalization (SATAQ-3) • Eating pathology (EAT-26) • Male body dissatisfaction (MBAS) • Physical activity (IPAQ) and BMI	• No significant effects for men on any variable in completer sample
Internet-based programs targeting both weight and ED symptoms							
Doyle et al. [66]	Student Bodies 2 (16 weeks; expected range 60–120 min-utes)	Usual care WL	12–17-year olds; 14.9 (1.7)	80 (37.5%)	Indicated (>= 85th percentile weight) Mixed gender	• BMI • Body image and eating pathology (EDEQ)	• Did not examine gender as a potential moderator of treatment • Adolescents in SB2 achieved modest reduction in BMI at post, not at follow-up • Dietary restraint increased in SB2 at post Shape concerns decreased in WL control group at follow-up • Body image and eating pathology were not significantly improved
Jones et al. [67]	Student Bodies 2 – Binge ED (16 weeks, unknown)	WL	15.1 (1.0)	105 (30.5%)	Indicated (>= 85th percentile weight) Mixed gender	• BMI • Binge eating/ overeating (EBI) • Weight/shape concerns • Dietary fat and sugar intake • Depressive mood (CESDS)	• Did not examine gender as a potential moderator of treatment • Improvements in maintaining BMI and reduced weight and shape concerns (completer analysis) • No differences in dietary fat intake or depressive symptoms

Note. *BES* Body Esteem Scale, *BFFQ* Block Food Frequency Questionnaire, *BMI* body mass index, *CESDS* Center for Epidemiologic Studies Depression Scale, *ChEAT* Child Eating Attitudes Test, *EAT-26* Eating Attitudes Test, *EBI* Eating Behavior Inventory, *EDDI* Eating Disorder Diagnostic Interview, *EDE-*Q Eating Diagnostic Examination Questionnaire, *IPAQ* International Physical Activity Questionnaire (short version), *MBAS* Male Body Attitudes Scale, *PANAS* Positive and Negative Affect Schedule, *PAQ* Physical Activity Questionnaire, *SATAQ* Sociocultural Attitudes Towards Appearance Scale

Programs Targeting Weight and ED Symptoms in Adult Men

Three dual-focused mixed-gender programs have been evaluated in adults: *Healthy Weight* (*HW*; [59, 60]), *Project Health* (*PH*; [61]), and OBEyTA [62]. *HW* utilizes cognitive-behavioral strategies such as psychoeducation, goal setting, behavioral interventions, and body acceptance to assist participants in making small, incremental, lifestyle changes to improve their energy balance. *PH* includes cognitive dissonance-based activities making verbal commitments to participate, role-play, and exploring costs of obesity. OBEyTA focuses on raising awareness about appearance and media ideals and addresses other topics including one's self-concept, assertiveness, and perfectionism.

HW and *PH* had similar rates of ED symptom reductions and marginally lower rates of ED onset as compared to controls [61]. Analyzed as a combined intervention group, they had significantly lower body dissatisfaction than controls [63]. *PH* had superior outcomes regarding BMI and overweight and obesity onset as compared to *HW* and controls [61]. Of note, later analyses found that gender did not significantly moderate the effects of either program (*Project Health* or *Healthy Weight*) regarding body mass index or ED symptom changes [64]. Both programs had similar outcomes regarding ED pathology and body dissatisfaction, whereas *PH* outperformed *HW* in the obesity variables. Finally, in a study in which university students were non-randomly assigned to OBEyTA, study skills, or an assessment-only comparison group, post and 3-month follow-up completer analyses for men failed to find benefits for OBEyTA on any ED pathology or body image concern variables compared to either comparison condition [62].

Internet-Based Programs Targeting Both Weight and ED Symptoms

At its inception, *Student Bodies* [65] was designed as a cognitive-behavioral ED prevention program for women only; however, given their focus on reducing obesity and binge eating, concerns which both have a more equivalent gender ratio, two recent adaptations have included men: *Student Bodies 2* (*SB2*; [66]) and *Student Bodies 2 – Binge Eating Disorder* (*SB2-BED*; [67]). The programs use psychoeducation, behavioral activities (self-monitoring, goal setting), and cognitive exercises. Results from the full sample of men and women show that *SB2* did not improve shape and weight concern and temporarily increased dietary restraint. The full sample that received *SB2-BED* yielded modest reduction in body mass index and reduction in binge episodes, but did not improve shape and weight concern. Neither study considered gender as a moderator; thus a summary of the effects for men is not possible.

Conclusions and Future Directions

While the development and evaluation of ED prevention programs for boys and men have grown considerably in the recent years, there is still a dearth of information of efficacious and effective ED prevention programs for boys and men. Lack of funding for ED prevention in men has likely stalled the ability to determine whether current programs can actually prevent ED onset. Indeed, to date, only dual-focused obesity and ED prevention programs in mixed-gender samples (*Healthy Weight* and *Project Health* [61]) have evaluated effects on ED onset in men. Further, few programs for adolescents or adults have demonstrated efficacy in reducing ED symptoms in boys and men or mixed-gender samples, with male-specific variants of the *Body Project* (the *Body Project: MTM* [36] and the *PRIDE Body Project* [35]) and mixed-gender versions of *Healthy Weight*, *Project Health*, *Student Bodies 2*, and *Student Bodies 2 – Binge ED* demonstrating efficacy in this regard. However, the latter two did not examine whether gender moderated treatment effects.

Collapsing across age groups and consistent with Stice and colleagues [30, 31], larger benefits for men have occurred when using selected versus universal prevention approaches. Selected or indicated programs may be particularly relevant for boys and men, as they tend to score lower on traditional measures of ED psychopathology, which may limit the ability to find statistically significant improvements over time in universal samples. Further, female-centric measures may not accurately capture clinically significant symptoms or risk factors for boys and men, thus highlighting the need for future studies to assess constructs and use measures that have been validated in, and are relevant for, boys and men. Notably, although many school-based programs and some programs with young adults are implemented in mixed-gender group formats, it will be essential for future research to investigate whether gender moderates intervention effects. Indeed, most mixed-gender programs fail to report results for boys and men only and generally report weaker full sample effects than single gender programs. While Internet-based programs have promise to address barriers to treatment for boys and men, none of these programs have been primarily developed to address male-specific ED risk factors. Thus, more research in online interventions for men are needed. Overall, ED prevention programs for men have made notable progress in recent decades, and there are several programs that hold promise for preventing the onset of EDs. Continued research on this topic has the capacity to reduce the public health burden and stigma associated with EDs in boys and men.

Conflict of Interest Dr. Brown is a master trainer for the Body Project Collaborative.

References

1. Strother E, Lemberg R, Stanford SC, Turberville D. Eating disorders in men: underdiagnosed, undertreated, and misunderstood. Eat Disord. 2012;20(5):346–55.
2. Hudson JI, Hiripi E, Pope HG Jr, Kessler RC. The prevalence and correlates of eating disorders in the National Comorbidity Survey Replication. Biol Psychiatry. 2007;61(3):348–58.
3. Pope HG Jr, Gruber AJ, Choi P, Olivardia R, Phillips KA. Muscle dysmorphia. An underrecognized form of body dysmorphic disorder. Psychosomatics. 1997;38(6):548–57.
4. Olivardia R, Pope HG Jr, Hudson JI. Muscle dysmorphia in male weightlifters: a case-control study. Am J Psychiatry. 2000;157(8):1291–6.
5. Bramon-Bosch E, Troop NA, Treasure JL. Eating disorders in males: a comparison with female patients. Eur Eat Disord Rev. 2000;8(4):321–8.
6. Griffiths S, Hay P, Mitchison D, Mond JM, McLean SA, Rodgers B, et al. Sex differences in the relationships between body dissatisfaction, quality of life and psychological distress. Aust N Z J Public Health. 2016;40(6):518–22.
7. Griffiths S, Mond JM, Li Z, Gunatilake S, Murray SB, Sheffield J, et al. Self-stigma of seeking treatment and being male predict an increased likelihood of having an undiagnosed eating disorder. Int J Eat Disord. 2015;48(6):775–8.
8. Striegel-Moore RH, Leslie D, Petrill SA, Garvin V, Rosenheck RA. One-year use and cost of inpatient and outpatient services among female and male patients with an eating disorder: evidence from a national database of health insurance claims. Int J Eat Disord. 2000;27(4):381–9.
9. Brown TA, Keel PK. Current and emerging directions in the treatment of eating disorders. Subst Abus. 2012;6:33–61.
10. Keel PK, Brown TA. Update on course and outcome in eating disorders. Int J Eat Disord. 2010;43(3):195–204.
11. O'Connell ME, Boat T, Warner KE. Preventing mental, emotional, and behavioral disorders among young people: progress and possibilities. Washington, DC: National Academies Press; 2009.
12. Neumark-Sztainer D, Levine MP, Paxton SJ, Smolak L, Piran N, Wertheim EH. Prevention of body dissatisfaction and disordered eating: what next? Eat Disord. 2006;14(4):265–85.
13. Udo T, Grilo CM. Prevalence and correlates of DSM-5–defined eating disorders in a nationally representative sample of US adults. Biol Psychiatry. 2018;84(5):345–54.
14. Kater KJ, Rohwer J, Levine MP. An elementary school project for developing healthy body image and reducing risk factors for unhealthy and disordered eating. Eat Disord. 2000;8(1):3–16.
15. Smolak L, Levine MP, Schermer F. A controlled evaluation of an elementary school primary prevention program for eating problems. J Psychosom Res. 1998;44(3–4):339–53.
16. Bird EL, Halliwell E, Diedrichs PC, Harcourt D. Happy being me in the UK: a controlled evaluation of a school-based body image intervention with pre-adolescent children. Body Image. 2013;10(3):326–34.
17. O'Dea JA, Abraham S. Improving the body image, eating attitudes, and behaviors of young male and female adolescents: a new educational approach that focuses on self-esteem. Int J Eat Disord. 2000;28(1):43–57.
18. Varnado-Sullivan PJ, Zucker N, Williamson DA, Reas D, Thaw J, Netemeyer SB. Development and implementation of the Body Logic Program for adolescents: a two-stage prevention program for eating disorders. Cogn Behav Pract. 2001;8(3):248–59.
19. Stanford JN, McCabe MP. Evaluation of a body image prevention programme for adolescent boys. Eur Eat Disord Rev Prof J Eat Disord Assoc. 2005;13(5):360–70.
20. Warschburger P, Zitzmann J. The efficacy of a universal school-based prevention program for eating disorders among German adolescents: results from a randomized-controlled trial. J Youth Adolesc. 2018;47(6):1317–31.

21. Wilksch S, Paxton S, Byrne S, Austin S, McLean S, Thompson K, et al. Prevention across the spectrum: a randomized controlled trial of three programs to reduce risk factors for both eating disorders and obesity. Psychol Med. 2015;45(9):1811–23.
22. Wilksch SM, Wade TD. Reduction of shape and weight concern in young adolescents: a 30-month controlled evaluation of a media literacy program. J Am Acad Child Adolesc Psychiatry. 2009;48(6):652–61.
23. Darcy AM, Doyle AC, Lock J, Peebles R, Doyle P, Le Grange D. The Eating Disorders Examination in adolescent males with anorexia nervosa: how does it compare to adolescent females? Int J Eat Disord. 2012;45(1):110–4.
24. Buddeberg-Fischer B, Klaghofer R, Gnam G, Buddeberg C. Prevention of disturbed eating behaviour: a prospective intervention study in 14-to 19-year-old Swiss students. Acta Psychiatr Scand. 1998;98(2):146–55.
25. Gumz A, Weigel A, Daubmann A, Wegscheider K, Romer G, Löwe B. Efficacy of a prevention program for eating disorders in schools: a cluster-randomized controlled trial. BMC Psychiatry. 2017;17(1):293.
26. Goldberg L, Elliot DL, Clarke GN, MacKinnon DP, Zoref L, Moe E, et al. The Adolescents Training and Learning to Avoid Steroids (ATLAS) prevention program: background and results of a model intervention. Arch Pediatr Adolesc Med. 1996;150(7):713–21.
27. Goldberg L, MacKinnon DP, Elliot DL, Moe EL, Clarke G, Cheong J. The adolescents training and learning to avoid steroids program: preventing drug use and promoting health behaviors. Arch Pediatr Adolesc Med. 2000;154(4):332–8.
28. MacKinnon DP, Goldberg L, Clarke GN, Elliot DL, Cheong J, Lapin A, et al. Mediating mechanisms in a program to reduce intentions to use anabolic steroids and improve exercise self-efficacy and dietary behavior. Prev Sci. 2001;2(1):15–28.
29. Yager Z, McLean SA, Li X. Body image outcomes in a replication of the ATLAS program in Australia. Psychol Men Masc. 2019;20(3):418–28.
30. Stice E, Shaw H. Eating disorder prevention programs: a meta-analytic review. Psychol Bull. 2004;130(2):206–27.
31. Stice E, Shaw H, Marti CN. A meta-analytic review of eating disorder prevention programs: encouraging findings. Annu Rev Clin Psychol. 2007;3:207–31.
32. Festinger L, Carlsmith JM. Cognitive consequences of forced compliance. J Abnorm Soc Psychol. 1959;58(2):203.
33. Stice E. A prospective test of the dual-pathway model of bulimic pathology: mediating effects of dieting and negative affect. J Abnorm Psychol. 2001;110(1):124.
34. Becker CB, Stice E. From efficacy to effectiveness to broad implementation: evolution of the Body Project. J Consult Clin Psychol. 2017;85(8):767.
35. Brown TA, Keel PK. A randomized controlled trial of a peer co-led dissonance-based eating disorder prevention program for gay men. Behav Res Ther. 2015;74:1–10.
36. Brown TA, Forney KJ, Pinner D, Keel PK. A randomized controlled trial of The Body Project: more than muscles for men with body dissatisfaction. Int J Eat Disord. 2017;50(8):873–83.
37. Jankowski GS, Diedrichs PC, Atkinson MJ, Fawkner H, Gough B, Halliwell E. A pilot controlled trial of a cognitive dissonance-based body dissatisfaction intervention with young British men. Body Image. 2017;23:93–102.
38. Kilpela LS, Blomquist K, Verzijl C, Wilfred S, Beyl R, Becker CB. The body project 4 all: a pilot randomized controlled trial of a mixed-gender dissonance-based body image program. Int J Eat Disord. 2016;49(6):591–602.
39. Unikel-Santoncini C, De León-Vázquez CD, Rivera-Márquez JA, Bojorquez-Chapela I, Méndez-Ríos E. Dissonance-based program for eating disorders prevention in Mexican University students. Psychosoc Interv. 2019;28(1):29–35.
40. Sepulveda A, Carrobles J, Gandarillas A, Poveda J, Pastor V. Prevention program for disturbed eating and body dissatisfaction in a Spanish university population: a pilot study. Body Image. 2007;4(3):317–28.

41. Feldman MB, Meyer IH. Eating disorders in diverse lesbian, gay, and bisexual populations. Int J Eat Disord. 2007;40(3):218–26.
42. Kelly JS, Langdon D, Serpell L. The phenomenology of body image in men living with HIV. AIDS Care. 2009;21(12):1560–7.
43. Feldman MB, Torino JA, Swift M. A group intervention to improve body image satisfaction and dietary habits in gay and bisexual men living with HIV/AIDS. Eat Disord. 2011;19(5):377–91.
44. Blashill AJ, Safren SA, Wilhelm S, Jampel J, Taylor SW, O'Cleirigh C, et al. Cognitive behavioral therapy for body image and self-care (CBT-BISC) in sexual minority men living with HIV: a randomized controlled trial. Health Psychol. 2017;36(10):937.
45. Eisenberg D, Nicklett EJ, Roeder K, Kirz NE. Eating disorder symptoms among college students: prevalence, persistence, correlates, and treatment-seeking. J Am Coll Health. 2011;59(8):700–7.
46. Aardoom JJ, Dingemans AE, Spinhoven P, Van Furth EF. Treating eating disorders over the internet: a systematic review and future research directions. Int J Eat Disord. 2013;46(6):539–52.
47. Melioli T, Bauer S, Franko DL, Moessner M, Ozer F, Chabrol H, et al. Reducing eating disorder symptoms and risk factors using the internet: a meta-analytic review. Int J Eat Disord. 2016;49(1):19–31.
48. Moessner M, Minarik C, Ozer F, Bauer S. Effectiveness and cost-effectiveness of school-based dissemination strategies of an internet-based program for the prevention and early intervention in eating disorders: a randomized trial. Prev Sci. 2016;17(3):306–13.
49. Moessner M, Minarik C, Özer F, Bauer S. Can an internet-based program for the prevention and early intervention in eating disorders facilitate access to conventional professional healthcare? J Ment Health. 2016;25(5):441–7.
50. Lipson SK, Jones JM, Taylor CB, Wilfley DE, Eichen DM, Fitzsimmons-Craft EE, et al. Understanding and promoting treatment-seeking for eating disorders and body image concerns on college campuses through online screening, prevention and intervention. Eat Behav. 2017;25:68–73.
51. Winzelberg AJ, Eppstein D, Eldredge KL, Wilfley D, Dasmahapatra R, Dev P, et al. Effectiveness of an internet-based program for reducing risk factors for eating disorders. J Consult Clin Psychol. 2000;68(2):346.
52. Jones M, Lynch KT, Kass AE, Burrows A, Williams J, Wilfley DE, et al. Healthy weight regulation and eating disorder prevention in high school students: a universal and targeted web-based intervention. J Med Internet Res. 2014;16(2):e57.
53. Taylor C, Taylor K, Jones M, Shorter A, Yee M, Genkin B, et al. Obesity prevention in defined (high school) populations. Int J Obes Suppl. 2012;2(S1):S30.
54. Wilfley DE, Agras WS, Taylor CB. Reducing the burden of eating disorders: a model for population-based prevention and treatment for university and college campuses. Int J Eat Disord. 2013;46(5):529.
55. Boutelle K, Neumark-Sztainer D, Story M, Resnick M. Weight control behaviors among obese, overweight, and nonoverweight adolescents. J Pediatr Psychol. 2002;27(6):531–40.
56. Reas DL, Grilo CM. Timing and sequence of the onset of overweight, dieting, and binge eating in overweight patients with binge eating disorder. Int J Eat Disord. 2007;40(2):165–70.
57. Schwartz MB, Henderson KE. Does obesity prevention cause eating disorders?. J AM Child Adolesc Psychiatry. 2009;48(8):784–86.
58. Stock S, Miranda C, Evans S, Plessis S, Ridley J, Yeh S, et al. Healthy buddies: a novel, peer-led health promotion program for the prevention of obesity and eating disorders in children in elementary school. Pediatrics. 2007;120(4):e1059–e68.
59. Stice E, Shaw H, Burton E, Wade E. Dissonance and healthy weight eating disorder prevention programs: a randomized efficacy trial. J Consult Clin Psychol. 2006;74(2):263–75.
60. Stice E, Yokum S, Burger K, Rohde P, Shaw H, Gau JM. A pilot randomized trial of a cognitive reappraisal obesity prevention program. Physiol Behav. 2015;138:124–32.

61. Stice E, Rohde P, Shaw H, Gau JM. An experimental therapeutics test of whether adding dissonance-induction activities improves the effectiveness of a selective obesity and eating disorder prevention program. Int J Obes (Lond). 2018;42(3):462–8.
62. Castillo I, Solano S, Sepúlveda AR. A controlled study of an integrated prevention program for improving disordered eating and body image among Mexican University students: a 3-month follow-up. Eur Eat Disord Rev. 2019;27(5):541–56.
63. Rohde P, Desjardins CD, Arigo D, Shaw H, Stice E. Mediators of two selective prevention interventions targeting both obesity and eating disorders. Behav Res Ther. 2018;106:8–17.
64. Stice E, Desjardins CD, Shaw H, Rohde P. Moderators of two dual eating disorder and obesity prevention programs. Behav Res Ther. 2019;118:77–86.
65. Taylor CB, Bryson S, Luce KH, Cunning D, Doyle AC, Abascal LB, et al. Prevention of eating disorders in at-risk college-age women. Arch Gen Psychiatry. 2006;63(8):881–8.
66. Doyle AC, Goldschmidt A, Huang C, Winzelberg AJ, Taylor CB, Wilfley DE. Reduction of overweight and eating disorder symptoms via the internet in adolescents: a randomized controlled trial. J Adolesc Health. 2008;43(2):172–9.
67. Jones M, Luce KH, Osborne MI, Taylor K, Cunning D, Doyle AC, et al. Randomized, controlled trial of an internet-facilitated intervention for reducing binge eating and overweight in adolescents. Pediatrics. 2008;121(3):453–62.

Chapter 14
Psychotherapy with Men with Eating Disorders: The Influence of Gender Socialization and Masculine Gender Norms on Engagement and Treatment

Douglas W. Bunnell

Learning Objectives
1. Readers will review differences in the clinical presentations of EDs in men and women.
2. Readers will explore how adherence to masculine gender norms affects help-seeking and therapeutic engagement.
3. Readers will learn specific strategies for adapting the structure and language of psychotherapy to improve therapeutic engagement.

Key Points
- Clinical presentations of EDs in men and women are subtly but significantly different, and these differences may reflect the impact of gender socialization.
- Adherence to masculine gender norms interferes with detection, assessment, treatment planning, and treatment delivery for men with EDs.
- Treatment of men and women with EDs is largely similar, but addressing the impact of gender can facilitate effective treatment.
- Exploration of gender socialization and beliefs about masculinity helps clinicians develop an understanding of core beliefs and cognitions that maintain men's EDs and increase the risk for relapse.
- Clinicians need to be aware of their own gender biases about men and about men in psychotherapy.

D. W. Bunnell (✉)
Private Practice, Westport, CT, USA

J. M. Nagata et al. (eds.), *Eating Disorders in Boys and Men*,
https://doi.org/10.1007/978-3-030-67127-3_14

Psychotherapy with Men with Eating Disorders: The Influence of Gender Socialization and Masculine Gender Norms on Engagement and Treatment

What used to be uncertain is now incontrovertibly true. Men struggle with eating disorders (EDs) at rates that belie the persistent myth that these disorders only affect girls and women. In the past decade, we have developed greater awareness of the prevalence of EDs in non-typical populations including men, older individuals, people of color, and people in bodies that do not fit the underweight stereotype. We now recognize that many people dealing with EDs have been hiding in plain sight.

This chapter will focus on some of the unique aspects of the treatment of EDs in men. The fundamental components of the treatment of EDs are, as noted in a number of other chapters in this book, similar for both men and women. But there are critical differences in the clinical presentations of EDs across genders that need to shape treatment. Our conceptual models for both the etiology and maintenance of EDs remain highly gendered and reflect our wealth of information about EDs in women. Most of what we know about EDs remains grounded in what we know about women with EDs. We know much less about the temperamental vulnerability of men to EDs, the psychological motivations and underpinnings of men's ED psychopathology, and the developmental phenomenology of EDs in men across the lifespan. Retrofitting conceptual and treatment models based on the experiences of women with EDs can take us only part of the way.

Community sample surveys indicate that up to one in three individuals with EDs is a man but many fewer men actually present for treatment [1]. Men are also vastly underrepresented in ED research. Gorrell and Murray reported that only 1% of peer-reviewed articles focus exclusively on men [2]. There is a comparable gap in clinical training. Most clinicians have had little to no direct experience treating men with EDs, in some large part because men do not present for treatment as often [3]. The gap between community prevalence and referral for treatment remains substantial and reflects the lack of awareness about men with EDs as well as more general sociocultural phenomena such as mental health stigma and masculine gender socialization. This latter factor is a significant issue in understanding the unique treatment needs of men with EDs [4]. It has an enormous impact on men's perception and experience of treatment. Addressing the implications of masculine gender socialization represents one of the best opportunities for effectively adapting existing ED treatments for men with these disorders.

Following a brief overview of the unique aspects of the clinical presentations of men with EDs, this chapter will explore how gender influences treatment. These influences extend into our clinical and conceptual models and particularly into the language we use in treatment. They also shape the clinical relationship. Clinicians and patients bring their own gender expectations into treatment, and these expectations, left unexplored, can limit treatment engagement and effectiveness. The final section of this chapter addresses what clinicians need to know to best identify, engage, and treat men.

How Are Men with EDs Different Than Women with EDs?

The fundamental features of eating psychopathology are consistent across gender. Assessment and treatment for men and women are therefore quite similar in how they address the general core elements of nutrition, cognition, emotion, and development. However, clinicians also need to consider important differences in presentation to increase treatment engagement and efficacy, as outlined below:

Eating Behaviors While most eating disorder behaviors are consistent across gender, men are less likely to report a subjective sense of a loss of control, despite reporting similar rates of objective binge eating compared to women [5]. Men may also have different subjective standards about what constitutes "a large amount of food." Binge eating, or the failure to maintain strict control of eating, is less socially noteworthy in men than in women. It is more culturally normative for men to occasionally overeat, and this norm may contribute to lower rates of detection, referral, and diagnosis of men with this most common type of eating disorder.

Body Image and Weight Body dissatisfaction and the overvaluation of weight and shape are core features of most EDs. Men generally report lower levels of body dissatisfaction compared to women [6], but the nature of the dissatisfaction is gendered [7]. Whereas women generally report decreasing body dissatisfaction as they age, men's body dissatisfaction may increase with age [8]. Men with anorexia nervosa (AN) are more likely to describe a strong fear of weight gain rather than a clear intent to lose weight [9]. Their reluctance to gain weight often reflects concerns regarding the impact of weight gain on body image goals defined by leanness and muscularity but not thinness [10, 11]. Clinical experience suggests that men are less likely to explicitly endorse a desire to lose weight, and this complicates clinical detection and assessment. For many men, anxiety about their bodies is rooted more in concern about losing or lacking muscular definition and not in a clear concern about a particular weight or clothes size [9]. Given the considerable barriers to access to care, men may not enter treatment until their symptoms are especially severe, and they may be particularly medically compromised at the time of initial assessment [12].

Exercise Body-related goals and expectations are often couched in terms of exercise and fitness goals, and clinicians need to carefully explore motivations for exercise regimens. Dedication to exercise and fitness is still more socially consistent and acceptable for boys and men than for girls and women, so excessive exercise may be seen as normative and even admirable. Compulsive exercise can mask underlying anxiety about weight and shape and serves more of an affective regulation function in men than it does in women [13].

Age of Onset There is some discrepancy in the literature about the age of onset of EDs in men with some studies finding that boys and men have a younger age of onset of AN [14], while others report a later onset [15] or no differences between genders [16]. Notably, men may develop medically significant symptoms well before they seek treatment for the disorder [16]. Younger and less developmentally mature patients are often less able to articulate their motivations and feelings about their bodies, weight, shape, and exercise behaviors. This is often compounded by the relatively high rates of boys and men with avoidant/restrictive food intake disorder (ARFID) compared with rates for other EDs. Clinicians may find it difficult to elicit information about the motivations and goals of restricted eating with their patients who are men or young men.

Comorbidity EDs are associated with significant psychiatric comorbidity in populations of both men and women [17]. Depression and anxiety disorders are common [1]. Rates of comorbid PTSD in women with ED are significant, but less is known about comorbid PTSD/trauma reactions in men [18].

Traits and Temperament Traits such as perfectionism, emotional and experiential avoidance, and obsessionality are risk factors for the development and maintenance of AN [19]. Other traits such as impulsivity are thought to be risk factors for binge eating and bulimia nervosa (BN) [19, 20]. Most of the research on the role of traits and temperament is based on the study of women with EDs, but clinical evidence suggests that men with these traits also have a higher risk for EDs. Men in general are more likely to display externalizing trait-based behaviors such as aggression and impulsivity rather than internalizing traits such as perfectionism, which may help to explain the relatively lower rates of AN in men [21]. Emotional expression also differs across gender in that men are more likely to describe physical pain rather than emotional pain and are more likely to express anger and irritability than sadness and flat affect [22]. As such, it is likely that the common manifestations of ED-related temperamental factors that clinicians are familiar with in women may be less obvious or predictable with men.

Sexual Orientation Most men with EDs are heterosexual [23]. But there is strong evidence that the rates of EDs in gay and bisexual men are indeed higher than the rates in heterosexual men [24, 25].

How Does Gender Influence EDs?

The social construct of gender was a central element in early conceptual modes of EDs [26]. The field contested that there was something about being female that was associated with the development of these disorders. Then the pendulum swung toward biological models, and we now recognize that the gender disparity in ED prevalence reflects a mixed array of etiological factors. The following section discusses how gender influences EDs regarding stigma and barriers to treatment, seeking help, motivation, identity and personal meaning, and gender socialization.

Stigma and Barriers to Treatment There are significant structural barriers to the detection, diagnosis, and referral to treatment of men with EDs [27, 28]. The common misperception by professionals, carers, and patients that EDs are limited to young White and underweight women keeps men, older, non-White, and non-underweight people from receiving the care they need. It also limits what we know about people with EDs who do not fit the stereotype. The perception of EDs as "female" disorders can increase self-stigma for men, due to a perceived failure to comply with masculine gender expectations [29], which can in turn create another barrier to seeking treatment. Patients' families and loved ones also internalize these stigmas and stereotypes about EDs, which inevitably influence their perceptions of and reactions to their loved ones' struggles. As such, it is essential that psychoeducational curricula reflect the differences in the nature of family members' and loved ones' responses to men with these disorders.

Seeking Help In addition to the structural barriers to detection and referral, men are also less likely than women to seek mental health care even when they are in considerable distress [30, 31]. This discrepancy has enormous implications for research and clinical engagement of men with EDs. Men with EDs delay seeking help and are therefore often sicker for longer before entering treatment [16]. Men are still prone to perceive psychological treatment as an indication of personal defectiveness [32]. Men are also more likely to prematurely drop out of mental health treatment than women [33, 34].

Motivation Ambivalence about weight gain and recovery are cardinal features of EDs. Stigma and concerns about the implications for masculinity can coalesce into a lack of motivation or commitment to change. Clinicians need to adapt the content and language of psychoeducational material developed for women to reflect the gender-specific aspects of eating disorder dynamics and cognitions in men. Men with AN, as noted above, are less likely to articulate concerns about their actual weight or a desire to lose weight. Using conventional ED language and concepts to provide psychoeducation to men runs the risk of providing information that does not match up with their actual experience. This is risky on at least two fronts: the patient will not receive the information he may need, and the clinician may signal a lack of competency around factors relevant to men's EDs. Rather than pursuing detailed inquiry about weight loss goals, drive for thinness, and thinness-related body dissatisfaction, clinicians working with men should focus on concerns about body size and muscle definition. Clinicians can facilitate the exploration of men's motivations and objectives by adopting a "student" stance, asking the patient to "teach" the clinician about the unique aspects of his motivations and goals. This will also signal the clinician's openness to new perspectives that are not rooted in conventional wisdom about women with EDs.

Identity and Personal Meaning Patients, especially those with longer lengths of illness, often describe how their identity has become wrapped up in their ED. Thus, helping patients disentangle their sense of self from their ED is an essential clinical goal. For men with EDs, it is important that clinicians address how the eating disorder symptoms affect their sense of masculine identity. This requires an awareness of how men perceive their symptoms in the context of their masculinity. For men with EDs, the positive benefits often include a sense that their ED behaviors allay fears about softness, weakness, or lack of power. Compared to women, men may be less susceptible to concerns that their actual individual identity is wrapped up in their ED, as EDs may be more ego-dystonic for men. However, anxiety may peak as men gain weight or normalize their eating, and clinicians need to help men address what they are "losing" as they recover.

Gender Socialization There is increasing evidence that the degree of adherence to gender norms influences eating psychopathology [35]. By conventional codes of masculine gender socialization, defined as prioritizing self-reliance, stoicism, negative attitudes toward femininity, and higher levels of sexual objectification, men are prone to see the need for treatment or assistance as a sign of weakness and failure. Fear, or devaluation of "feminine" norms of things like emotional expression, need for interpersonal connection, and vulnerability, may reinforce the belief that their ED is shameful and embarrassing [36]. Masculine gender norms still emphasize stoicism and rationality. Indeed, masculine norms have been associated with specific types of clinical presentations [37–39]. A review on this topic found a strong link between higher levels of masculinity and emotional distress, including depression, substance abuse, and anger [40]. Masculinity norm adherence was also associated with negative attitudes toward help-seeking and with lower levels of mental health [41–43].

There is less research evidence about the impact of masculine gender norm adherence in EDs, but adherence to masculine gender norms was found to be associated with higher rates of AN in both men and women [28, 44]. This suggests that gendered norms such as self-reliance, stoicism, and aggression may reinforce the temperamental, nutritional, and interpersonal maintaining factors for EDs. Further, adherence to masculine norms is particularly associated with muscularity-oriented disordered eating in men [4]. These gendered trait-based maintenance factors are important treatment targets in psychotherapy. Clinicians need to attend to the implications of masculine gender identity on issues such as intimacy, communication, power, health care, parenthood, sexuality, and performance [45, 46]. Each of these areas can shape each individual's unique constellation of factors that caused and that maintain his ED.

Many men with EDs describe experiences of teasing and bullying [47], including being bullied for their weight, shape, or level of muscularity. Kindlon, Thompson, and Barker described the "culture of cruelty" that can characterize the masculine social-developmental milieu, a milieu in which bullying and shaming reinforce avoidance of emotion and that fosters competition and control [48]. These experiences also foster the development of shame-based rules about emotions, vulnerability, and dependence. More specifically, these experiences can become internalized and concretized in men's perceptions of their bodies and their nutritional needs. As men enter treatment for disordered eating, it is essential that clinicians develop an understanding of that individual's history and experience of teasing.

Treatment Outcomes

Variations in the precise definition of recovery from EDs continue to complicate the evaluation of treatment outcomes. Defining recovery as behavioral symptom remission yields vastly different outcomes than using a standard that incorporates robust cognitive, emotional, and nutritional improvement [49]. Research on treatment outcomes for men with EDs has a host of other limitations including small sample sizes, inadequate follow-up periods, and reliance on women-centric assessment instruments that underreport eating psychopathology in men. Table 14.1 summarizes some of the existing outcome research. A host of smaller sample studies yielded a wide range of outcome rates and gender differences [50–53].

Some studies found lower rates of ED diagnoses at follow-up [54]. Others noted nuanced gender differences between men and women with AN related to body dissatisfaction [55] and drive for thinness [56]. Yet, a thorough review concluded that the existing research provided no clear evidence of gender differences in treatment response [57].

The best empirical data on treatment outcomes for men come from studies of inpatient populations. Strobel and colleagues reported on the longer-term outcomes of inpatient treatments of 119 men with AN and 60 men with BN [58]. Remission was defined by no diagnosis of AN, BN, or eating disorder not otherwise specified

Table 14.1 Treatment outcome studies including males

Authors	Year	N	Diagnoses	Length of follow-up
Bardone-Cone et al. [49]	2019	36	Mixed	12 months
Oyebode et al. [51]	1988	13	AN	9.22 years
Herpertz-Dahlmann et al. [52]	2001	7	AN	3, 7, 10 years
Støving et al. [53]	2011	17	Mixed	AN – 4.6 years EDNOS – 4.6 years BN – 6.2 years
Deter et al. [54]	1998	12	AN	12 years
Bean et al. [55]	2004	7	AN	15 months
Strobel et al. [58]	2019	119 – AN 60 – BN	AN, BN	AN – 5.80 years BN – 7.50 years
Fernandez-Aranda et al. [59]	2009	19	BN	12 months
Weltzin et al. [60]	2012	111	Mixed	n/a
Grabhorn et al. [61]	2013	13	AN	2.5 years

(EDNOS) at the time of the follow-up assessment. Men with AN had higher body weights at the end of inpatient treatment, but the remission rates at follow-up were indistinguishable from remission rates for samples of women: 40% vs 41%, respectively. Men with AN had a higher incidence of EDNOS at follow-up and had significantly lower scores on psychological measures of eating disorder cognitions, obsessive-compulsive symptoms, and depression. Men with BN had remission rates comparable to women with BN but did not show higher rates of EDNOS at follow-up. Men with BN, however, did report lower scores on perfectionism and higher scores on interpersonal distrust. The outcome measures did not address cognitions related to the drive for muscularity; however, as noted earlier, this distinction may have skewed the estimate of the severity of eating disorder cognitions and anxiety in men. The authors noted that while treatment appeared to be effective for approximately 40% of men and women, there were important differences in the psychological factors that influence treatment response and risk for relapse. These findings were consistent with prior research [59–61].

The research on treatment outcomes for men with BN is especially limited. Fernandez-Aranda and colleagues reported that 29% of men and 26% of women still had a diagnosis of BN or subthreshold BN 1 year after completing treatment [59]. Earlier studies showed no gender differences in outcome for BN patients [60].

Thus, overall, treatment outcomes appear to be comparable for men and women. It is noteworthy that existing treatments help less than 50% of people of either gender achieve a lasting remission. Strobel and colleagues noted that gendered differences may be disguised in the general findings [58]. They suggest that some men with AN are indistinguishable from women with AN in their focus on a drive for thinness. There appears to be another substantial subgroup of men with AN for whom the driving motivation is related to muscularity rather than thinness [57]. There is a compelling need for further research into these nuanced gender differences and into the particular psychiatric comorbidities of men with both AN and BN.

The expansion of the definition of recovery to include psychological and cognitive maintaining factors complicates research but also enhances clinical conceptualization and treatment planning. Our best existing treatments are not helping at least 50% of men, and women, seeking care. Can a focus on the gendered aspects of EDs help clinicians improve the effectiveness of the treatments they are delivering?

Psychotherapy with Men

Before turning to specific adaptations for the psychotherapeutic treatment of men with EDs, it is useful to briefly review what is known about men in psychotherapy for general mental health concerns. Men are likely to approach treatment with considerable skepticism about the process and goals [62]. They resist, avoid, and drop out of treatment more often and more quickly than women [34, 63]. However, specific clinical "micro skills" or "man-friendly" adjustments may help improve clinical engagement [62, 64]. These include judicious use of clinician self-disclosure, normalization of men's experience and symptoms, deliberate use of masculine-centric language and metaphors (e.g., sports references), and a collaborative treatment relationship that is action oriented, transparent, and focused on clear, behaviorally measurable goals [62].

In addition to these recommendations, there are online mental health resources for men that provide good examples of how psychoeducation crafted with a sensitivity to masculine language and emphasis on positive aspects of traditionally masculine characteristics can minimize stigma and treatment avoidance. One, https://headsupguys.org/mens-depression/, directly challenges common myths and misperceptions that men have about depression (e.g., the myth that "Real men are in control of their emotions and don't let things get to them" is countered with "Real strength is facing whatever challenges arise") [65]. It is important that clinicians avoid a "deficit-based" perspective on how men approach psychotherapeutic engagement [62] and instead look for opportunities to leverage the positive aspects of masculinity in order to improve treatment engagement and outcomes.

Mahalik and colleagues have also written extensively on the issue of men's engagement in psychotherapy [38]. They also emphasize the importance of clinician awareness and knowledge about the influence of gender socialization. Gender issues need to be addressed in the clinical assessment of men seeking mental health care, and the clinical conceptualization and treatment planning should incorporate interventions to address ways that gender beliefs may be influencing symptoms and treatment [38]. The authors stress the importance of helping men find role models, suggesting that men benefit from having access and connection to other men who are dealing with similar issues.

Psychotherapy for Men with Eating Disorders

Most of the psychotherapeutic approaches to the treatment of EDs, particularly CBT (cognitive-behavioral therapy), DBT (dialectical behavior therapy), ACT (acceptance and commitment therapy), IPT (interpersonal psychotherapy), and psychodynamic therapies, emphasize the development of mental perspective and focus on increasing awareness of the connections between thoughts, feelings, and ED behaviors. They also help patients activate affective expression and decrease avoidance of emotion. Attunement to inner experience and affect, and the capacity to communicate that attunement to others, is the essential process of psychotherapy. Men, who may be less socialized and less practiced at the recognition and communication of inner psychological experience, may benefit from adaptations to standard psychotherapy protocols. Clinicians who are more familiar working with women with EDs need to be attuned to how men express and communicate distress, need, anger, and intimacy. Signs of grief, sadness, irritability, and anxiety are often gendered.

If we examine the core components of the current evidence-based treatments for EDs, there are concepts, language, and interventions that clearly reflect a gendered model of the ED. Below are some considerations for how these treatments may be adapted to be more relevant for men with EDs.

Cognitive-Behavioral Therapy The core dimensions of the cognitive model of EDs are dietary restraint, the overvaluation of shape and weight, and the control of eating. Events and associated mood changes are less central features of the model, but they often contribute to the etiology and maintenance of the ED cycles [66]. What does the overvaluation of weight, shape, and control look like for men? Men with EDs are less likely to endorse the concept that their eating concerns are related to conscious concerns about their weight. Their shape concerns are less likely to be focused on a thin ideal; concerns about muscularity are likely to be more prominent. While the general cognitive model may apply to men, it is important for clinicians to explore how the conventional explanations and teaching points in CBT-E can be adapted to better speak to the unique aspects of men's ED behaviors and cognitions.

Interpersonal Psychotherapy IPT is based on a conceptualization of eating psychopathology that emphasizes the role of relationships. The four key modules are grief, interpersonal disputes, interpersonal deficits, and role transitions. Less directive than CBT-E, IPT protocols encourage the patient to drive the process. Men may be less familiar with the language of relationships, so they may feel less adept at directing the therapy process. Grief, for instance, can be experienced as a sign of weakness. Interpersonal disputes and social isolation may be perceived as normative based on masculine gender norms. The notion that his social relationships have an impact on his psychological functioning can threaten the masculine norm of stoicism, emotional control, and self-sufficiency. Clinicians working with men in IPT should be alert to unintentional gender bias that presumes agreement about the centrality of relationships. Men may need additional gender-nuanced education about the underlying rationale of IPT.

Dialectical Behavior Therapy With its emphasis on developing a personalized understanding of each individual's adaptation to their unique biological endowment and environmental experiences, DBT creates a space for a thorough exploration of gender influences. EDs, from a DBT perspective, reflect difficulties in managing intense emotion or, in the case of AN, difficulties with the overcontrol of emotions. Masculine socialization directly influences men's capacity for distress tolerance, their vulnerability to impulsivity, and their view of themselves in their personal relationships. Emotional constriction remains more culturally normative and ego-syntonic for men than it is for women. Many of the standard DBT assignments, educational materials, and coping strategies tend to reflect feminine values such as openness, vulnerability, trust, compromise, and desirability of empathic connection. While these values can and do have deep meaning for many men, their comfort and familiarity with these concepts may be relatively limited, particularly if they strongly conform with masculine gender norms.

Psychodynamic Psychotherapy Psychodynamic models for eating psychopathology emphasize the adaptive functions of the ED behaviors. This approach usually incorporates a focus on the relationship patterns, early attachment experiences, separation-individuation, exploration of psychological conflict, identity development, and capacity for mentalization and mature relatedness. Dynamic models provide an obvious space for the careful consideration of the role of gender socialization. But, as is true with most psychotherapies, psychodynamic concepts and language reflect a bias toward feminine gender norms of emotional expressiveness, intimacy, empathy, relatedness, and vulnerability. Clinicians also value these characteristics and run the risk of subtly communicating that men are somehow less emotionally evolved. This communication can be subtle, although not always, and make it even more difficult for men to settle in and engage in psychotherapy.

The existing ED therapies, from a more general perspective, make use of a variety of concepts that, while relevant for men, may be less personally significant or even discordant. Some of these phrases and concepts have become embedded in our day-to-day ED treatment language. "Fat is not a feeling," "Reach out to people not to your ED," and "Tell me what you think triggered your binge," as examples, have subtle but significant gender implications. Men are less likely to identify with the concept that "fat" is a proxy for an emotional reaction. They are less likely to experience their perceived body imperfections as representative of their emotional state or of their general self-worth. This reflects the reality that men have not historically been as socialized to equate body status with self-esteem as have women. Encouraging men to use their personal relationships as resources for symptom delay works against masculine norms that value self-sufficiency. Even basic interventions such as the exploration of antecedents, behaviors, and consequences, a core feature of virtually all ED treatments, incorporate language that may not click for men. Asking men to identify "triggers" or to elaborate on "how did you feel when that happened" presumes that men are experienced and comfortable with the expression of emotions and that they accept the idea that they are personally affected by interpersonal interactions. It is helpful for clinicians working with men to evaluate men's familiarity with these concepts before moving too quickly into active interventions.

Other common psychotherapeutic terms can gloss over gendered differences. Encouraging patients to be "vulnerable" or to express their "needs" or "fears," while intuitively valid and in many cases strongly supported by research evidence, has potentially different meanings for men. Vulnerability and need violate the masculine code and can evoke defensive withdrawal or avoidance. Pushing for an emotionally charged therapeutic relationship can activate similar reactions from men. Consider some of the terms therapists might use to encourage emotional activation in their work with ED patients: "trust," "open up," "share," "connect," "feel," "emotionally touched," or "moved." While these concepts and terms describe a process that encourages emotional expression, men may not intuitively grasp their relevance for treatment.

What Can Clinicians Do? As noted above, attending to gender issues in the treatment of men with ED is arguably more essential than it may be in the treatment of men with other psychiatric illnesses. Clinicians need to educate themselves about the role of gender socialization on the development of masculine identity. Returning to Seidler's and colleagues' set of recommendations for optimizing psychotherapy with men [62], here are some specific adaptations to conventional ED treatment techniques that can facilitate therapeutic engagement of men with these disorders:

1. *Use therapeutic techniques that have clear, measurable, and attainable goals.* Setting and meeting specific goals will help build motivation and engagement.
2. *Emphasize collaboration.* A hierarchical, therapist-as-expert, stance can activate shame and competition.
3. *Avoid the use of jargon.* Conventional psychotherapy language is gendered and may further activate men's concerns that their ED reveals something about their gender identity.
4. *Explore gender norm expectations as a framework for discussion about core beliefs.* Gender norms influence and reinforce ED thoughts and behaviors.
5. *Discuss connections between adherence to gender norms and ED thoughts, feelings, and behaviors.* This discussion also helps to minimize emotional and experiential avoidance.
6. *Decrease rigidity about gender norm expectations.* Replacing rigid beliefs about what makes him a man with more fluid and adaptive beliefs about masculinity can help to soften rigid beliefs about the body, emotional expression, and vulnerability [67].
7. *Explore personal assumptions about men and men with EDs.* Does the clinician view men as less emotionally evolved than women? Are masculine norms about emotion and vulnerability inherently limiting and destructive? Do they have different emotional reactions to the men they work with than to the women in their practice? Exploring these issues is particularly important when working with men with EDs. Most ED clinicians are women, and most, if not all, of their training experiences have involved working with women with EDs. There is an inevitable pressure, conscious, or otherwise, to understand men with EDs through the lens of one's own personal and professional experiences. These biases show up in a variety of subtle ways from the office design and décor to the way clinicians address their patients. What might it mean, for instance, if one tends to address men by their last name but women by their first name?
8. *Explore how gender influences the therapeutic relationship.* Men may feel less immediately comfortable working with clinicians who are women given the potential for shame and avoidance. These reactions can be minimized by proactively introducing the issue of the gender difference and exploring the patient's experience of requesting help from a woman. Clinicians who are men, by virtue of their own gender socialization, are prone to their own avoidance of emotionality. They should ensure that they do not communicate a "C'mon be a man" reaction or a reaction of discomfort with men's emotionality [68]. They may be particularly prone to avoid deeper emotional content and should be alert to tendencies to steer the discussion to neutral or safe topics.

Countertransference Implicit biases about gender influence the clinician's emotional response as well. Countertransference, defined as the full range of the clinicians' emotional responses to their patient, is an important source of information in psychotherapy [69]. Since most clinicians have only limited experience working with men with EDs, it is more difficult to detect atypical or significant emotional reactions. Developing countertransferential sensitivity to men with EDs often requires additional consultation and supervision.

Implications for Clinical Program Design

Residential and partial hospital programs still have limited capacity to treat men with EDs. This is changing but these treatment resources are still difficult to access for many men. For the time being, men, even if they can access higher levels of care, will often be a small minority of the patients in a particular program. Even in gender-specific programs, the clinical protocols will be largely based on the experience of what has worked well for women in the programs. In programs that mix men and women, specialized group therapy sessions, specific sessions and family protocols for dads and sons, and deliberate inclusion of men's friends, partners, and spouses can help minimize a sense of marginalization within the milieu. Gender-focused training for clinical staff is essential as well. Men with EDs, particularly if they are in the minority in a given patient cohort, need the experience of talking with other men, ideally other men who have dealt with these disorders. Hiring men for the clinical staff can also help to minimize the sense of "otherness." Men working in these programs may need additional supervision and support as they join clinical teams typically comprised of a majority of women. Clinical leadership needs to be sure that issues of gender are addressed in team meetings and clinical trainings.

Conclusions

Clinicians specializing with EDs must become more familiar with the unique issues related to the assessment, treatment planning, engagement, and delivery of treatment to men. While the basic outlines of treatment are similar for men and women, clinicians should expect that issues related to the gender socialization of masculinity will influence detection, referral, and treatment. Gender socialization issues are likely to most relevant as men enter treatment. Concerns about help-seeking, violations of internalized gender norms, and concerns about "having a woman's disease" can chip away at motivation for treatment and recovery. Clinicians can mitigate some of these forces by adapting their conceptualizations of ED to incorporate gender-related factors such as the intersection of the ED behaviors and cognitions with men's experience of their masculinity. The language of psychotherapy, from dynamic to cognitive models, is loaded with gendered terms and concepts that can also heighten the discomfort of men seeking assistance. Finally, it is crucial that clinicians explore and manage their own internal gender biases that can be activated when working with men with EDs.

This chapter has focused on some of the ways that men struggle to engage and make use of our existing treatments for ED. It is important to close with an acknowledgment of how important treatment can be for men, most of whom may not have had previous psychological treatments. Men are eager to be heard, and they may be especially surprised that a clinician is able to understand and accept their thoughts, feelings, and concerns without judgment. With relatively minor but thoughtful adaptations to our standard treatment approaches, we can facilitate that experience. Men will respond with openness, gratitude, and relief if we do.

References

1. Hudson JI, Hiripi E, Pope HG, et al. The prevalence and correlates of eating disorders in the national comorbidity survey replication. Biol Psychiatry. 2007;61:349–58.
2. Gorrell S, Murray SB. Eating disorders in males. Child Adolesc Psychiatr Clin N Am. 2019;28:641–51. https://doi.org/10.1016/j.chc.2019.05.012.
3. Sweeting H, Walker L, MacLean A, et al. Prevalence of eating disorders in males: a review of rates reported in academic research and UK mass media. Int J Mens Health. 2015;14(2). doi:https://doi.org/10.3149/jmh.1402.86.
4. Griffiths S, Murray SB, Touyz S. Extending the masculinity hypothesis: an investigation of gender role conformity, body dissatisfaction, and disordered eating in young heterosexual men. Psychol Men Masc. 2015a;16(1):108–14.
5. Striegel-Moore RH, Rosselli F, Perrin N, et al. Are there gender differences in the core symptoms, temperament, and short-term prospective outcome in anorexia nervosa? Int J Eat Disord. 2009;39(7):570–5.
6. Quittkat HL, Hartmann AS, Dusing R, Buhlmann U, Vocks S. Body dissatisfaction, importance of appearance, and body appreciation in men and women over the lifespan. Front Psych. 2019;10:864. https://doi.org/10.3389/fpsyt.2019.00864.
7. Talbot D, Smith E, Cass J. Male body dissatisfaction, eating disorder symptoms, body composition, and attentional bias to body stimuli evaluated using visual search. J Exp Psychopathol. 2019. https://doi.org/10.1177/2043808719848292.
8. Baker JH, Higgins Neyland MK, Thornton LM, Runfola CD, Larsonn H, Lichtenstein P, Bulik C. Body dissatisfaction in adolescent boys. Dev Psychol. 2019;55(7):1566–78. https://doi.org/10.1037/dev0000724.
9. Olivardia R. Body image and muscularity. In: Grant JE, Potenza MN, editors. Textbook of men's mental health. Washington, DC: American Psychiatric Publishing; 2007. p. 307–24.
10. Calzo JP, Sonneville KR, Haines J, et al. The development of associations among body mass index, body dissatisfaction, and weight and shape concern in adolescent boys and girls. J Adolesc Health. 2012;51(5):517–23.
11. Murray SB, Rieger E, Hildebrandt T, et al. A comparison of eating, exercise, shape and weight related symptomatology in males with muscle dysmorphia and anorexia nervosa. Body Image. 2012;9(2):193–200.
12. Coelho JS, Lee T, Karnabi P, et al. Eating disorders in biological males: clinical presentation and consideration of sex difference in a pediatric sample. J Eat Disord. 2018;6:40. https://doi.org/10.1186/s0337-018-0226-y.
13. Murray SB, Griffiths S, Rieger E, Touyz S. A comparison of compulsive exercise in male and female presentations of anorexia nervosa: what is the difference? Adv Eat Disord. 2014;2:65–70.
14. Zerwas S, Larsen JT, Petersen L, et al. The incidence of eating disorders in a Danish register study: associations with suicide risk and mortality. J Psychiatr Res. 2015;65:16–22. https://doi.org/10.1016/j.jpsychires.2015.03.003.
15. Forman-Hoffman VL, Watson TL, Andersen AE. Eating disorder age of onset in males: distribution and associated characteristics. Eat Weight Disord. 2008;13(2):28–31.
16. Carlat DJ, Camargo CA, Herzog DB. Eating disorders in males: a report on 135 patients. Am J Psychiatry. 1997;154:1127–32.
17. Gadalla TM. Psychiatric comorbidity in eating disorders: a comparison of men and women. J Mens Health. 2008;5(3):209–17. https://doi.org/10.1016/j.jomh.2008.06.033.
18. Brewerton TB. Eating disorders, trauma and comorbidity: focus on PTSD. Eat Disord. 2007;15:285–304.
19. Schmidt U, Treasure J. Anorexia nervosa: valued and visible. A cognitive-interpersonal maintenance model and its implications for research and practice. Br J Clin Psychol. 2006;45:343–66.
20. Treasure J, Schmidt U. The cognitive-interpersonal maintenance model of anorexia nervosa revisited: a summary of the evidence for cognitive, socio-emotional and interpersonal pre-

disposing and perpetuating factors. J Eat Disord. 2013;1:13. https://doi.org/10.1186/2050-2974-1-13.
21. Kendler KS, Myers J. The boundaries of the internalizing and externalizing genetic spectra in men and women. Psychol Med. 2014;44(3):647–55. https://doi.org/10.1017/S0033291713000585.
22. Cavanagh A, Wilson CJ, Caputi P, Kavanagh DJ. Symptom endorsement in men versus women with a diagnosis of depression: a differential item functioning approach. Int J Soc Psychiatry. 2016;62:549–59.
23. Feldman M, Meyer I. Eating disorders in diverse lesbian, gay and bisexual populations. Int J Eat Disord. 2007;40:218–26.
24. Brown TA, Keel PK. The impact of relationships on the association between sexual orientation and disordered eating in men. Int J Eat Disord. 2012;45(6):792–9.
25. Brown TA, Keel PK. Relationship status predicts lower restrictive eating pathology for bisexual and gay men across 10-year follow-up. Int J Eat Disord. 2015;48(6):700–7.
26. Fallon P, Katzman M, Wooley SC. Feminist perspectives on eating disorders. New York: Guilford Press; 1994.
27. Griffiths S, Mond JM, Li Z, Gunatilake S, Murray SB, Sheffield J, Touyz S. Self-stigma of seeking treatment and being male predict an increased likelihood of having an undiagnosed eating disorder. Int J Eat Disord. 2015b;48(6):775–8.
28. Griffiths S, Mond JM, Murray SB, Touyz S. The prevalence and adverse associations of stigmatization in people with eating disorders. Int J Eat Disord. 2015c;48(6):767–74.
29. Kierski W, Blazina C. The male fear of the feminine and its effects on counseling and psychotherapy. J Mens Stud. 2009;17(2):155–72. https://doi.org/10.3149/jms.1702.155.
30. Seidler ZE, Rice SM, Oliffe JL, et al. Men in and out of treatment for depression: strategies for improved engagement. Aust Psychol. 2017;1:1–11. https://doi.org/10.1111/ap.12331.
31. Sierra Hernandez CA, Han C, Oliffe JL, Ogrodniczuk JS. Understanding help-seeking among depressed men. Psychol Men Masc. 2014;15(3):346–54. https://doi.org/10.1037/a0034052.
32. Staczan P, Schmuecker R, Koehler M, et al. Effects of sex and gender in ten types of psychotherapy. Psychother Res. 2017;27(1):74–88.
33. Pederson EL, Vogel DL. Male gender role conflict and willingness to seek counseling: testing a mediation model on college-aged men. J Couns Psychol. 2007;54(4):373–84. https://doi.org/10.1037/0022-0167.54.4.373.
34. Spendelow JS. Cognitive–behavioral treatment of depression in men: tailoring treatment and directions for future research. Am J Mens Health. 2015;9(2):94–102. https://doi.org/10.1177/1557988314529790.
35. Siegel JA, Sawyer KB. "We don't talk about feelings or struggles like that": white men's experiences of eating disorders in the workplace. Psychol Men Masc. 2019; doi:https://doi.org/10.1037/men0000253.
36. Mahalik JR, Good GE, Tager D, et al. Developing a taxonomy of helpful and harmful practices for clinical work with boys and men. J Couns Psychol. 2012;59(4):591–603. https://doi.org/10.1037/a0030130.
37. Levant RF, Richmond K. A review of research on masculinity ideologies using the male role norms inventory. J Mens Stud. 2008;15(2):130–46. https://doi.org/10.3149/jms.1502.130.
38. Mahalik J, Good GE, Englar-Carlson M. Masculinity scripts, presenting concerns and help-seeking: implications for practice and training. Prof Psychol Res Pr. 2003;34:123–31.
39. O'Neil JM. Summarizing 25 years of research on men's gender role conflict using the Gender Role Conflict Scale: new research paradigms and clinical implications. Couns Psychol. 2008;36(3):358–445. https://doi.org/10.1177/0011000008317057.
40. O'Neil JM. The psychology of men. In: Altmaier EM, Hansen JIC, editors. Oxford library of psychology: the Oxford handbook of counseling psychology. Oxford: Oxford Press; 2012. p. 375–408.
41. Seidler ZE, Dawes AJ, Rice SM, et al. The role of masculinity in men's help-seeking for depression: a systematic review. Clin Psychol Rev. 2016;49:106–18. https://doi.org/10.1016/j.cpr.2016.09.002.

42. Wong YJ, Ho MR, Wang S, et al. Meta-analyses of the relationship between conformity to masculine norms and mental health-related outcomes. J Couns Psychol. 2017;64(1):80–93.
43. Owen J, Wong YJ, Rodolfa E. The relationship between clients' conformity to masculine norms and their perceptions of helpful therapist actions. J Couns Psychol. 2010;57(1):68–78. https://doi.org/10.1037/a00117870.
44. Murnen SK, Smolak L. Femininity, masculinity and disordered eating: a meta-analytic review. Int J Eat Disord. 1997;22(3):231–42.
45. Vogel DL, Heath PJ. Men, masculinities, and help-seeking patterns. In: Wong YJ, Wester SR, editors. APA handbooks in psychology series. APA handbook of men and masculinities. Washington, DC: American Psychological Association; 2016. p. 685–707.
46. O'Neil JM. Gender role journey therapy with men. In: O'Neil JM, editor. Men's gender role conflict: psychological costs, consequences, and an agenda for change. Washington, DC: American Psychological Association; 2015. p. 249–78.
47. Puhl RM, Wall MM, Chen C, et al. Experiences of weight teasing in adolescence and weight-related outcomes in adulthood: a 15-year longitudinal study. Prev Med. 2017;100:173–9. https://doi.org/10.1016/j.ypmed.2017.04.023.
48. Kindlon DJ, Thompson M, Barker T. Raising Cain: protecting the emotional life of boys. New York: Ballantine Books; 1999.
49. Bardone-Cone AM, Johnson S, Raney TJ, Zucker N, Watson H, Bulik C. Eating disorder recovery in men: a pilot study. Int J Eat Disord. 2019;1:1–10. https://doi.org/10.1002/eat23153.
50. Morgan HG, Russell GF. Value of family background and clinical features as predictors of long-term outcome in anorexia nervosa: Four-year follow-up study of 41 patients. Psychol Med. 1975;5:355–71. https://doi.org/10.1017/s0033291700056981.
51. Oyebode F, Boodhoo JA, Schapira K. Anorexia nervosa in males: clinical features and outcome. Int J Eat Disord. 1988;7:121–4. https://doi.org/10.1002/1098-108X(198801)7:1<121::AID-EAT2260070113>3.0.CO;2-U.
52. Herpertz-Dahlmann B, Müller B, Herpertz S, Heussen N, Hebebrand J, Remschmidt H. Prospective 10-year follow-up in adolescent anorexia nervosa course, outcome, psychiatric comorbidity, and psycho- social adaptation. J Child Psychol Psychiatry. 2001;42(5):603–12. https://doi.org/10.1111/1469-7610.00756.
53. Støving RK, Andries A, Brixen K, Bilenberg N, Hørder K. Gender differences in outcome of eating disorders: A retrospective cohort study. Psychiatry Res. 2011;186:362–6. https://doi.org/10.1016/j.psychres.2010.08.005.
54. Deter HC, Köpp W, Zipfel S, Herzog W. Männliche anorexia nervosa—Patienten im Langzeitverlauf. Neurologist. 1998;69:419–26. https://doi.org/10.1007/s001150050291.
55. Bean P, Loomis CC, Timmel P, Hallinan P, Moore S, Mammel J, Weltzin T. Outcome variables for anorexic males and females one year after discharge from residential treatment. J Addict Dis. 2004;23(2):83–94. https://doi.org/10.1300/J069v23n02_06.
56. Murray SB, Nagata JM, Griffiths S, Calzo JP, Brown TA, Mitchison D, et al. The enigma of male eating disorders: a critical review and synthesis. Clin Psychol Rev. 2017;57:1–11.
57. Strobel C, Quadflieg N, Voderholzer U, Naab S, Fichter M. Short- and long-term outcome of males treated for anorexia nervosa: a review of the literature. Eat Weight Disord. 2018;23:541–52. https://doi.org/10.1007/s40519-018-0538-6.
58. Strobel C, Quadflieg N, Naab S, Voderholzer U, Fichter MM. Long-term outcomes in treated males with anorexia nervosa and bulimia nervosa—a prospective, gender-matched study. Int J Eat Disord. 2019;52:1353–64. https://doi.org/10.1002/eat.23151.
59. Fernández-Aranda F, Krug I, Jiménez-Murcia S, Granero R, Núñez A, Penelo E, et al. Male eating disorders and therapy: a controlled pilot study with one year follow-up. J Behav Ther Exp Psychiatry. 2009;40:479–86.
60. Weltzin T, Cornella-Carlson T, Fitzpatrick ME, Kennington B, Bean P, Jefferies C. Treatment issues and outcomes for males with eating disorders. Eat Disord. 2012;20(5):444–59. https://doi.org/10.1080/10640266.2012.715527.

61. Grabhorn R, Köpp W, Gitzinger I, von Wietersheim J, Kaufhold, J. Differences between female and male patients with eating disorders-results of a multicenter study on eating disorders (MZ-Ess). Psychotherapie, Psychosomatik, Medizinische Psychologie. 2003;53:15–22. https://doi.org/10.1055/s-2003-36479.
62. Seidler ZE, Rice SM, Orgrdniczuk JS, et al. Engaging men in psychological treatment: a scoping review. Am J Mens Health. 2018;12(6):1882–900.
63. Calear AL, Batterham PJ, Christensen H. Predictors of help-seeking for suicidal ideation in the community: risks and opportunities for public suicide prevention campaigns. Psychiatry Res. 2014;219(3):525–30. https://doi.org/10.1016/j.psychres.2014.06.027.
64. Englar-Carlson M, Evans MP, Duffey T. A counselor's guide to working with men. Alexandria: Wiley; 2014.
65. Heads ups Guys.: https://headsupguys.org/mens-depression(2020). Accessed 15 February 2020.
66. Fairburn CG. Cognitive behavior therapy and eating disorders. New York: The Guilford Press; 2008.
67. Cochran SV, Rabinowitz FE. Gender-sensitive recommendations for assessment and treatment of depression in men. Prof Psychol Res Pr. 2003;34(2):132–40. https://doi.org/10.1037/0735-7028.34.2.132.
68. Smart R. A man with a "woman's problem": male gender and eating disorders. In: Englar-Carlson M, Stevens MA, editors. In the room with men: a casebook of therapeutic change. Washington, D.C.: American Psychological Association; 2006. p. 319–38.
69. Bunnell DW. Gender socialization, countertransference and the treatment of men with eating disorders. Clin Soc Work J. 2015;44(1):99. https://doi.org/10.1007/s10615-015-1564-z.

Part V
Specific Populations and Social Cultural Considerations

Chapter 15
Racial and Ethnic Considerations in the United States

Kimberly Yu and Marisol Perez

Learning Objectives

1. Summarize current literature on eating disorders among racial and ethnic minority men in the United States.
2. Recognize how implicit biases have influenced studies within this literature.
3. Understand key culture-specific variables that may be important in the assessment, etiology, and treatment of eating disorders in men.

Key Points

- Certain racial/ethnic minority groups may engage in more extreme body and weight change strategies and binge eating compared with White men.
- Body image varies substantially across racial/ethnic minority men.
- An implicit bias of the literature is the assumption that etiological models based on White samples are normative.
- Race and ethnicity are often viewed and treated as static variables, when they can be dynamic and context-specific.
- There is no research on prevention and treatments specifically for racial/ethnic minority men.

Introduction

Recently, disordered eating pathology among racial/ethnic minority men has gained critical attention, initiating newfound interest in prevalence, etiology, assessment, and treatment within these populations. In the past, studies addressing the relation

K. Yu · M. Perez (✉)
Department of Psychology, Arizona State University, Tempe, AZ, USA
e-mail: KimberlyYu@asu.edu; Marisol.Perez@asu.edu

J. M. Nagata et al. (eds.), *Eating Disorders in Boys and Men*,
https://doi.org/10.1007/978-3-030-67127-3_15

of race and ethnicity to disordered eating have disproportionately excluded men [1, 2]. As such, it is of great importance to incorporate the study of racial/ethnic minority groups in the eating disorder literature. The integration of these groups is essential in identifying disparities in eating disorder prevalence and presentation across groups and elucidating the roles of racial/ethnic minority-related variables such as acculturation, discrimination, socioeconomic status, body composition, and cultural norms in the conceptualization, etiology, prevention, and treatment of disordered eating pathology in diverse populations. For the purpose of this chapter, we focus here on four racial/ethnic groups: Black, Asian American, Latino, and Native American/First Nations men. The majority of the reviewed research is based on samples from the United States. However, a more detailed examination of disordered eating pathology across additional racial/ethnic minority groups is greatly warranted. For this review of the literature, keyword searches were conducted in Google Scholar, PubMed, and PsycINFO using the following words in combination: eating disorders, male, men, boys, race, ethnicity, Black, Asian American, Latino, Native American, disordered eating, eating pathology, binge eating, body dissatisfaction, muscle, and muscularity.

Implicit Bias of the Literature

In the history of eating disorder research, the vast majority of information contributing to etiological models, the clustering of symptoms that developed the diagnostic criteria informing assessments and screeners, and the empirically supported treatments have been based on middle-class and upper-class White women. This has contributed to an implicit bias within the current literature suggesting that etiological models, prevalence rates, and clustering of symptomatology developed based on Whites are normative. Thus, studies within the existing literature on racial/ethnic minority men have predominantly examined the degree to which White models generalize to racial/ethnic minority groups and the extent to which minorities deviate. This has serious implications for racial/ethnic minority health and is a common problem in the mental health field reflecting the history of racism in the United States, perpetuating the view of minorities being "subordinates" to Whites [3]. Indeed, most of the literature reviewed here uses Whites in a referent manner, and research has not taken an exploratory and broad approach to develop assessments and screeners for racial/ethnic minorities. Thus, as it stands, key symptoms and behaviors of disordered eating pathology exhibited by racial/ethnic minority groups but not Whites may be largely underrecognized in the field of eating disorder research.

Another weakness of the eating disorder literature is the treatment of race and ethnicity as static and stable variables [4]. Within the United States, race and ethnicity are socially constructed variables. Consequently, individuals who immigrate to and enter the United States are labeled per the country's definition (e.g., "Black"), despite potentially not identifying with the specified culture. Further, research demonstrates that the degree of racial/ethnic self-identification fluctuates across time and context [5, 6], and the dynamic nature of identity should be considered in this work.

Prevalence Rates

The Collaborative Psychiatric Epidemiology Surveys consists of 3 nationally representative samples from the United States comprising over 14,000 adults (more than 8000 racial/ethnic minorities), which were collected by the University of Michigan Research Center. All individuals received a diagnostic assessment consistent with the *Diagnostic and Statistical Manual of Mental Disorders*, 4th edition (DSM-IV; [7]), criteria. Marques and colleagues [8] published prevalence rates across racial/ethnic minority men and conducted group comparisons, summarized in Table 15.1.

Among racial/ethnic minority men, there were higher prevalence rates of bulimia nervosa and binge eating disorder than anorexia nervosa. There were significant group differences between Latino men and non-Latino White men, where Latinos reported significantly ($p < 0.05$) greater rates of bulimia nervosa [8]. There were no other significant group differences.

Eating Disorder Symptoms and Behaviors

Black Men

Broadly, it seems that racial/ethnic minority men may engage in more extreme body change strategies compared with White men [9]. However, some nuances exist among specific racial/ethnic groups. For example, Black boys and men have been shown to engage in more extreme weight loss strategies (e.g., chronic dieting and use of diet pills, laxatives, and diuretics) compared with White boys and men [10–16]. Additionally, compared with Whites, Black boys have also been shown to use more weight or muscle gain strategies such as supplements or exercise [11, 13, 14, 17]. In terms of steroid use, the literature is mixed with some findings suggesting higher rates [18], lower rates [19], and similar rates of use [20]. Finally, findings

Table 15.1 Lifetime prevalence rates of DSM-IV eating disorder diagnoses across race/ethnicity

Lifetime history	Non-Latino White	Latinos	Asian American	African American
Anorexia nervosa	0.14 (0.12)	0.03 (0.07)	0.07 (0.12)	0.18 (0.14)
Bulimia nervosa	0.08 (0.08)	1.73 (0.50)	1.14 (0.50)	0.90 (0.32)
Binge eating disorder	0.94 (0.33)	1.54 (0.45)	0.84 (0.42)	0.78 (0.31)

Data presented as weighted percent mean (standard error percent)

indicate that, compared with White men and boys, Black men and boys also engage in more binge eating [10, 12, 14, 18, 21, 22].

Interestingly, although Black men may engage in more binge eating, extreme weight loss strategies, and weight/muscle strategies, previous work suggests Black men have more positive body image compared with White men. Indeed, a meta-analysis found that 21 out of 27 studies that examined body image supported this association across both adolescent boys and adult men [9]. This may be due to the fact that Black men report greater preference for larger body sizes, which may be protective against body dissatisfaction [23]. Increased body positivity may be also attributed to positive weight and body size perception [16, 24] and familial attitudes about diverse body sizes [9].

Asian American Men

Among Asian Americans, the literature on disordered eating pathology is largely inconsistent. Specifically, some evidence indicates the presence of higher levels of weight loss strategies among Asian Americans compared with Whites (e.g., [12, 16]), while other evidence indicates no difference [25, 26]. Similarly, regarding the use of weight/muscle gain strategies, previous work indicates that Asian Americans are either less likely [16] or more likely to want to gain muscle compared with Whites [27]. Despite these inconsistencies, it is possible that Asian American men may be more likely to use strategies oriented toward the development of greater muscularity compared with Whites [27, 28]. Similarly, mixed findings have emerged with regard to steroid use among Asian Americans. Indeed, existing work indicates Asian Americans may be more likely [18, 29], less likely [19], and equally likely to use steroids when compared with Whites [30]. Discrepancies are also present in the literature on binge eating. While some research suggests that Asian American men and boys are more likely to binge eat than men and boys from other racial/ethnic groups [16, 27, 31], this finding has not been universal [32]. Interestingly, one study found that compulsive exercise was particularly high among Asian American men who binge eat compared to White and Black men [27]; however, this finding has not been replicated. Compulsive exercise, paired with binge eating, may be illustrative of muscularity-oriented eating [28, 33], supporting previous findings highlighting the potentially heightened use of muscle-building strategies among Asian American men.

Findings regarding body image among Asian American men are also inconsistent. While some findings suggest that Asian Americans are less likely (e.g., [34, 35]) or equally likely [12, 34, 36] to endorse body image concerns when compared to Whites, other work suggests that Asian American boys and men may be particularly susceptible to body image concerns [16, 37], especially those focused on muscularity [27, 38]. Overall, much more work is needed to elucidate these discrepancies. Notably, intragroup variability among Asian Americans in body size and weight may account for some of the inconsistencies found among Asian American men [27, 39]. For example, Filipino men, who may have a higher body mass index than other Asian American groups (e.g., Chinese and Japanese men), also endorse greater body dissatisfaction [40]. Alternatively, acculturation, exposure to media, and body image ideals and perceptions of masculinity may also account for some of the discrepancies found among Asian American men [9, 27, 39].

Latino Men

In regard to Latino boys and men within the United States, previous work indicates greater use of extreme weight loss strategies including chronic dieting, vomiting, and use of diet pills compared to Whites [9, 12, 16]. Latinos have also been shown to engage in more binge eating [12, 14, 31] and purging than Whites [8]. Very little work exists on the use of strategies to build muscle or gain weight among Latinos, and existing research is largely inconsistent, indicating Latinos may be more [11, 13] or equally likely to use weight/muscle gain strategies compared with Whites [29]. Similarly, findings on steroid use among Latinos have been largely mixed with some studies suggesting that Latinos are more likely to use steroids than Whites [18] and other findings indicating no differences [29]. More work is needed to clarify these inconsistencies.

Notably, while some mixed findings exist (e.g., [16, 41]), evidence suggests that Latinos do not differ in their body image when compared with Whites [9]. However, some findings suggest that Latinos endorse more positive attitudes toward larger body sizes compared with White boys and men [11, 16, 24]. Indeed, some work has found that Latinos are less likely to perceive themselves as overweight compared with Whites [24]. In light of similar body image perceptions and dissimilar rates of binge eating and weight loss strategies compared with Whites, it is possible that familial conflict, acculturation, and marginalization may account for some of the disparities highlighted with regard to disordered eating pathology among Latinos [9]. However, more work is needed to examine these factors among Latino populations.

Native American and Other First Nations Men

Native American and other First Nations men have been largely neglected in the literature on disordered eating. However, the limited existing work has indicated that Native American and other First Nations boys and men report greater incidence of extreme weight loss behaviors [12, 16, 31, 42, 43]. Native Americans also report greater prevalence of binge eating compared to Whites [12, 16, 31, 42, 43]. The extant research demonstrates no difference between Native American/First Nation boys and men and Whites on weight gain/muscle gain strategies [16, 18]. However, the existing literature on steroid use is mixed with some findings indicating higher likelihood of use among Native American/First Nations men [44] and others indicating no difference in steroid use when compared with Whites [16, 18].

Evidence also suggests that Native American/First Nations people endorse more body image concerns compared with Whites [12, 16, 42, 43, 45]. High rates of overweight and obesity within Native American/First Nations populations coupled with greater likelihood of perception of overweight [16] may contribute to these elevated rates of body dissatisfaction. Higher rates of binge eating and extreme weight loss behaviors may be attributed to cultural conflict and familial pressures [43]. Family seems to play a unique role among Native American men. Interestingly, Native American adolescents with one Native parent have also been found to be less likely to report body image concerns and disordered eating behaviors, compared to their peers with two Native American parents, highlighting the potential role of acculturation in impacting disordered eating pathology within this population [43].

Summary

Overall, it appears that men belonging to a range of racial/ethnic minority groups may engage in more extreme body and weight change strategies and binge eating compared with Whites [9]. However, some inconsistencies exist, and more work is needed to elucidate these findings. In particular, body image seems to vary substantially across racial/ethnic minority groups [9], highlighting the necessity of examining additional mediating and moderating variables such as acculturation, discrimination, socioeconomic status, body mass index (BMI), and cultural norms.

Relevant Culture-Specific Variables

Here, we review acculturation and discrimination as potentially salient cultural factors warranting greater consideration in the examination of disordered eating pathology among racial/ethnic minority populations. First, acculturation has been found to be associated with disordered eating pathology and is noteworthy when considering racial/ethnic minority populations. However, much of the literature on acculturation and disordered eating pathology addresses populations of women, and more work is needed to expand this literature to groups of men. The extant body of literature provides some evidence for the association between acculturation and disordered eating pathology among Black men [46]. Among Asian Americans, findings are mixed, with some indicating an association between acculturation, disordered eating, and body image concerns [22, 39] and others reporting no association [34, 47]. Among Latinos, acculturative stress, rather than acculturation, has been found to be associated with body image concerns [48]. Acculturative stress is the daily stress of balancing two different cultures and has been found to be unique from general daily stress [49]. Interestingly, among Native American men, acculturation to Western values was associated with fewer body image concerns as well as less disordered eating symptomatology [43]. It seems that, in some cases, acculturation to Western ideals may be protective against disordered eating pathology, whereas in others, greater adherence to Western ideals can be detrimental. Future research should examine the role of acculturative stress as an important factor in the consideration of disordered eating pathology.

Previous research asserts that racism contributes to mental and physical health issues [50]. Research has found that Black fathers and their adolescent sons, who report more everyday discrimination relative to other Black father-son dyads, also report more emotional eating [51]. Further, emotional eating has been found to mediate the relationship between everyday discrimination and BMI among Black adolescent boys [51]. Yet, for Black fathers, everyday discrimination has been shown to have an indirect effect on BMI through emotional eating [51]. Among Asian American college men, perceived perpetual racism significantly predicts drive for muscularity above and beyond internalization of Western standards for masculine physiques [39]. These findings highlight the importance of understanding racial contexts as they relate to eating disorder behaviors. Furthermore, these findings are consistent with other research that has found everyday discrimination to be associated with negative coping, depression, low self-esteem, and anxiety among Black adolescent boys [52, 53]. To date, no studies have specifically examined the effects of discrimination on disordered eating pathology among Latino, Asian American, and Native American/First Nations men. Additional work is needed to determine the effects of discrimination on eating disorder behaviors and symptomatology among ethnic/racial minority men.

Summary

Further research should continue to examine the extent to which acculturation, acculturative stress, and discrimination play a role in disordered eating pathology among racial/ethnic minority men. Additionally, more nuanced research using multi-contextual frameworks integrating diverse biological, psychological, developmental, and environmental perspectives to determine conditional and differential susceptibility to disordered eating pathology is greatly needed.

Future Directions in Assessment, Prevention, and Treatment

It is noteworthy to highlight gaps in this literature. Currently, there is no research examining the psychometric properties of screeners and assessments for eating disorders and correlates among racial/ethnic minority men. This is important as knowledge and assumptions about eating disorder assessment and treatment rely on valid and reliable assessment measures. Further, there is no research examining prevention of eating disorders, drive for muscularity, or other correlates specifically within racial/ethnic minority men. However, one study conducted a cognitive dissonance-based prevention program for eating disorder behaviors and risk factors specific for sexual minority men [54]; the sample consisted of 43% racial/ethnic minority men, and, although minority-specific analyses were not conducted, overall the intervention group had significant decreases in body dissatisfaction, drive for muscularity, dietary restraint, and bulimic symptoms [54]. A second study conducted a comparison of a cognitive dissonance-based prevention program for women compared to a group consisting of men and women [55]. Although no racial-/ethnic-specific analyses were conducted, the sample did consist of 23.8% racial/ethnic minorities. For men, the prevention program produced significant decreases in body dissatisfaction and body attitudes toward low fat and muscularity [55]. Although both cognitive dissonance prevention programs yielded significant decreases in a racially and ethnically diverse sample of men, both studies were underpowered to examine minority men specifically. Thus, the extent to which these findings generalize to racial/ethnic minority men remains unclear.

Within the treatment literature, there are no studies examining the extent to which empirically supported treatments generalize to racial/ethnic minority men. Further, we were unable to locate any case studies. Future research is therefore crucial to explore the extent to which current treatments are efficacious and if any cultural modifications are required to make treatments more appropriate for use within ethnic/racial minority groups of men.

Conclusion

There is a paucity of research on disordered eating pathology among racial/ethnic minority men at all levels of clinical science. Although some research has emerged on the prevalence of eating disorder symptoms and behaviors among racial/ethnic minority men, it remains in its infancy stage. In particular, a noted weakness of the existing literature is the tendency to examine the extent to which racial/ethnic minority men deviate from the "norm" (i.e., White men). Additionally, research has not taken an exploratory and broad approach to develop assessments and screeners for racial/ethnic minority men. Consequently, disordered eating symptoms that are uniquely exhibited by racial/ethnic minorities may be largely underrecognized in the field of eating disorder research. The literature on prevalence of disordered eating highlights that, in general, racial/ethnic minority men exhibit more extreme body change strategies than their White counterparts. Preliminary research has found associations between disordered eating symptoms and acculturation and discrimination among Black men and disordered eating and acculturative stress among Latinos. Finally, the empirical literature addressing assessment psychometrics and efficacy/effectiveness of eating disorder prevention and treatment programs among racial/ethnic minority men is extremely limited.

Echoed throughout this chapter is the critical need for more research incorporating a racial and ethnic minority perspective. Existing etiological models of eating disorders need to be generalized to men and integrated within existing racial and ethnic minority stress frameworks (see, e.g., [56]). Further, examining the intersectionality of minority identity and the potential additive role of being a racial or ethnic minority man may provide a more nuanced understanding of eating disorder development, treatment, and prevention.

References

1. Mehler PS, Sabel AL, Watson T, Andersen AE. High risk of osteoporosis in male patients with eating disorders. Int J Eat Disord. 2008;41:666–72. https://doi.org/10.1002/eat.20554.
2. Kimber M, Couturier J, Georgiades K, Wahoush O, Jack SM. Ethnic minority status and body image dissatisfaction: a scoping review of the child and adolescent literature. J Immigr Minor Health. 2015;17:1567–79. https://doi.org/10.1007/s10903-014-0082-z.
3. Vega WA, Rumbaut RG. Ethnic minorities and mental health. Annu Rev Sociol. 1991;17:351–83. https://doi.org/10.1146/annurev.so.17.080191.002031.
4. Perez M, Plasencia M. Psychological perspectives on ethnic-minority eating behavior and obesity. In: Blume A, editor. Social issues in living color: challenges and solutions from the perspective of ethnic minority psychology. New York: Praeger Books; 2016.
5. Kiang L, Fuligni AJ. Ethnic identity in context: variations in ethnic exploration and belonging within parent, same-ethnic peer, and different-ethnic peer relationships. J Youth Adolesc. 2009;38:732–43. https://doi.org/10.1007/s10964-008-9278-7.
6. Saylor ES, Aries E. Ethnic identity and change in social context. J Soc Psychol. 1999;139:549–66. https://doi.org/10.1080/00224549909598416.
7. American Psychiatric Association. Diagnostic and statistical manual of mental disorders. 4th ed. Text Revision. Washington, D.C.: American Psychiatric Association Publishing; 2000.
8. Marques L, Alegria M, Becker AE, Chen CN, Fang A, Chosak A, et al. Comparative prevalence, correlates of impairment, and service utilization for eating disorders across US ethnic groups: implications for reducing ethnic disparities in health care access for eating disorders. Int J Eat Disord. 2011;44:412–20. https://doi.org/10.1002/eat.20787.
9. Ricciardelli LA, McCabe MP, Williams RJ, Thompson JK. The role of ethnicity and culture in body image and disordered eating among males. Clin Psychol Rev. 2007;27:582–606. https://doi.org/10.1016/j.cpr.2007.01.016.
10. Gray JJ, Ford K, Kelly LM. The prevalence of bulimia in a black college population. Int J Eat Disord. 1987;6:733–40. https://doi.org/10.1002/1098-108X(198711)6:6<733::AID-EAT2260060606>3.0.CO;2-U.
11. Serdula MK. Weight control practices of U.S. adolescents and adults. Ann Intern Med. 1993;119:667. https://doi.org/10.7326/0003-4819-119-7_Part_2-199310011-00008.
12. Story M, French SA, Resnick MD, Blum RW. Ethnic/racial and socioeconomic differences in dieting behaviors and body image perceptions in adolescents. Int J Eat Disord. 1995;18:173–9. https://doi.org/10.1002/1098-108X(199509)18:2<173::AID-EAT2260180210>3.0.CO;2-Q.
13. Neumark-Sztainer D, Story M, Falkner NH, Beuhring T, Resnick MD. Sociodemographic and personal characteristics of adolescents engaged in weight loss and weight/muscle gain behaviors: who is doing what? Prev Med. 1999;28:40–50. https://doi.org/10.1006/pmed.1998.0373.
14. Neumark-Sztainer D, Hannan PJ. Weight-related behaviors among adolescent girls and boys: results from a national survey. Arch Pediatr Adolesc Med. 2000;154:569–77. https://doi.org/10.1001/archpedi.154.6.569.
15. Barry DT, Grilo CM. Eating and body image disturbances in adolescent psychiatric inpatients: gender and ethnicity patterns. Int J Eat Disord. 2002;32:335–43. https://doi.org/10.1002/eat.10082.
16. Neumark-Sztainer D, Croll J, Story M, Hannan PJ, French SA, Perry C. Ethnic/racial differences in weight-related concerns and behaviors among adolescent girls and boys: find-

ings from project EAT. J Psychosom Res. 2002;53:963–74. https://doi.org/10.1016/S0022-3999(02)00486-5.
17. Nagata JM, Bibbins-Domingo K, Garber AK, Griffiths S, Vittinghoff E, Murray SB. Boys, bulk, and body ideals: sex differences in weight-gain attempts among adolescents in the United States. J Adolesc Health. 2019;64:450–3. https://doi.org/10.1016/j.jadohealth.2018.09.002.
18. Irving LM, Wall M, Neumark-Sztainer D, Story M. Steroid use among adolescents: findings from project EAT. J Adolesc Health. 2002;30:243–52. https://doi.org/10.1016/S1054-139X(01)00414-1.
19. Komoroski EM, Rickert VI. Adolescent body image and attitudes to anabolic steroid use. Am J Dis Child. 1992;146:823–8. https://doi.org/10.1001/archpedi.1992.02160190055019.
20. Yesalis CE, Kennedy NJ, Kopstein AN, Bahrke MS. Anabolic-androgenic steroid use in the United States. JAMA. 1993;270:1217–21. https://doi.org/10.1001/jama.1993.03510100067034.
21. Johnson WG, Rohan KJ, Kirk AA. Prevalence and correlates of binge eating in white and African American adolescents. Eat Behav. 2002;3:179–89. https://doi.org/10.1016/S1471-0153(01)00057-5.
22. Aruguete MS, Nickleberry LD, Yates A. Acculturation, body image, and eating attitudes among black and White college students. N Am J Psychol. 2003;6:393–404.
23. Russell W. Comparison of self-esteem, body satisfaction, and social physique anxiety across males of different exercise frequency and racial background. J Sport Behav. 2002;25:74–90.
24. Paeratakul S, White MA, Williamson DA, Ryan D, Bray GA. Sex, race/ethnicity, socioeconomic status, and BMI in relation to self-perception of overweight. Obes Res. 2012;10:345–50. https://doi.org/10.1038/oby.2002.48.
25. Barr SI. Dieting attitudes and behavior in urban high school students: implications for calcium intake. J Adolesc Health. 1995;16:458–64. https://doi.org/10.1016/1054-139X(94)00092-S.
26. Mintz LB, Kashubeck S. Body image and disordered eating among Asian American and Caucasian college students: an examination of race and gender differences. Psychol Women Q. 1999;23:781–96. https://doi.org/10.1111/j.1471-6402.1999.tb00397.x.
27. Kelly NR, Cotter EW, Tanofsky-Kraff M, Mazzeo SE. Racial variations in binge eating, body image concerns, and compulsive exercise among men. Psychol Men Masculinity. 2015;16:326–36. https://doi.org/10.1037/a0037585.
28. Murray SB, Nagata JM, Griffiths S, Calzo JP, Brown TA, Mitchison D, et al. The enigma of male eating disorders: a critical review and synthesis. Clin Psychol Rev. 2017;57:1–11. https://doi.org/10.1016/j.cpr.2017.08.001.
29. Eisenberg ME, Wall M, Neumark-Sztainer D. Muscle-enhancing behaviors among adolescent girls and boys. Pediatrics. 2012;130:1019–26. https://doi.org/10.1542/peds.2012-0095.
30. Radakovich J, Broderick P, Pickell G. Rate of anabolic-androgenic steroid use among students in junior high school. J Am Board Fam Pract. 1993;6:341–5. https://doi.org/10.3122/jabfm.6.4.341.
31. Croll J, Neumark-Sztainer D, Story M, Ireland M. Prevalence and risk and protective factors related to disordered eating behaviors among adolescents: relationship to gender and ethnicity. J Adolesc Health. 2002;31:166–75. https://doi.org/10.1016/S1054-139X(02)00368-3.
32. Striegel RH, Bedrosian R, Wang C, Schwartz S. Why men should be included in research on binge eating: results from a comparison of psychosocial impairment in men and women. Int J Eat Disord. 2012;45:233–40. https://doi.org/10.1002/eat.20962.
33. Griffiths S, Murray SB, Touyz S. Disordered eating and the muscular ideal. J Eat Disord. 2013;1:15. https://doi.org/10.1186/2050-2974-1-15.
34. Cachelin FM, Rebeck RM, Chung GH, Pelayo E. Does ethnicity influence body-size preference? A comparison of body image and body size. Obes Res. 2002;10:158–66. https://doi.org/10.1038/oby.2002.25.
35. Yang CF, Gray P, Pope HG. Male body image in Taiwan versus the West: Yanggang Zhiqi meets the Adonis Complex. Am J Psychiatry. 2005;162:263–9. https://doi.org/10.1176/appi.ajp.162.2.263.

36. Wang Z, Byrne NM, Kenardy JA, Hills AP. Influences of ethnicity and socioeconomic status on the body dissatisfaction and eating behaviour of Australian children and adolescents. Eat Behav. 2005;6:23–33. https://doi.org/10.1016/j.eatbeh.2004.05.001.
37. Edman JL, Yates A. A cross-cultural study of disordered eating attitudes among Filipino and Caucasian Americans. J Eat Disord. 2005;13:279–89. https://doi.org/10.1080/10640260590932887.
38. Keum BT, Wong SN, DeBlaere C, Brewster ME. Body image and Asian American men: examination of the drive for muscularity scale. Psychol Men Masculinity. 2015;16:284–93. https://doi.org/10.1037/a0038180.
39. Cheng HL, McDermott RC, Wong YJ, La S. Drive for muscularity in Asian American men: sociocultural and racial/ethnic factors as correlates. Psychol Men Masculinity. 2016;17:215–27. https://doi.org/10.1037/men0000019.
40. Yates A, Edman J, Aruguete M. Ethnic differences in BMI and body/self-dissatisfaction among Whites, Asian subgroups, Pacific Islanders, and African-Americans. J Adolesc Health. 2004;34:300–7. https://doi.org/10.1016/j.jadohealth.2003.07.014.
41. Frederick DA, Forbes GB, Grigorian KE, Jarcho JM. The UCLA Body Project I: gender and ethnic differences in self-objectification and body satisfaction among 2,206 undergraduates. Sex Roles. 2007;57:317–27. https://doi.org/10.1007/s11199-007-9251-z.
42. Smith JE, Krejci J. Minorities join the majority: eating disturbances among Hispanic and Native American youth. Int J Eat Disord. 1991;10:179–86. https://doi.org/10.1002/1098-108X(199103)10:2%3C179::AID-EAT2260100206%3E3.0.CO;2-S.
43. Lynch WC, Heil DP, Wagner E, Havens MD. Ethnic differences in BMI, weight concerns, and eating behaviors: comparison of Native American, White, and Hispanic adolescents. Body Image. 2007;4:179–90. https://doi.org/10.1016/j.bodyim.2007.01.001.
44. Handelsman DJ, Gupta L. Prevalence and risk factors for anabolic-androgenic steroid abuse in Australian high school students. Int J Androl. 1997;20:159–64. https://doi.org/10.1046/j.1365-2605.1997.d01-285.x.
45. Ricciardelli LA, McCabe MP, Ball K, Mellor D. Sociocultural influences on body image concerns and body change strategies among Indigenous and Non-Indigenous Australian Adolescent girls and boys. Sex Roles. 2004;51:731–41. https://doi.org/10.1007/s11199-004-0722-1.
46. Marais DL, Wassenaar DR, Kramers AL. Acculturation and eating disorder symptomatology in black men and women. Eat Weight Disord St. 2003;8:44–54. https://doi.org/10.1007/BF03324988.
47. Kwan MY, Gordon KH, Minnich AM. An examination of the relationships between acculturative stress, perceived discrimination, and eating disorder symptoms among ethnic minority college students. Eat Behav. 2018;28:25–31. https://doi.org/10.1016/j.eatbeh.2017.12.003.
48. Warren CS, Rios RM. The relationships among acculturation, acculturative stress, endorsement of Western media, social comparison, and body image in Hispanic male college students. Psychol Men Masculinity. 2013;14:192–201. https://doi.org/10.1037/a0028505.
49. Kroon Van Diest AM, Tartakovsky M, Stachon C, Pettit JW, Perez M. The relationship between acculturative stress and eating disorder symptoms: is it unique from general life stress? J Behav Med. 2014;37:445–57. https://doi.org/10.1007/s10865-013-9498-5.
50. Brondolo E, Gallo LC, Myers HF. Race, racism, and health: disparities, mechanisms, and interventions. J Behav Med. 2009;32:1–8. https://doi.org/10.1007/s10865-008-9190-3.
51. Coleman A, O'Neil J, Ferris AM. The mediation effect between everyday discrimination, gender role conflict, emotional eating, and obesity in African American fathers and sons. Psychol Men Masc. 2019;20(2):182–93. https://doi.org/10.1037/men0000201.
52. Mereish EH, N'cho HS, Helms JE. Discrimination and depressive symptoms among Black American men: moderated-mediation effects of ethnicity and self-esteem. Behav Med. 2016;42(3):190–6. https://doi.org/10.1080/08964289.2016.1150804.

53. Assari S, Moazen-Zadeh E, Caldwell CH, Zimmerman MA. Racial discrimination during adolescence predicts mental health deterioration in adulthood: gender differences among Blacks. Front Public Health. 2017;29(5):104. https://doi.org/10.3389/fpubh.2017.00104.
54. Brown TA, Keel PK. A randomized controlled trial of a peer co-led dissonance-based eating disorder prevention program for gay men. Behav Res Ther. 2015;74:1–10. https://doi.org/10.1016/j.brat.2015.08.008.
55. Kilpela LS, Blomquist K, Verzijl C, Winfred S, Beyl R, Becker CB. The body project 4 all: a pilot randomized controlled trial of a mixed-gender dissonance-based body image program. Int J Eat Disord. 2016;49:591–602. https://doi.org/10.1002/eat.22562.
56. Mason TB, Lewis RJ. Minority stress, body shame, and binge eating among lesbian women: social anxiety as a linking mechanism. Psychol Women Q. 2016;40:428–40.

Chapter 16
Cross-Cultural Considerations in Latin American Boys and Men

Emilio J. Compte and Eva Trujillo

Learning Objectives

1. To describe the prevalence of eating disorders and disordered eating among Latin American boys and men
2. To highlight the characteristics of eating disorders among Latin American boys and men
3. To summarize the eating disorder, muscle dysmorphia, and body image assessment measures that have been validated among Latin American boys and men

Key Points

- Features of disordered eating among Latin American men are similar to those observed in men from developed countries.
- More recently, a wide variety of disordered eating and body image-related measures have been validated across different Latin American male populations.
- Research in clinical samples of Latin American boys and men remains a gap in the literature.

E. J. Compte (✉)
Research Department, Comenzar de Nuevo Treatment Center, Monterrey, Nuevo León, Mexico

School of Psychology, Universidad Adolfo Ibáñez, Peñalolén Santiago, Chile
e-mail: emilio.compte@comenzardenuevo.net; emilio.compte@uai.cl

E. Trujillo
Psychiatry Department, Comenzar de Nuevo Treatment Center, Monterrey, Nuevo León, Mexico
e-mail: eva.trujillo@comenzardenuevo.net

J. M. Nagata et al. (eds.), *Eating Disorders in Boys and Men*,
https://doi.org/10.1007/978-3-030-67127-3_16

Introduction

Despite that men[1] in Latin America have been an understudied population in the eating disorder (ED) field, fortunately, an increasing body of evidence that has developed over the last several years has allowed us to enhance our understanding of the ED experience in this population. In the current chapter, we first aim to describe the prevalence of ED in Latin American males, as well as potential risk factors in this population. Cross-cultural research including Latin American males will also be discussed. Specific features of ED and the availability of assessment measures in this population are also described. Finally, evidence-based knowledge on sociocultural influences in ED among Latin American men is presented.

Prevalence of ED in Latin American Boys and Men

The majority of studies investigating the prevalence of ED in Latin American populations have used a survey-based cross-sectional design and present rates of ED risk and risky eating behaviors, as opposed to full threshold ED diagnosed through a clinical interview (see Table 16.1). The screening instruments vary across studies, and the nature of the measures should be taken into consideration while comparing results. For example, despite potentially lacking sensitivity to detect specific features of disordered eating among males, the Brief Risky Eating Behaviors Screening Questionnaire has been widely used across studies with Mexican samples.

As part of the Drug and Alcohol Prevalence in Student Population Survey in Mexico City conducted in 1997, 2000, and 2013, two studies report data from ED survey items based on criteria from the fourth edition of the *Diagnostic and Statistical Manual of Mental Disorders* (DSM-IV) [1]. The prevalence of ED risk in those studies ranged from 1.3% to 4.3% among males, which was lower compared to the prevalence of ED risk in females [2, 3]. A higher proportion of boys presented with binge eating episodes, purging behaviors, and weight gain concerns in 1997 versus 2003, whereas a lower proportion presented with body weight overestimation and dietary restraint [3]. A number of studies have used the Brief Risky Eating Behaviors Screening Questionnaire [4], a ten-item questionnaire based on DSM-IV ED criteria. For example, Barriguete et al. [5] used data from the 2006 Mexican National Health and Nutrition Survey, which included the participation of 12,456 teenage boys. Among males, 0.4% were found to be at risk for an ED, which is a small rate compared to 1.0% found in females. Males from urban locations had double the prevalence of risk for an ED compared to those from rural areas. In this study, the prevalence of ED behaviors among males across age groups was not found to significantly differ, whereas Unikel et al. [1] reported that binge eating was more common among older versus younger adolescent boys. In another study, 2.9%

[1] In this chapter, we use the terms males and boys/men interchangeably.

Table 16.1 Studies of eating disorder prevalence among Latin American boys and men

Author (year)	Country	Population (sample size, mean age)	Design	ED instruments	Criteria	Results
Unikel, Saucedo-Molina, Villatoro, and Fleiz (2002)	Mexico	Adolescent students from Mexico City (boys 47.9%, $n = 3640$, age range 13–18)	Cross-sectional, survey-based	DSM-based questions included in the 1997 Drug and Alcohol Prevalence in Student Population Survey of Mexico City	DSM-IV	Girls showed higher means of clinical symptoms compared to boys; 1.5% and 2.2% of boys between age 13–15 and 16–18, respectively, met risk criteria for developing an ED, compared to 5.4% and 16.1% of girls from age 13–15 and 16–18, respectively. Boys aged 16–18 had a significantly higher proportion of binge eating (7.3%) compared to boys aged 13–15 (4.6%). No age differences were observed for boys in self-induced vomiting (0.6%, 0.4%), dietary restraint (1.0%, 0.9%), excessive exercise (16.4%, 18.6%), laxative misuse (0.7%, 0.2%), or weight gain concerns (5.0%, 5.9%)
Unikel, Bojórquez, Villatoro, Fleiz, and Medina (2006)	Mexico	Student population in Mexico City in 1997 (boys 47.9%, $n = 4676$, mean age = 14.5), in 2000 (boys 50.9%, $n = 1675$, mean age = 14.6), and in 2003 (boys 50.1%, $n = 1533$, mean age = 14.5)	Cross-sectional, survey-based	DSM-based questions included in the Drug and Alcohol Prevalence in Student Population Survey of Mexico City	DSM-IV	A higher proportion of boys presented with the following in 1997 versus 2003: weight gain concerns (5.4% versus 11.5%), binge episodes (2.6% versus 6.5%), and purging behaviors (1.3% versus 6.1%); a lower proportion of boys presented with body weight overestimation (18.2% to 11.0%) and dietary restraint (18.9% to 11.9%). Presence of at least 3 ED risk indicators was 1.3% in 1997, 4.3% in 2000, and 3.8% in 2003. Across years, boys aged 12–13 showed a higher proportion of presence of at least 3 ED risk indicators (2.2%–5.7%) compared to boys from other age groups
Barriguete et al. (2009)	Mexico	Adolescents from the Mexican Health and Nutrition Survey 2006 (49.7% males, $n = 12{,}456$, age range 10–10)	Cross-sectional, survey-based	Brief Risky Eating Behaviors Screening Questionnaire (scores >10 considered risk for ED)	Cutoff score-based	Males showed lower ED risk than females (0.4% vs. 1.0%). No differences on frequency of ED behaviors among males across ages were observed. ED risk prevalence in urban locations was double that of rural ones. With the exception of binge eating, for which adolescent men from rural settings were less likely to binge eat compared to males from urban and metropolitan areas, no differences were observed in ED behaviors across settings

(continued)

Table 16.1 (continued)

Author (year)	Country	Population (sample size, mean age)	Design	ED instruments	Criteria	Results
Nuño, Celis, and Unikel (2009)	Mexico	High school freshmen students in Guadalajara (40.8% boys, *n* = 463, mean age = 15.3)	Cross-sectional, survey-based	Brief Risky Eating Behaviors Screening Questionnaire (scores >10 considered risk for ED)	Cutoff score-based	2.9% of males were at risk for an ED (compared to 10.3% of females). Males showed lower weight concerns, binge eating episodes, and dietary restraint and were less likely to be following a diet compared to females. Among males, ED behaviors were associated with impulsivity traits, depressive symptoms, suicide ideation, and stress
Rutsztein, Murawski, Elizathe, and Scappatura (2010)	Argentina	High school students in Buenos Aires and metropolitan areas (37.7% men, *n* = 171, mean age = 14.7)	Two-stage, cross-sectional study	1st stage: risk for ED – (a) EDI-2 subscale cutoff scores (drive for thinness >14, bulimia >7, body dissatisfaction >16) or (b) presence of weight control purging behaviors 2nd stage: EDE-based interview	DSM-IV and ICD-10	Almost 6% of males were found to be at risk for an ED, and 2.9% (*n* = 5) were diagnosed with an ED. All cases were identified as EDNOS. No differences among genders were observed for sociocultural variables. Although both males and females wanted to lose weight, differences between current and desired weight were significantly lower for males. No males showed high levels of body dissatisfaction or body image distortions. Among ED behaviors, males showed significantly less dietary restraint and self-induced vomiting than females, and no differences were observed for laxative and diuretic misuse. Males also tended to score lower on EDI-2 subscales
Saucedo-Molina and Unikel (2010)	Mexico	Adolescents and young adult students from Pachuca City, in Hidalgo, Mexico (45.1% males, *n* = 381, mean age = 17.8)	Cross-sectional, survey-based	Brief Risky Eating Behaviors Screening Questionnaire (scores >10 considered risk for ED)	Cutoff score-based	Males showed a lower prevalence of risky eating behaviors compared to females (2.9% versus 8.4%). Among males, high school students showed higher frequency of binge eating episodes, loss of control eating, excessive exercise, and diet pill use, while undergraduate students presented with higher weight gain concerns, dietary restraint, and laxative misuse. Self-induced vomiting and diuretic misuse were not observed among high school and undergraduate male students. Male gender was identified as a protective factor for risky eating behaviors

Reyes-Rodríguez et al. (2012)	Puerto Rico	Male university students from 11 campuses ($N = 709$, mean age = 18.26)	Cross-sectional, survey-based	Risk for ED: (a) BULIT-R > 85 or (b) EAT-26 > 20	Cutoff score-based	Among male college students, 2.3% and 5.1% scored above the cutoff point on the BULIT-R and on the EAT-26, respectively. Precisely 4.4% reported sufficient frequency and severity to approximate DSM-IV criteria for BN. Over one-fifth (21.3%) of participants were dieting with the intention to lose weight. Males at risk for an ED were more likely to engage in binge eating episodes and compensatory behaviors. Depressive symptoms and stressful events were more frequent among males at risk for an ED compared to those who scored below the cutoff values
Benjet, Mendez, Borges, and Medina-Mora (2012)	Mexico	Participants ($N = 3005$) from the Mexican Adolescents Mental Health Survey from Mexico City and 16 metropolitan areas (proportion of males not specified, age range 12–17)	Cross-sectional, interview-based	Composite International Diagnostic Interview (CIDI)	DSM-IV	Prevalence rates overall were 0.5% for AN, 1.0% for BN, and 1.4% for BED. There were no gender differences in the proportion of AN cases; 30.5% of BN cases were male, and 24.9% of BED cases were male
Silva, Silva, Silva, Pedrino, and Rosa (2013)	Brazil	Non-athlete population with exercise dependence symptoms (60.3% males, $n = 105$, age range 18–62)	Cross-sectional, survey-based	Risk for ED: EAT-26 > 21	Cutoff score-based	Proportion of men at risk for ED was lower than that observed for women (40% versus 60%). Men in the sample presented with exercise dependence symptoms without ED attitudes

(continued)

Table 16.1 (continued)

Author (year)	Country	Population (sample size, mean age)	Design	ED instruments	Criteria	Results
Compte, Sepulveda, and Torrente (2015)	Argentina	Male university students from Buenos Aires (*N* = 472, mean age = 22.5)	Two-stage, cross-sectional study	1st stage: risk for ED, EAT-26 > 15; risk for MD, DMS > 31 2nd stage: EDE 12.0 interview (for ED cases) and DMS > 52 (possible cases of MD)	DSM-IV	Prevalence of ED among male university students was 1.9%; all cases were identified as EDNOS. Prevalence of possible cases of MD was 6.9%. Men with ED reported desiring a BMI lower than their current BMI, while men with possible MD reported desiring a higher BMI than their current BMI. No differences were observed between cases of ED and possible cases of MD in body dissatisfaction, frequency of physical exercise, and food supplement intake. Both ED and MD risks were associated with a higher frequency of physical exercise, muscularity concerns, body dissatisfaction, and social anxiety. MD risk was also associated with higher levels of worry and lower levels of self-esteem
Unikel, Díaz de León, and Rivera-Márquez (2016)	Mexico	Freshmen university students with overweight or obesity (43.7% males, *n* = 390, mean age = 20.4)	Cross-sectional, survey-based	Brief Risky Eating Behaviors Screening Questionnaire (scores >10, high risk for ED; scores <10 and > 7, moderate risk for ED)	Cutoff score-based	Proportion of males with overweight or obesity and risky eating behaviors was 18.2% for moderate risk and 3.8% for high risk, lower to what has been observed among females (37.8% and 10.8%, respectively). Muscularity concerns were associated with an increased risk of risky eating behaviors among males (OR = 4.4 [2.1, 12.7 95% CI])
Zapata et al. (2018)	Chile	Adolescent students from Concepción City, Chile (37.5% male, *n* = 396, age range 13–18).	Cross-sectional, survey-based	Risk for ED: EAT-40 > 30	Cutoff score-based	Lower proportion of ED risk in males versus females (6.6% versus 21.8%). Among males, those 17 years of age showed greater ED risk (9.3%). Males with obesity showed higher ED risk (14.7%) compared to males with overweight (8.3%) or normal weight (5.2%)

Notes: *ED* eating disorders, *DSM-IV Diagnostic and Statistical Manual of Mental Disorders* (4th ed.), *ICD-10* International Statistical Classification of Diseases and Related Health Problems, *AN* anorexia nervosa, *BN* bulimia nervosa, *BED* binge eating disorders, *EDNOS* eating disorders not otherwise specified, *MD* muscle dysmorphia, *EAT-26* Eating Attitudes Test-26, *EAT-40* Eating Attitudes Test-40, *BULIT-R* Bulimia Test – Revised, *DMS* Drive for Muscularity Scale of teenage boys from Guadalajara were classified as at risk for an ED which is a small rate compared to 10.3% found in females, and ED behaviors among boys were found to be associated with impulsivity traits, depressive symptoms, suicidal ideation, and stress [6]. The same instrument was used in a study of adolescents and young adults in the city of Pachuca, located in the state of Hidalgo, Mexico [7]. Males showed a 2.9% prevalence of risky eating behaviors, consistent with findings from the Guadalajara study [6]. Similarly, 3.8% male freshmen university students from Mexico City with overweight or obesity were found to be at a high risk for an ED [8]. Of interest, this study also assessed concerns about muscularity, which were found to be associated with a four times greater likelihood of reporting risky eating behaviors.

Among cross-sectional survey-based studies, both 40-item and 26-item versions of the Eating Attitudes Test (EAT) [9] have also been used as screening instruments in studies of Latin American men. For example, Reyes-Rodríguez et al. [10] observed that 5.1% of male university students presented at risk for an ED, and those at risk also showed higher levels of depressive symptoms and stressful life events. Also, in a sample of individuals with exercise dependence symptoms from the city of Goiânia (Brazil), Silva et al. [11] reported that 40% of men (versus 60% of women) were identified as at risk by the EAT-26. Finally, in a recent study of students from Concepción, Chile, 6.6% of adolescent boys scored were identified as at risk on the EAT-40. Across the weight spectrum, male high school students with obesity showed higher ED risk (14.7%) compared to males with overweight (8.3%) or normal weight (5.2%) [12].

Few studies have conducted a clinical interview to establish the prevalence of ED among Latin American men [13–15]. Rutsztein et al. [14] studied the prevalence of ED among male and female adolescent students from four high schools in Buenos Aires and metropolitan areas (Argentina). Participants were first classified as at risk or not at risk based on cutoff criteria for the drive for thinness, bulimia, and body dissatisfaction subscales of the Eating Disorder Inventory-2 [16] or if they presented with any weight control purging behavior. Participants then completed a face-to-face interview based on the Eating Disorder Examination interview [17]. Findings from this study showed that almost 6% of adolescent boys were identified as at risk for an ED and 2.9% were diagnosed with an ED, which in all cases was categorized as eating disorder not otherwise specified (EDNOS). Also in Argentina, Compte et al. [15] conducted a two-stage epidemiological study in a representative sample of exclusively male participants from six different universities in Buenos Aires. Participants were screened for an ED using the EAT-26 [18] and for muscle dysmorphia (MD) using the Drive for Muscularity Scale (DMS) [19]. For the second stage, the Eating Disorder Examination interview was used to identify cases of ED based on DSM-IV; in the absence of a validated structured interview for MD, a threshold of 52 on the DMS was considered for possible cases of MD. Consistent with previous findings in Argentinian adolescent boys [14], all cases of ED were EDNOS, with a prevalence of almost 2%. Of particular interest, the prevalence of possible cases of MD among male college students in Argentina was 6.9%, which resembles the total prevalence of ED among female university students [20]. Those identified as at risk of ED or MD exhibited greater social anxiety, body dissatisfaction, concerns with muscularity, and frequency of physical exercise. Of particular interest, individuals with an ED reported desiring a body mass index (BMI) lower than their current BMI, whereas possible cases of MD reported desiring a BMI higher than their current BMI [15]. Finally, Benjet et al. [13] used the Composite International Diagnostic Interview, a structured interview for the assessment of mental disorders according to the ICD-10 and DSM-IV developed by the World Health Organization [21], to assess the prevalence of ED among a large sample of male and female adolescents from the Mexican Adolescent Mental Health Survey in Mexico City and metropolitan areas. The lifetime prevalence among all adolescents was 0.5% for anorexia nervosa (AN), 1.0% for bulimia nervosa (BN), and 1.4% for binge eating disorder (BED). No gender differences for AN cases were observed; males accounted for 30.5% of BN cases and 24.9% of BED cases (Table 16.1).

Potential Risk Factors for ED in Latin American Boys and Men

Among the associated ED risk factors in males from Latin American countries, data from the 2014 Mexican National Survey of Drug Use in Students revealed that maternal education was associated with weight control practices among boys [22]. It has been suggested elsewhere that mothers are important agents of socialization in terms of weight control practices and that adult women with more education are more likely to engage and transmit weight control practices as a value to their children [22]. Also, among Venezuelan adolescents, BED was associated with male gender [23]. Recent evidence further suggests that, among Mexican adolescent boys, high levels of drive for muscularity are associated with disordered eating behaviors as well as higher BMI scores and higher levels of physical activity [24]. Also, Brazilian teenage boys with high levels of ideal body internalization were twice as likely to report restrictive eating compared to peers with low levels of ideal body internalization [25].

Among young adult men in Latin American countries, in addition to internalization of the aesthetic thin ideal, self-esteem, and body dissatisfaction, the drive for muscularity is also associated with disordered eating behaviors among male university students [26]. Among male university students, Compte et al. [27] described an integrated model of associated factors for ED and MD. For both conditions, body dissatisfaction is posited to function as an underlying psychological dimension that reinforces the drive to engage in body change behaviors associated with the ideal body. Physical exercise as a weight control behavior and appearance comparison as an indicator of ideal body internalization and body checking behavior are conceptualized as representing part of the behavioral spectrum associated with the development of ED and MD among Argentinian young men.

Cross-Cultural Studies

To our knowledge, Acosta-Garcia and Gómez-Peresmitre [28] conducted the first report on cross-cultural ED research that studied differences in body dissatisfaction among Spanish and Mexican girls and boys. Results suggested a significant interaction between factors (gender and nationality). Mexican participants showed some degree of body dissatisfaction; Mexican girls presented a significant desire to be thinner, and Mexican boys showed a desire to increase body size. Spanish participants from both genders, however, tend to be satisfied with their body image. Nevertheless, among Spanish and Mexican university students, the latest evidence suggested no differences between the countries in terms of sociocultural influences on appearance, with women showing higher levels than men [29]. Further, Mexican men were more likely to engage in physical exercise aimed at losing weight and follow more than two weight-loss diets in the last year compared to Spanish men [29]. On the other hand, a recent study conducted with community samples from Spain and Chile observed that male and female participants with overweight from both countries were more dissatisfied with their figure than normal weight individuals; however, effect sizes were stronger for women [30].

Giardino and Procidano [31] conducted a cross-sectional study to examine the nature and correlates of MD among men and weightlifters recruited from university gyms in Mexico and the United States. Results among men showed that weightlifters in the United States did not present with higher symptoms of MD or engage in more bodybuilding behaviors as hypothesized. Further, exposure to Western culture (acculturation) did not explain MD symptomatology among Mexican males, as expected. Among men from both countries, MD was found to be associated with bodybuilding behavior, exercise dependence, and eating pathology. Men from both countries also reported higher levels of MD compared to women from the United States and Mexico.

Features of ED Among Latin American Boys and Men

Similar to previous research in Western cultures [32], weightlifters and athletes from Latin American countries have been considered a target population. In one study, weightlifters from Valparaiso, Chile, showed significantly higher levels of interest in appearance and scored higher on the EDI and EDI-40 compared to medical school students; however, no differences in body dissatisfaction were observed among groups [33]. Weightlifters also reported checking their appearance and weight more frequently than university students. Similarly, in a study of gym users and non-gym user university students from Guadalajara, Mexico, there were no significant group differences in body dissatisfaction; however, compared to university students, gym users reported greater symptoms of disordered eating and risky physical exercise behaviors driven by a desire to increase their muscularity [34]. Similarly, among Argentinian men who exercise (50.1% weightlifters and 49.9% CrossFit users), MD was found to be positively associated with body dissatisfaction, disordered eating, and frequency of training days while negatively correlated with the frequency of resting days. Of particular interest, one-third of participants used food supplements as a way to improve their appearance, more than 30% of the sample reported exercise-related injuries, and around 34% trained without the supervision of a healthcare professional [35, 36].

Additionally, a socio-sport model in Brazilian male athletes posits that sociocultural factors and body fat dissatisfaction contribute to the development of disordered eating [37]. Among the sociocultural factors, specific sport-related pressures toward weight are particularly important to consider among male athletes. For example, in rugby-football, a large body size is considered an advantage for sports performance. In this regard, a recent study among 203 collegiate rugby players in Argentina [38] suggests that regardless of the player's position, all participants reported desiring a higher BMI compared to their actual BMI. Additionally, a study conducted with over 150 Brazilian athletes from weight-class sports, sports where leanness improves performance, and sports with aesthetic focus compared differences in percent body fat, ED psychopathology, and body dissatisfaction [39]. No significant differences across groups were found for the main variables; however, athletes with (versus without) body image dissatisfaction had a higher percent body fat. Finally, also among Brazilian athletes, food supplement intake was associated with the male gender, the use of pharmacological substances, and the risk for MD [40]. Food supplement intake was observed to be associated with ED, including muscularity-oriented forms of disordered eating, across the different male samples, suggesting that supplement use is highly relevant with regard to ED psychopathology in men.

There remain subpopulations that are understudied among Latin American males. Few studies to our knowledge have directly assessed features of disordered eating and body dissatisfaction across rural Latin American populations. In this regard, Penelo et al. [41] compared scores on the Eating Disorder Examination Questionnaire (EDE-Q) [42] among teenage boys and girls from urban and rural areas in Mexico. Results showed that adolescent girls from rural and urban areas, and boys from urban areas, scored higher in the attitudinal subscales than adolescent boys from rural settings. Similarly, Miranda et al. [43] studied body image concerns among adolescents from rural cities. Results suggested a higher risk for body dissatisfaction among females and participants with obesity, as well as for those in early adolescence. Additionally, ED among sexual minorities has been understudied across Latin American men. According to a study conducted in a large community sample of cisgender gay men from ten Latin American countries, gay men tend to show a slightly higher prevalence of risk for ED compared to previous studies in community heterosexual male samples, ranging from 6.4% to 15.0% [36]. Finally, clinical populations remain relatively understudied within Latin American studies. In this regard, a study described features of ED in a clinical sample of teenage boys in Chile [44, 45]. The mean age of males with an ED ($N = 33$) was 14 years, with an average symptom duration of 9.5 months prior to diagnosis; 55.2% of boys were identified with AN restricting type and 23.6% with BN purging type. Additionally, 37% of boys presented with a history of being overweight. Finally, 63.1% presented with psychiatric comorbidity at the time of assessment, mostly comprised of mood disorders and obsessive-compulsive personality traits.

ED, MD, and Body Image Assessment in Latin American Boys and Men

Table 16.2 reports the psychometric properties of validation studies that used male samples in Latin American countries. Among the ED measures, Escoto and Camacho [46] validated the Children's Eating Attitudes Test (ChEAT) [47] using a large sample of boys and girls in Mexico. The five-factor underlying structure was similar to that observed in the original version, and psychometric properties were adequate. Also, the SCOFF questionnaire [48] was validated in a large sample of university students from Mexico [49]. Through an exploratory and confirmatory approach, a two-factor structure exhibited the best fit for male participants. The Eating Disorder Examination Questionnaire (EDE-Q) [42] was also validated in a sample of Mexican male and female adolescents [41], as well as in four adult community samples from Argentina [50]. Studies followed a similar methodology, with factor structures tested through confirmatory factor analysis (CFA) and measurement invariance analyses carried out among subset samples. Among Mexican teenagers, a 2-factor EDE-Q solution was invariant across genders and retained all 22 items. Adequate internal consistency and test-retest reliability were also found for the EDE-Q in a sample of Mexican adolescent boys [41]. On the other hand, among Argentinian university students, athletes, weightlifters, and CrossFit users [50], a CFA failed to support previous models including all 22 attitudinal items, and a previously described brief 8-item single-factor model provided the best fit to the data. Internal consistency was adequate, and factor structure remained invariant for this eight-item EDE-Q across the four community subsamples of Argentinian men. Finally, the psychometric properties for the EAT-26 [18] were assessed among Colombian young adult men with and without an ED [51]. Through exploratory factor analysis (EFA), a four-factor model was described, contrary to the original three-factor solution. However, the internal consistency of two of the four derived subscales was less than acceptable.

Measures of MD also have been validated in Latin American samples. For the Muscle Appearance Satisfaction Scale (MASS) [52], Escoto et al. [53] conducted a series of CFAs using data from 258 Mexican bodybuilders and arrived at a 17-item, 5-factor solution similar to the original measure, but with 2 items removed. Significant positive correlations with drive for muscularity, together with adequate internal consistency and evidence of test-retest reliability, support the psychometrics of this Mexican version of the MASS. Recently, Compte et al. [35] conducted an EFA and CFA among separate subset samples of men who exercise to validate

Table 16.2 Eating disorders, body dissatisfaction, muscle dysmorphia, and related measures validated in Latin American boys and men

Author (year)	Scale	Country	Populations (sample sizes)	Factor analysis method and solution (total items)	Measurement invariance	Internal consistency	Test-retest reliability
Escoto and Camacho (2008)	ChEAT (Children's Eating Attitudes Test)	Mexico	Elementary and high school students aged 9–15 (boys = 607, girls = 634)	PCA – 5-factor (motivation to lose weight, avoid fattening foods, concern for food, compensatory behaviors, and perceived social pressure) (25 items)	–	Cronbach's alpha: 0.63–0.77	$r = 0.84$–0.85 (4-week)
Sánchez-Armass et al. (2008)	SCOFF (Sick, Control, One stone, Fat, Food)	Mexico	University applicants aged 16 to 21 (males = 1596, females = 1998)	EFA and CFA – male version: 2-factor (loss of control over food and purging behavior) (5 items)	–	Kuder and Richardson Formula 20 (KR20): 0.40–0.18	–
Campana et al. (2013)	DMS (Drive for Muscularity Scale); SMAQ (Swansea Muscularity Attitudes Questionnaire); MBIDS (Male Body Ideal Distress Scale)	Brazil	Brazilian army ($n = 254$), university students ($n = 88$), industry workers ($n = 66$), athletes ($n = 62$), non-military candidates for a temporary position in the Brazilian army ($n = 408$), age 18–39	CFA – DMS, 2-factor (muscularity attitudes and muscularity behaviors) (15 items); SMAQ, 3-factor (investment in muscularity, masculinity and muscularity and muscularity general benefit) (15 items); 1-factor (Masculine Body Ideal Distress) (6 items)	–	DMS: Cronbach's alpha – 0.80–0.87. SMAQ: Cronbach's alpha – 0.64–0.90. MBIDS: Cronbach's alpha – 0.84	–

Campana et al. (2013b)	BBACS (Brief Body Avoidance and Checking Scale)	Brazil	Male gym users and track and field events participants ($N = 325$). Mean age = 23.0	CFA – 2-factor (muscle and fat checking, body avoidance) (12 items)	–	Cronbach's alpha: 0.71–0.72	–
Carvalho et al. (2013)	MBDS (Male Body Dissatisfaction Scale)	Brazil	Male ED patients ($n = 10$), male college students ($n = 74$), mean age = 23.5	No factor analysis was conducted (25 items)	–	Cronbach's alpha: 0.92	–
Cervantes-Luna et al. (2013)	BMS (Body Modification Scale)	Mexico	Male adolescent students: study 1 – $n = 270$, age 11–15; study 2, $n = 200$, age 12–16	EFA and CFA – 3-factor (weight loss, increment in muscle mass or tone, and weight gain) (20 items)	–	Cronbach's alpha: 0.74–0.89, across studies	$r = 0.63–0.92$, across subscales and studies
Escoto et al. (2013)	DMS (Drive for Muscularity Scale)	Mexico	Male university students ($N = 569$), age 17–26	EFA and CFA – 3-factor (attitudes, supplement consumption, training adherence) (15 items)	–	Cronbach's alpha: 0.68–0.86	–
Penelo et al. (2013)	EDE-Q (Eating Disorder Examination Questionnaire)	Mexico	Elementary and high school students from urban and rural areas, age 11–18 (boys = 1384, girls = 1544)	CFA – 2-factor (restraint and eating, weight and shape concerns) (22 items)	Metric and scalar invariance across genders and area of residence was achieved	Cronbach's alpha: 0.80–0.94	$r = 0.84–0.88$ (2-week)

(continued)

Table 16.2 (continued)

Author (year)	Scale	Country	Populations (sample sizes)	Factor analysis method and solution (total items)	Measurement invariance	Internal consistency	Test-retest reliability
Carvalho et al. (2014)	MBCQ (Male Body Checking Questionnaire)	Brazil	Male university students ($N = 287$), age 18–30	PCA and CFA – 4-factor (global muscle checking, chest and shoulder checking, other-comparative checking, and body testing) (19 items)	–	Cronbach's alpha: 0.71–0.90	–
Compte et al. (2015)	DMS (Drive for Muscularity Scale) and MBAS (Male Body Attitudes Scale)	Argentina	Male university students ($N = 423$), age 18–73	CFA – DMS: 2-factor (muscularity attitudes and muscularity behaviors) (15 items). MBAS: 2-factor (muscularity and low body fat) (22 items)	–	Cronbach's alpha: DMS – 0.86–0.91; MBAS, 0.91 across subscales	–
Castillo et al. (2016)	MBAS (Male Body Attitudes Scale)	Mexico	Male university students ($N = 148$), age 17–27	EFA – 3-factor (muscularity, low body fat, and height) (20 items)	–	Cronbach's alpha: 0.68–0.88	–
Constaín et al. (2017)	EAT-26 (Eating Attitudes Test-26)	Colombia	Males with EDs ($n = 21$), median age = 21, and controls ($n = 114$), median age = 22	EFA – 4-factor (diet and bulimia and concerns about food, diet, oral control and diet, oral control and bulimia) (25 items)	–	Cronbach's alpha: 0.27–0.89	–

da Silva et al. (2017)	MBDS (Male Body Dissatisfaction Scale)	Brazil and Portugal	Male Brazilian ($n = 513$) and Portuguese ($n = 419$) higher education students, age 18–35	CFA – 2-factor (musculature, general body appearance) (12 items)	Weak invariance indicates the adequacy of the model for both samples; however, the absence of the intercept invariance indicates mean differences	Cronbach's alpha: 0.85 and 0.86 (Brazil), 0.84 and 0.88 (Portugal)	–
Escoto et al. (2018)	MASS (Muscle Appearance Satisfaction Scale)	Mexico	Gym users ($N = 258$), age 15–57	CFA – 5-factor (muscle checking, substance use, bodybuilding dependence, muscle dissatisfaction, injury risk) (17 items)	–	Omega: 0.77–0.89	$r = 0.75$–0.91 (2-week)
Compte et al. (2019)	EDE-Q (Eating Disorder Examination Questionnaire)	Argentina	Male university students ($n = 232$), weightlifters ($n = 277$), CrossFit users ($n = 275$), athletes ($n = 202$), age 18–68	CFA – Brief 1-factor (8 items)	Configural, metric, and scalar invariance suggested that the model, factor loadings, and intercepts were invariant across samples	Omega: range from 0.86 to 0.91 across samples	–

(continued)

Table 16.2 (continued)

Author (year)	Scale	Country	Populations (sample sizes)	Factor analysis method and solution (total items)	Measurement invariance	Internal consistency	Test-retest reliability
Compte et al. (2019b)	MDDI (Muscle Dysmorphic Disorder Inventory)	Argentina	Weightlifters (*n* = 276) and CrossFit users (*n* = 275), mean age = 29.7	EFA and CFA – 3-factor (drive for size, appearance intolerance, functional impairment) (13 items)	The model structure, magnitude of the factor loadings, and item intercepts were invariant across weightlifters and CrossFit users	Omega: ranged from 0.72 to 0.84, across 1st and 2nd split-half samples	–
Costa et al. (2019)	BAS-2 (Body Appreciation Scale-2)	Brazil	Adult student and staff population at two universities (men = 430, women = 560), age 18–50	EFA (conducted separately across genders) and CFA – 1-factor (10 items)	Results supported scalar invariance across genders	Among men, omega coefficient was acceptable across EFA and CFA subset samples: 0.86 and 0.92	$r = 0.81$ (3-week)

Notes: *PCA* principal component analysis, *EFA* exploratory factor analysis, *CFA* confirmatory factor analysis, *ED* eating disorder the Muscle Dysmorphic Disorder Inventory (MDDI) [54] among Argentinian men. Data supported the original three-factor solution, and adequate psychometric properties were observed. Validity was further supported through positive associations with male body dissatisfaction, disordered eating, and frequency of training days.

Numerous body dissatisfaction scales have been validated in Latin American men. The Drive for Muscularity Scale (DMS) [19], a 15-item 2-factor measure that assesses muscularity-oriented body image concerns and behaviors, has been validated in samples from Brazil [55], Mexico [45], and Argentina [56]. However, the CFA supported the original factor structure only among Argentinian university students and Brazilian men, whereas among Mexican male university students, an EFA revealed a three-factor solution (i.e., attitudes, substance intake, and training adherence). Furthermore, in a sample of Brazilian men, Campana et al. [55] translated and examined the factor structure of the 20-item 2-factor Swansea Muscularity Attitudes Questionnaire (SMAQ) [57] and the 8-item single-factor Male Body Ideal Distress Scale (MBIDS) [58]. While the unitary factor structure for the MBIDS was confirmed among Brazilian men, the original factor structure of the SMAQ showed poor fit, and a 15-item 3-factor model was better supported. Also among Brazilian men, the Male Body Dissatisfaction Scale (MBDS) [59], an originally 25-item 3-factor measure, was validated. First Carvalho et al. [60] assessed the conceptual, semantic, and instrumental equivalences in an initial attempt to translate the scale into Brazilian-Portuguese, and more recently, da Silva et al. [61] presented evidence supporting a reduced 12-item 2-factor version of the MBDS in a large sample of male college students from Brazil and Portugal ($N = 932$).

Tylka et al. [62] developed the 3-factor 24-item Male Body Attitudes Scale (MBAS), which assesses concerns about muscularity, height, and low body fat, with a total score reflecting general attractiveness. In Latin American men, the MBAS has been validated among male university students from Argentina [56] and Mexico [63]. The Argentine validation confirmed a two-factor structure with ten items loading on the Muscularity Concerns factor and eight items loading on the Low Body Fat factor, as well as on four additional items contributing to the total score; the Height subscale was not considered for the analysis, as it was comprised of only two items. Psychometric support for the Argentine version of the MBAS was evidenced by adequate internal consistency and positive associations with disordered eating, body checking behaviors, and social anxiety. In a sample of Mexican college students, an EFA revealed a 3-factor 24-item solution similar to the original MBAS, with scores found to be positively associated with disordered eating. Similar to the MBAS, the Body Modification Scale (BMS) [64] was developed to simultaneously assess pro-thin and pro-muscle body change behaviors. A Spanish-language version of the BMS was evaluated among adolescent boys in Mexico City through using EFA and CFA [65]. A final 3-factor model that resembles the original version, though retaining only 20 of the 24 original items, was supported. Adequate internal consistency and evidence of test-retest reliability also suggested that the BMS is a reliable instrument to assess body change strategies in adolescent boys in Mexico.

Other body image-related measures also have been validated among samples of Latin American men. Campana et al. [66] developed and validated the Brief Body Avoidance and Checking Scale (BBACS) among physically active men in Brazil. A CFA that supported the theoretical 2-factor structure (Muscle and Fat Checking and Body Avoidance) comprised of 12 items. The BBACS also showed adequate internal consistency and was also found to be associated with male body ideal distress, drive for muscularity, and exercise intensity and frequency. Additionally, a Brazilian version of the Male Body Checking Questionnaire (MBCQ) [67] was validated by Carvalho et al. [68] among male university students using EFA and CFA. Similar to the original version, a 19-item 4-factor structure was supported. However, among Brazilian university male students, items corresponding to each factor were grouped according to different types of body checking behaviors (e.g., body comparison with others, use of reflective surfaces). Adequate internal consistency and positive associations with body dissatisfaction also suggested that MBCQ is a reliable and valid tool to assess body checking among Brazilian men. Lastly, the Brazilian version of the Body Appreciation Scale-2 (BAS-2) [69] focuses on positive aspects of body image. The ten-item BAS-2 was developed to avoid sex-specific bias, and a single-factor solution invariant across genders was described for the original version. A ten-item single-factor structure that is invariant across sex was also supported within a large sample of Brazilian men and women. Further psychometric support was evidenced by adequate internal consistency, test-retest reliability, positive associations with satisfaction with life and self-esteem, and negative associations with appearance dissatisfaction, drive for muscularity, and disordered eating [70] (Table 16.2).

Sociocultural Influences

Few studies have addressed sociocultural influences for the development and maintenance of ED among males in Latin America. In this regard, a study conducted in adolescent boys and girls in the city of Temuco, Chile, aimed to examine how perceived sociocultural influences were related to body dissatisfaction and body change behaviors [71]. No differences between genders were observed for perceived pressures to lose weight from adults or older siblings/cousins in the family. However, compared to girls, boys reported greater perceived pressure to lose weight from peers and higher perceived pressure from family, peers, and the media to increase their muscularity. Findings from this study suggest not only that boys were under social pressure to lose weight but also that the perceived pressure from peers may relate to messages focused on leanness and muscle tone, which may at times be conflated with the idea of weight loss more generally. Similarly, Mexican male university students were more likely to engage in disordered eating behaviors if they perceived criticism from both parents, had obesity, and desired a slimmer body [72]. Also in this line, a large cohort study ($N = 2486$) of male and female adolescents in Brazil found that in adolescents with a normal BMI, perceived parental opinions on their weight at age 11 were associated with body dissatisfaction at age 15 and disordered eating behaviors in later adolescence, although effect sizes were larger for girls than for boys [73]. Additionally, a study that investigated maternal dissatisfaction with their child's body size among 548 mother-child dyads in Brazil found that mothers of boys were more likely to desire a larger body size for their son, compared to mothers of girls. There was also a positive correlation between the mothers' body dissatisfaction and dissatisfaction with their child's body size, suggesting that mothers may generalize their body dissatisfaction to the perception of their own child's body size [74].

Conclusion

In conclusion, conducting epidemiological studies of ED, MD, and body dissatisfaction in males remains a challenge in Latin America, mainly due to the lack of appropriate assessment instruments, perceived stigma, shame associated with disclosure of mental health issues, and female-centric nature of the current classification schemes. The impairment in quality of life and psychosocial well-being, and the loss of productivity seen in ED and related forms of psychopathology, seems to be comparable in males and females. It is imperative to address barriers like shame, stigma, and female-centric services, to allow people to access treatment in a timely way. It is also crucial that future epidemiological studies conducted in Latin America be more inclusive of males and male-relevant variables.

References

1. American Psychiatric Association, editor. Diagnostic and statistical manual of mental disorders. 4th ed. Washington, DC: American Psychiatric Association; 1994.
2. Unikel C, Saucedo-Molina T, Villatoro J, Fleiz C. Conductas alimentarias de riesgo y distribución del Indice de Masa Corporal en estudiantes de 13 a 18 años. Salud Ment [Internet]. 2002 [cited 2020 Jan 13];25(2):49–57.
3. Unikel C, Bojórquez-Chapela L, Villatoro-Velázquez J, Fleiz-Bautista C, Medina-Mora Icaza ME. Risky eating behaviors in student population in México City: trends 1997–2003. Rev Investig clínica. 2006;58(1):15–27.
4. Unikel C, Bojórquez I, Carreño S. Validación de un cuestionario breve para medir conductas alimentarias de riesgo. Salud Publica Mex. 2004;46(6):509–15.
5. Barriguete-Melendez J, Unikel-Santoncini C, Aguilar-Salinas C, Cordova-Villalobos J, Shamah T, Barquera S, et al. Prevalencia de conductas alimentarias anormales de adolescentes en México: Encuesta Nacional de Salud y Nutrición ENSANUT 2006. Salud Publica Mex. 2009;51:S638–44.
6. Nuño-Gutiérrez BL, Celis-de la Rosa A, Unikel-Santoncini C. Prevalence and associated factors related to disordered eating in student adolescents of Guadalajara across sex. Rev Investig Clin. 2009;61(4):286–93.

7. Saucedo–Molina T de J, Unikel Santoncini C. Disordered eating, internalization of the body thin–ideal and body mass index in high school and college students from a private institution in Hidalgo, Mexico Salud Ment 2010;33(1):11–19.
8. Unikel C, Díaz C, Rivera JA. Conductas alimentarias de riesgo y correlatos psicosociales en estudiantes universitarios de primer ingreso con sobrepeso y obesidad. Salud Ment. 2016;39(3):141–8.
9. Garfinkel PE, Newman A. The eating attitudes test: twenty-five years later. Eat Weight Disord. 2001;6(1):1–24.
10. Reyes-Rodriguez ML, Sala M, Von Holle A, Unikel C, Bulik CM, Camara-Fuentes L, et al. A description of disordered eating behaviors in Latino males. J Am Coll Heal. 2011;59(4):266–72.
11. da Silva EF, da Silva AR, da Silva AD, Pedrino GR, Rosa DA. Prevalence of eating disorder attitudes among men and women with exercise dependence symptoms: a non-athlete population study. Rev Bras Ciências do Esporte. 2013;35(3):599–610.
12. Zapata D, Granfeldt G, Muñoz S, Celis M, Vicente B, Sáez K, et al. Risk of eating disorders in Chilean adolescents of different types educational establishments. Arch Latinoam Nutr. 2018;68(3):217.
13. Benjet C, Méndez E, Borges G, Medina-mora ME. Epidemiología de los trastornos de la conducta alimentaria en una muestra representativa de adolescentes. Salud Ment. 2012;35(6):483–90.
14. Rutsztein G, Murawski B, Elizathe L, Scappatura ML. Eating disorders: Detection in female and male adolescents in Buenos Aires. A two-stage study / Trastornos alimentarios: Detección en adolescentes mujeres y varones de Buenos Aires. Un estudio de doble fase. Rev Mex Trastor Aliment / Mex J Eat Disord. 2010;1(1):48–61.
15. Compte EJ, Sepulveda AR, Torrente F. A two-stage epidemiological study of eating disorders and muscle dysmorphia in male university students in Buenos Aires. Int J Eat Disord. 2015;48(8):1092–101.
16. Garner DM. Eating disorder Inventory-2. Professional manual. Psychological Assessment Resources: Odessa; 1991.
17. Fairburn CG, Cooper Z. The eating disorder examination. In: Binge eating: nature, assessment and treatment. 12th ed. New York: Guilford Press; 1993. p. 317–60.
18. Garner DM, Olmsted MP, Bohr Y, Garfinkel PE. The eating attitudes test: psychometric features and clinical correlates. Psychol Med. 1982;12(04):871.
19. McCreary DR, Sasse DK, Saucier DM, Dorsch KD. Measuring the drive for muscularity: factorial validity of the drive for muscularity scale in men and women. Psychol Men Masc. 2004;5(1):49–58.
20. Eisenberg D, Nicklett EJ, Roeder K, Kirz NE. Eating disorder symptoms among college students: prevalence, persistence, correlates, and treatment-seeking. J Am Coll Heal. 2011;59(8):700–7.
21. Kessler RC, Üstün TB. The World Mental Health (WMH) survey initiative version of the World Health Organization (WHO) composite international diagnostic interview (CIDI). Int J Methods Psychiatr Res. 2004;13(2):93–121.
22. Bojorquez I, Villatoro J, Delgadillo M, Fleiz C, Fregoso D, Unikel C. Social factors, weight perception, and weight control practices among adolescents in Mexico. J Health Psychol. 2018;23(7):939–50.
23. Morales Pernalete AR, Gordillo Gutierrez CA, Pérez Alvarado CJ, Marcano Flores DA, Pérez Pérez FA, Flores Navas HL, et al. Risk factors for binge eating disorders and its association with obesity in adolescents. Gac Med Mex. 2014;150(1):125–31.
24. Arellano-Pérez OG, Vázquez-Cervantes MJ, Fernández Cortés TL, Saucedo-Molina T d J. Drive for muscularity and disordered eating behaviors and its relationship with anthropometric indicators and physical activity in Mexican adolescent men. Eat Weight Disord - Stud Anorexia, Bulim Obes. 2019;24(4):661–70.
25. Fortes L de S, Morgado FF da R, Ferreira MEC. Fatores associados ao comportamento alimentar inadequado em adolescentes escolares. Arch Clin Psychiatry (São Paulo). 2013;40(2):59–64.

26. Díaz de León-Vázquez C, Rivera-Márquez JA, Bojorquez-Chapela L, Unikel-Santoncini C. Variables associated with disordered eating behaviors among freshman students from Mexico City. Salud Publica Mex. 2017;59:258.
27. Compte EJ, Sepúlveda AR, Torrente F. Approximations to an integrated model of eating disorders and muscle dysmorphia among university male students in Argentina. Men Masc. 2018:1–18.
28. Acosta Garcia MV, Gómez PG. Valoración de la delgadez. Un estudio transcultural (México/España). Psicothema. 2002;14(2):221–6.
29. Mancilla-Díaz JM, Lameiras-Fernández M, Vázquez-Arévalo R, Alvarez-Rayón G, Franco-Paredes K, López-Aguilar X, et al. Sociocultural influences and disordered eating behaviors in men and woman of Spain and Mexico. Rev Mex Trastor Aliment / Mex J Eat Disord. 2010;1(1):36–47.
30. Varela C, Oda-Montecinos C, Saldaña C. Estudio transcultural de los diferentes componentes de la insatisfacción corporal en muestras comunitarias de España y Chile. Nutr Hosp. 2019;36(3):691–7.
31. Giardino JC, Procidano ME. Muscle dysmorphia symptomatology: a cross-cultural study in Mexico and the United States. Int J Mens Health. 2012;11(1):83–103.
32. Murray SB, Nagata JM, Griffiths S, Calzo JP, Brown TA, Mitchison D, et al. The enigma of male eating disorders: a critical review and synthesis. Clin Psychol Rev. 2017;57:1–11.
33. Behar R, Molinari D. Dismorfia muscular, imagen corporal y conductas alimentarias en dos poblaciones masculinas. Rev Med Chile. 2010:1386–94.
34. Baile Ayensa J, Gonzales Díaz A, Ramírez Ortiz C, Suarez AP. Imagen corporal, hábitos alimentarios y hábitos de ejercicio físico en hombres usuarios de gimnasio y hombres universitarios no usuarios. Rev Psicol del Deport. 2011;20(2):353–66.
35. Compte EJ, Nagata JM, Sepúlveda AR, Rivas A, Sbdar LS, Menga S, et al. Assessment and validation of a Spanish version of the muscle dysmorphia disorder inventory in Argentinian men who exercise: Inventario de Dismorfia muscular. Body Image. 2019;31:24–34.
36. Toro-Alfonso J, Urzúa Morales A, Sánchez CI. El Cuerpo del Delito: La imagen corporal e indicadores de trastornos alimentarios en una muestra de hombres gay de diez países latinoamericanos. Rev Arg Clínica Psic. 2012;21(2):101–12.
37. Fortes L de S, Ferreira MEC, de Oliveira SMF, Cyrino ES, Almeida SS. A socio-sports model of disordered eating among Brazilian male athletes. Appetite. 2015;92:29–35.
38. Compte EJ, Murray SB, Sepúlveda AR, Schweiger S, Bressan M, Torrente F. What position do you play? Eating disorder pathology among rugby players, and the understudied role of player position. Int J Eat Disord. 2018;51(8):1015–9.
39. Goltz FR, Stenzel LM, Schneider CD, Goltz FR, Stenzel LM, Schneider CD. Disordered eating behaviors and body image in male athletes. Rev Bras Psiquiatr. 2013;35(3):237–42.
40. Garcez Nabuco HC. Factores asociados con la suplementación de la dieta entre los atletas brasileños. Nutr Hosp. 2016;33(3):678–84.
41. Penelo E, Negrete A, Portell M, Raich RM. Psychometric Properties of the Eating Disorder Examination Questionnaire (EDE-Q) and Norms for Rural and Urban Adolescent Males and Females in Mexico. Tomé D, editor. PLoS One. 2013;8(12):e83245.
42. Fairburn CG, Beglin SJ. Assessment of eating disorders: interview or self-report questionnaire? Int J Eat Disord. 1994;16(4):363–70.
43. Miranda VPN, Conti MA, Bastos RR, Laus MF, Almeida S. de S, Ferreira MEC. Imagem corporal de adolescentes de cidades rurais. Cien Saude Colet. 2014;19(6):1791–801.
44. Salas F, Hodgson MI, Figueroa D, Urrejola P. Clinical features of adolescent males with eating disorders. Rev Med Chil. 2011;139(2):182–8.
45. Escoto C, Alvarez-Rayón G, Mancilla-Díaz JM, Camacho Ruiz EJ, Franco Paredes K, Juárez Lugo CS. Psychometric properties of the drive for muscularity scale in Mexican males. Eat Weight Disord - Stud Anorexia, Bulim Obes. 2013;18(1):23–8.
46. Escoto C, Camacho E. Propiedades psicométricas del Test Infantil de Actitudes Alimentarias en una muestra mexicana. Rev Mex Psicol. 2008;25:99–106.

47. Maloney MJ, McGuire JB, Daniels SR. Reliability testing of a children's version of the eating attitude test. J Am Acad Child Adolesc Psychiatry. 1988;27(5):541–3.
48. Morgan JF, Reid F, Lacey JH. The SCOFF questionnaire: assessment of a new screening tool for eating disorders. BMJ. 1999;319(7223):1467–8.
49. Sánchez-Armass O, Drumond-Andrade FC, Wiley AR, Raffaelli M, Aradillas-García C. Evaluation of the psychometric performance of the SCOFF questionnaire in a Mexican young adult sample. Salud Publica Mex. 2008;54(4):375–82.
50. Compte EJ, Nagata JM, Sepúlveda AR, Schweiger S, Sbdar LS, Silva BC, et al. Confirmatory factor analysis and measurement invariance of the eating disorders examination-questionnaire across four male samples in Argentina. Int J Eat Disord. 2019;52(6):740–5.
51. Constaín GA, Rodríguez-Gázquez M de los Á, Ramírez Jiménez GA, Gómez Vásquez GM, Mejía Cardona L, Cardona Vélez J. Validez y utilidad diagnóstica de la escala Eating Attitudes Test-26 para la evaluación del riesgo de trastornos de la conducta alimentaria en población masculina de Medellín, Colombia. Atención Primaria 2017;49(4):206–213.
52. Mayville SB, Williamson DA, White MA, Netemeyer RG, Drab DL. Development of the muscle appearance satisfaction scale: a self-report measure for the assessment of muscle dysmorphia symptoms. Assessment. 2002;9(4):351–60.
53. Escoto Ponce de León M del C, Bosques-Brugada LE, Camacho Ruiz EJ, Alvarez-Rayón G, Franco Paredes K, Rodríguez Hernández G. Psychometric evaluation of the muscle appearance satisfaction scale in a Mexican male sample. Eat Weight Disord - Stud Anorexia, Bulim Obes. 2018;23(5):695–703.
54. Hildebrandt T, Langenbucher J, Schlundt DG. Muscularity concerns among men: development of attitudinal and perceptual measures. Body Image. 2004;1(2):169–81.
55. Campana ANNB, Tavares MDCGCF, Swami V, da Silva D. An examination of the psychometric properties of Brazilian Portuguese translations of the drive for muscularity scale, the Swansea muscularity attitudes questionnaire, and the masculine body ideal distress scale. Psic Men Masc. 2013;14(4):376–88.
56. Compte EJ, Sepúlveda AR, de Pellegrin Y, Blanco M. Confirmatory factor analysis of the Drive for Muscularity Scale-S(DMS-S) and Male Body Attitudes Scale-S (MBAS-S) among male university students in Buenos Aires. Body Image. 2015;14:13–9.
57. Morrison TG, Morrison MA. Psychometrics properties of the Swansea Muscularity Attitudes Questionnaire (SMAQ). Body Image. 2006;3(2):131–44.
58. Kimmel S, Mahalik J. Measuring masculine body ideal distress: development of a measure. Int J Mens Health. 2004;3(1):1–10.
59. Ochner CN, Gray JA, Brickner K. The development and initial validation of a new measure of male body dissatisfaction. Eat Behav. 2009;10(4):197–201.
60. de Carvalho PHB, Ferreira MEC, Kotait M, Teixeira PC, Hearst N, Cordás TA, et al. Conceptual, semantic, and instrumental equivalences: preliminary analysis of the Brazilian Portuguese version of the Male Body Dissatisfaction Scale (MBDS). Cad Saude Publica. 2013;29(2):403–9.
61. da Silva WR, Marôco J, Ochner CN, Campos JADB. Male body dissatisfaction scale (MBDS): proposal for a reduced model. Eat Weight Disord - Stud Anorexia, Bulim Obes. 2017;22(3):515–25.
62. Tylka TL, Bergeron D, Schwartz JP. Development and psychometric evaluation of the Male Body Attitudes Scale (MBAS). Body Image. 2005;2(2):161–75.
63. Castillo I, Solano S, Sepúlveda AR. Validación mexicana de la escala de actitudes masculinas sobre el cuerpo en estudiantes universitarios varones. Rev Iberoam Diagnóstico y Evaluación. 2018;46(1):51–65.
64. Mccabe MP, Vincent MA. Development of body modification and excessive exercise scales for adolescents. Assessment. 2002;9(2):131–41.
65. Cervantes-Luna BS, Alvarez-Rayón G, Gómez-Peresmitré G, mancilla-díaz J manuel. Reliability and constuct validity of the body modification scale in adolescent males. Salud Menta 2013;36:487–492.

66. Campana. ANNB, Swami V, Morgado FF da R, Campana MB, Morgado JJ, Ferreira L, et al. The brief body avoidance and checking scale for physically active men development and initial validation. Int J Sport Psychol 2013;44(6):531–545.
67. Hildebrandt T, Walker DC, Alfano L, Delinsky S, Bannon K. Development and validation of a male specific body checking questionnaire. Int J Eat Dis. 2010;43:77–87.
68. de Carvalho PHB, Conti MA, Ribeiro MS, Amaral ACS, Ferreira MEC. Psychometric assessment of the Male Body Checking Questionnaire (MBCQ). Psicol Reflexão e Crítica. 2014;27(4):700–9.
69. Tylka TL, Wood-Barcalow NL. The body appreciation scale-2: item refinement and psychometric evaluation. Body Image. 2015;12:53–67.
70. Junqueira ACP, Laus MF, Sousa Almeida S, Braga Costa TM, Todd J, Swami V. Translation and validation of a Brazilian Portuguese version of the body appreciation scale-2 in Brazilian adults. Body Image. 2019;31:160–70.
71. Mellor D, McCabe M, Ricciardelli L, Merino ME. Body dissatisfaction and body change behaviors in Chile: the role of sociocultural factors. Body Image. 2008;5(2):205–15.
72. de León-Vázquez CD, Villalobos-Hernández A, Rivera-Márquez JA, Unikel-Santoncini C. Effect of parental criticism on disordered eating behaviors in male and female university students in Mexico City. Eat Weight Disord - Stud Anorexia, Bulim Obes. 2019;24(5):853–60.
73. Abdalla S, Buffarini R, Weber AM, Cislaghi B, Costa JC, Menezes AMB, et al. Parent-related normative perceptions of adolescents and later weight control behavior: longitudinal analysis of cohort data from Brazil. J Adolesc Health. 2020;66(1):S9–16.
74. Pedroso J, Toral N, Bauermann Gubert M. Maternal dissatisfaction with their children's body size in private schools in the Federal District, Brazil. Wiley AS, editor. PLoS One. 2018;13(10):e0204848.

Chapter 17
Eating Disorders and Related Symptomatology in Sexual Minority Men and Boys

Alexandra D. Convertino, Christopher A. Albright, and Aaron J. Blashill

Learning Objectives
1. To understand how current theoretical models of eating pathology can include sexual minority-specific influences relevant for sexual minority men and boys
2. To incorporate this understanding and apply to theoretical models of prevention and treatment for eating pathology and how these might be adapted for sexual minority men and boys

Key Points
- Sexual minority men and boys (e.g., gay, bisexual) are at greater risk of developing eating pathology than their heterosexual peers.
- While some hypothesized mechanisms for the development and maintenance of eating pathology are similar among sexual minority men and boys as compared to heterosexual women and girls, it appears that sexual minority-specific influences (e.g., internalized homophobia, sexual orientation concealment) may also contribute to greater eating pathology.
- Very little adaption of existing treatment and prevention protocols has been conducted for sexual minority men and boys.
- Future research should seek to determine the extent to which current models, evidence-based treatment, and prevention protocols should be altered to fit the needs of sexual minority men and boys.

A. D. Convertino · C. A. Albright
San Diego State University/University of California San Diego Joint Doctoral Program in Clinical Psychology, San Diego, CA, USA
e-mail: aconvertino@ucsd.edu; calbright@sdsu.edu

A. J. Blashill (✉)
Department of Psychology, San Diego State University, San Diego, CA, USA

Department of Psychology, San Diego State University/University of California San Diego Joint Doctoral Program in Clinical Psychology, San Diego, CA, USA
e-mail: ajblashill@sdsu.edu

J. M. Nagata et al. (eds.), *Eating Disorders in Boys and Men*,
https://doi.org/10.1007/978-3-030-67127-3_17

Introduction

In recent years, considerable research efforts have been directed toward addressing eating disorders in sexual minority men and boys (i.e., individuals who identify as gay, bisexual, or any sexual identity other than heterosexual, as well as men and boys who experience attraction to and/or engage in sexual behavior with other men). In this chapter, we will begin by reviewing disparities in eating disorders and pathology in sexual minority men and boys. We will then review theoretical models, including adaptations of well-known developmental models of eating pathology specific to the experiences of sexual minority men and boys, that attempt to explain noted disparities. Next, we will discuss evidence-based prevention and treatment protocols in sexual minority men, as well as relevant adaptations of existing protocols for this group. Finally, we discuss future directions in eating disorder research for sexual minority men and boys.

Prevalence of Eating Disorders in Sexual Minority Men and Boys

Clear disparities in both eating disorder diagnoses and behaviors have emerged for sexual minority men and boys. Research in both adolescent boys and adult men have found increased rates of eating pathology, specifically anabolic steroid misuse [1], dieting for weight loss [2], fasting to lose weight [3], diet pill use [2–5], purging (i.e., vomiting and laxative use) [2–5], and binge eating [5, 6]. Furthermore, prior studies of self-reported eating disorder diagnoses have demonstrated increased prevalence in national college samples of gay, bisexual, and men unsure of their sexual orientation as compared to heterosexual cisgender men and women [3, 4].

Studies examining prevalence utilizing objective diagnostic assessment (rather than self-report) are rare. However, one study found higher lifetime prevalence rates of eating disorders in gay and bisexual men as compared to heterosexual men in New York (any eating disorder, 8.8% vs. 1.5%; anorexia nervosa, 1% vs. 0%; bulimia nervosa, 6.2% vs. 0%; binge eating disorder, 5.2% vs. 1.5%) [7]. Furthermore, a recent, nationally representative study of US adults found elevated rates of all eating disorder diagnoses in sexual minority individuals as compared to heterosexual men and women (any eating disorder, 3.6% vs. 1.6%; anorexia nervosa, 1.71% vs. 0.77%; bulimia nervosa, 1.25% vs. 0.24%; binge eating disorder, 2.17% vs. 0.81%) [8], though this study did not examine differences in diagnoses by sexual identity subgroups or gender. Taken together, there is a clear evidence of increased eating pathology in sexual minority men and boys.

Theoretical Models

The observed disparities in eating pathology are likely the result of a confluence of factors both unique and specific to sexual minority men and boys. Thus far, three models with strong theoretical support have been proposed to explain the development and maintenance of eating pathology in sexual minority men and boys: the tripartite influence model [9, 10], objectification theory [11], and sexual minority stress theory [12]. While the tripartite influence model and objectification theory were first proposed and tested in heterosexual women to explain elevated eating pathology, sexual minority stress theory was first proposed in sexual minorities to explain elevated psychopathology overall.

Tripartite Influence Model

The tripartite influence model [9, 10] posits that family, peers, and media communicate messages about the ideal body to individuals. While some individuals do not internalize (or believe) these messages, others do and compare themselves to this ideal. Since the ideal body is unattainable for most, individuals that compare themselves to the ideal typically find themselves falling short of the body ideal, creating body dissatisfaction. Body dissatisfaction will then lead some individuals to engage in disordered eating behaviors in order to achieve the body ideal.

Researchers have modified this model to include sexual minority-specific influences. At the social influence level, sexual minority communities and romantic partners have been implicated as further sources of sociocultural pressures for sexual minority men. A lean and muscular physique consistent with the mesomorphic ideal is widely acknowledged as the most attractive physical form in the sexual minority men community and may lead to greater pressure to conform to this ideal [13]. The effect of this pressure may be heightened for sexual minority men, as perceived social pressure to conform to appearance ideals has been found to be more strongly linked to social appearance anxiety and drive for thinness among sexual minority men as compared to heterosexual men [14]. In preliminary support of the tripartite influence model, gay community involvement and romantic partners were found to be additional significant predictors of internalization of the mesomorphic ideal and social comparison, which then predicted body dissatisfaction in a sample of primarily White gay men [15]. Since this is one of the few studies that examines the tripartite influence model in sexual minority men, further research is needed to expand this finding to other sexual minority men, particularly in bisexual and other sexual minority populations, and ethnically and racially diverse men.

Objectification Theory

Another model of disordered eating is objectification theory [11]. Objectification theory posits that women, through repeated experiences of objectification or reduction of their worth to the body or body parts, learn to internalize and perpetuate this observer's viewpoint onto themselves. This perspective results in increased self-monitoring of their appearance and experiencing body shame, leading to increased engagement in body modification behaviors such as eating pathology to meet cultural standards of appearance.

As standards of beauty for men have become increasingly salient and unattainable, the increased bodily scrutiny to which women are subject may also be placed onto men. Indeed, previous research has demonstrated that gay men experience objectification at similar rates to heterosexual women [16] and demonstrate a greater tendency to objectify themselves and other men as compared to heterosexual men [17]. Theoretically, these experiences and tendencies may be related to pursuing men as sexual partners, similar to heterosexual women, and the emphasis on physical attractiveness in sexual relationships that men often endorse [18]. Two studies have attempted to experimentally manipulate self-objectification with mixed results; while Michaels, Parent, and Moradi [19] found no increased body dissatisfaction following exposure to muscularity-idealizing images, Martins, Tiggemann, and Kirkbride [20] found that gay men experienced greater body dissatisfaction, body shame, and dietary restraint following the self-objectification condition as compared to heterosexual men. With these mixed results, future research should seek to examine these findings with different experimental conditions and with different sexual minority populations, including bisexual men.

Minority Stress Theory

Minority stress theory proposes that sexual minority men and boys are subjected to chronic stress based on their sexual orientation in a heterosexist society which leads to greater physical and mental illness [12]. Stressors are categorized into distal (direct discrimination, harassment, and victimization) and proximal stressors (internalized homophobia, concealment of sexual identity, and expectations of stigma-based rejection) [21]. Some minority stressors have been included in models of disordered eating development for sexual minorities. For example, some studies have found internalized homophobia to be associated with eating pathology [22, 23], while others have not [24]. Other predictors that have been tested included sexual orientation concealment [24] and discrimination [8, 24–26]. However, research on the influence of sexual minority-specific stressors on eating pathology has been mixed, and limited research has examined these stressors longitudinally, as sexual minority stress theory would imply, to examine whether proximal and distal stressors precede eating pathology development.

Summary

The tripartite influence model, objectification theory, and minority stress theory all have some research support in various capacities. Furthermore, these models may also interact or overlap with each other. For example, internalized homophobia, a sexual minority stressor, has been linked to body shame, a mediator in objectification theory [27, 28], and body dissatisfaction, a mediator in the tripartite model [29].

An additional complication for examining the development of eating pathology in sexual minority men is that most relevant self-report measures have not yet been psychometrically examined in this population or only segments of the population (see Table 17.1 for review).

In sum, these models theorize that sexual minority men and boys are subject to specific, culturally relevant factors that heighten their risk of eating pathology as compared to their heterosexual peers, such as less attainable beauty standards in the sexual minority community [13], as well as factors specific to the sexual minority community, including internalized homophobia and other stressors. Future research should consider conducting measurement invariance analyses comparing sexual minority men to heterosexual men and women for commonly used eating pathology and related predictors. Additionally, researchers have yet to test all hypothesized predictors in a single, integrated model, potentially omitting valuable explanatory mechanisms.

Table 17.1 Self-report measures that have been examined in sexual minority men

Measure	Symptomatology assessed	Psychometric research
Eating Disorder Examination Questionnaire [30]	Largely thinness-based eating disordered behaviors (e.g., restriction, purging) and body dissatisfaction	Acceptable internal consistency and convergent validity across subscales; factor structure confirmed in sexual minority men [31]
Drive for Muscularity Scale [32]	Attitudes and behaviors toward having a more muscular body	Acceptable internal consistency and convergent validity across subscales; factor structure confirmed in sexual minority men [33] Translation into Italian has been examined in gay men only [34]
Male Body Attitudes Scale [35]	Body dissatisfaction	Acceptable internal consistency across subscales and factor structure confirmed in gay men only [36]
Social Appearance Anxiety Scale [37, 38]	Anxiety about being evaluated by others based on appearance, including body shape	Acceptable internal consistency and convergent validity; factor structure confirmed in sexual minority men of color [38]
Sociocultural Attitudes Towards Appearance Questionnaire [39]	Pressures toward and internalization of the body ideal	Acceptable internal consistency and convergent validity across subscales; factor structure confirmed in sexual minority men [40]

Prevention and Treatment of Eating Disorders Among Sexual Minority Men

Although a considerable disparity in eating disorder pathology among sexual minority men is well-documented in the literature, little research attention has been devoted to evaluating eating disorder prevention efforts and treatments within this population to date. In fact, men remain underrepresented in eating disorder research broadly, which makes identifying the best treatments for sexual minority men somewhat challenging. Therefore, it is useful to first identify the few programs that have been tailored to sexual minority men specifically and subsequently examine how sexual minority men can be better served using existing treatments. From there, we can outline future research directions and how this population can be better served by prevention and treatment efforts moving forward.

Prevention of Eating Disorders

At the time of publication, the PRIDE Body Project is the only prevention program to the authors' knowledge that has been specifically adapted to the needs of sexual minority men. The PRIDE Body Project is a two-session group intervention derived from the Body Project, an eating disorder prevention project designed for adolescent girls, youth, and young adult women [41–43]. The program employs elements from cognitive dissonance theory in order to enact attitudinal and behavioral change. According to cognitive dissonance theory, people experience psychological discomfort when their behavior does not reflect their beliefs, leading people to change their beliefs to be concordant with their actions [44]. Thus, the activities contained within the PRIDE Body Project are designed to challenge the lean, muscular body ideal that many men internalize in order to reduce eating disorder attitudes and behaviors.

The PRIDE Body Project is a noteworthy prevention program in several regards. Firstly, the intervention is co-led by peers within the sexual minority community, which may increase the acceptability of the content of the program to those participating and ease of implementation in the community due to the reduced cost of employing peer facilitators. The intervention also addresses stressors that are specific to men within the LGBTQ+ community, which may be more salient targets for intervention than discussion surrounding more general body image concerns. Indeed, the results of a preliminary randomized controlled trial seem promising, with participants in the PRIDE Body Project demonstrating significant and large reductions in body ideal internalization, body dissatisfaction, dietary restraint, drive for muscularity, self- and partner objectification, and bulimic symptoms as compared to individuals in a waitlist control [45]. A large randomized controlled trial is currently underway testing the intervention as compared to a time- and attention-matched control group (NIH grant number R01MD012698). After more empirical support for the PRIDE Body Project has been established, other avenues of delivery can be explored (e.g., an online intervention), further increasing the feasibility and accessibility of the program.

Eating Disorder Treatments

There are currently no treatments for eating disorders that have been specifically designed for use within sexual minority men. However, there are several treatments for eating disorders that have strong empirical support, including enhanced cognitive-behavioral therapy, interpersonal psychotherapy, family-based treatment, and dialectical behavior therapy, and these treatments can be adapted to be more specific to the needs of sexual minority men. Using the aforementioned theoretical models, practitioners can integrate the sociocultural and interpersonal pressures unique to sexual minority man as treatment targets into existing eating disorder treatments to make these interventions more relevant and effective for this population.

Enhanced cognitive-behavioral therapy (CBT-E) is grounded in the transdiagnostic cognitive-behavioral theory of eating disorders, which asserts that perfectionism, low self-esteem, and interpersonal difficulties lead individuals to engage in maladaptive behaviors to change their body image and maintain eating disorder symptoms [46, 47]. Broadly, CBT-E involves understanding the client's history that led to eating disorder development, identifying and addressing factors that maintain eating disorder symptoms, and relapse prevention. At each of these stages, there are opportunities to adapt the protocol specifically to the experiences of sexual minority men. Environmental stressors, such as minority stress experiences and the sociocultural pressure from within the LGBTQ+ community to attain a lean physique, may contribute to both the etiology and relapse of eating disorder symptoms. Additionally, the interpersonal difficulties related to coming out, experiencing harassment and discrimination, and simply existing in a non-affirming society should all be considered as potential contributing factors to the maintenance of eating disorder symptomology.

These stressors would also be important to consider for sexual minority clients engaged in interpersonal therapy (IPT), in which the relationship between social dysfunction and psychological symptoms is a central focus [48]. The role that peers play in maintaining body image disturbance could be an important consideration using this treatment modality, as is consistent with the tripartite model of eating disorders [9, 10]. More specifically, treatment can address pressures from both sexual partners and the broader LGBTQ+ community to meet physical attractiveness standards and the influence that has on eating behaviors. Many interpersonal difficulties related to sexual minority identity, such as lack of social support from one's family and stress related to coming out, may lead to a desire to fit in with the LGBTQ+ community and the subsequent internalization of these standards of attractiveness and body image ideals. These social comparison behaviors may then lead to the incidence and maintenance of eating disorder symptoms. Indeed, IPT may be an especially useful treatment for sexual minority men, due to the fact that stress related to adhering to socially defined body ideals and stigma from both within and outside the LGBTQ+ community is so ubiquitous among sexual minority men. At this time, the efficacy of IPT among sexual minority men has not been empirically tested, but the use of IPT within this population certainly warrants further study.

Family-based therapy has empirical support for the treatment of anorexia nervosa and bulimia nervosa among adolescents [49]. Adolescence is an especially critical developmental period for sexual minority individuals, as many important milestones related to sexual minority identity (e.g., coming out) occur during this period. Additionally, a lack of familial social support related to sexual orientation is associated with psychological distress and poor mental health outcomes broadly [21, 50]. Practitioners can address the sociocultural influences that lead to body image disturbance and eating disorder symptoms in treatment and present ways that these influences can be challenged in the home. Additionally, therapists can provide psychoeducation to parents regarding sexual minority identity development and its relationship to body image concerns and eating pathology. Thus, involving families in the treatment of eating disorders among sexual minority adolescents could address these needs simultaneously, as parents will become better equipped to aid their child with both body image concerns and the development of their sexual identity.

Dialectical behavior therapy (DBT) has been used as a treatment for binge eating disorder and bulimia nervosa, operating under the theory that emotional dysregulation is the primary cause of binge eating and purging [51]. Minority stress theory posits that distress intolerance and emotional dysregulation among sexual minority individuals stem in part from minority stressors, such as experiences of prejudice and discrimination [21]. Mindfulness-based DBT techniques can be employed to help clients accept the reality of these stressors and offer coping strategies to replace maladaptive eating behaviors. Additionally, interpersonal effectiveness skills may help clients communicate more effectively with sexual partners and the broader LGBTQ+ community related to expectations regarding physical appearance. DBT might be an especially useful treatment modality for sexual minority individuals struggling with emotional dysregulation, as the distress tolerance skills learned in treatment can be applied to both eating disorder symptomology and the stress experienced due to their minority identity.

Although there are no eating disorder treatments specifically adapted to sexual minority men, it is worth mentioning two related interventions that have been adapted to sexual minority men and have shown promising empirical support. ESTEEM (Effective Skills to Empower Effective Men) is a transdiagnostic intervention derived from the unified protocol that addresses gay and bisexual men's experiences through the lens of minority stress and provides cognitive, behavioral, and emotional skills to cope with these stressors [52]. While the treatment is not specific to eating disorders, many of the underlying issues addressed in treatment (e.g., emotional dysregulation, avoidance behaviors) as well as the skills provided (e.g., mindfulness techniques) have many commonalities with existing eating disorder treatments, which suggests that integrating elements of eating disorder treatments into ESTEEM may be effective for sexual minority individuals with body image concerns and eating pathology. This intervention is currently being tested in a multisite trial (NIH grant number R01MH109413) and, should it prove efficacious, may be an important resource for practitioners looking to provide evidence-based, culturally competent care.

Cognitive-behavioral therapy for body image and self-care (CBT-BISC) is a treatment for sexual minority men living with HIV that addresses body image disturbance in the context of poor HIV self-care (i.e., poor antiretroviral therapy [ART] adherence) [53]. CBT-BISC integrates an empirically supported intervention for ART adherence (Life-Steps) [54] with prior CBT interventions addressing body image disturbance [55, 56]. Results of a randomized controlled trial comparing CBT-BISC to an enhanced treatment as usual condition found the treatment efficacious at improving body image disturbance, ART adherence, depressive symptoms, and global functioning [53], suggesting that CBT-BISC might be a beneficial avenue of treatment for sexual minority men living with HIV.

Conclusion

The fact that men and boys have been largely absent from past research into eating disorders makes evaluating prevention and treatment among eating disorders among sexual minority men challenging. Sexual minority men need to first be represented in broader eating disorder treatment research to assess if a moderating effect of sexual orientation on treatment outcomes exists; from there, efforts can be directed toward tailoring interventions for this population. Until there is sufficient evidence to conclude that sexual minority men have differential treatment success using existing interventions, efforts are best directed toward integrating elements of prevailing theories discussed in this chapter into existing treatments. By conducting further research among sexual minority populations and adapting existing treatments to sexual minority men, we can work to reduce this disparity and ameliorate the burden of eating pathology on this population.

References

1. Blashill AJ, Calzo JP, Griffiths S, Murray SB. Anabolic steroid misuse among US adolescent boys: disparities by sexual orientation and race/ethnicity. Am J Public Health. 2017;107:319–21.
2. Matthews-Ewald MR, Zullig KJ, Ward RM. Sexual orientation and disordered eating behaviors among self-identified male and female college students. Eat Behav. 2014;15:441–4.
3. Watson RJ, Adjei J, Saewyc E, Homma Y, Goodenow C. Trends and disparities in disordered eating among heterosexual and sexual minority adolescents. Int J Eat Disord. 2017;50:22–31.

4. Diemer EW, Grant JD, Munn-Chernoff MA, Patterson DA, Duncan AE. Gender identity, sexual orientation, and eating-related pathology in a national sample of college students. J Adolesc Health. 2015;57:144–9.
5. Laska MN, VanKim NA, Erickson DJ, Lust K, Eisenberg ME, Rosser BRS. Disparities in weight and weight behaviors by sexual orientation in college students. Am J Public Health. 2015;105:111–21.
6. Von Schell A, Ohrt TK, Bruening AB, Perez M. Rates of disordered eating behaviors across sexual minority undergraduate men and women. Psychol Sex Orientat Gend Divers. 2018;5:352–9.
7. Feldman MB, Meyer IH. Eating disorders in diverse lesbian, gay, and bisexual populations. Int J Eat Disord. 2007;40:218–26.
8. Kamody RC, Grilo CM, Udo T. Disparities in DSM-5 defined eating disorders by sexual orientation among U.S. adults. Int J Eat Disord. 2020;53:278–87. https://doi.org/10.1002/eat.23193.
9. Polivy J, Herman CP. Causes of eating disorders. Annu Rev Psychol. 2002;53:187–213.
10. Thompson JK, Heinberg LJ, Altabe M, Tantleff-Dunn S. Exacting beauty: theory, assessment, and treatment of body image disturbance. [Internet]. Washington: American Psychological Association; 1999 [cited 2018 Dec 5]. Available from: http://content.apa.org/books/10312-000.
11. Fredrickson BL, Roberts T-A. Objectification theory: toward understanding women's lived experiences and mental health risks. Psychol Women Q. 1997;21:173–206.
12. Meyer IH. Minority stress and mental health in gay men. J Health Soc Behav. 1995;36:38.
13. Parent MC. Clinical considerations in etiology, assessment, and treatment of men's muscularity-focused body image disturbance. Psychol Men Masculinity. 2013;14:88–100.
14. Carper TLM, Negy C, Tantleff-Dunn S. Relations among media influence, body image, eating concerns, and sexual orientation in men: a preliminary investigation. Body Image. 2010;7:301–9.
15. Tylka TL, Andorka MJ. Support for an expanded tripartite influence model with gay men. Body Image. 2012;9:57–67.
16. Engeln-Maddox R, Miller SA, Doyle DM. Tests of objectification theory in gay, lesbian, and heterosexual community samples: mixed evidence for proposed pathways. Sex Roles. 2011;65:518–32.
17. Kozak M, Frankenhauser H, Roberts T-A. Objects of desire: objectification as a function of male sexual orientation. Psychol Men Masculinity. 2009;10:225–30.
18. Siever MD. Sexual orientation and gender as factors in socioculturally acquired vulnerability to body dissatisfaction and eating disorders. J Consult Clin Psychol. 1994;62:252–60.
19. Michaels MS, Parent MC, Moradi B. Does exposure to muscularity-idealizing images have self-objectification consequences for heterosexual and sexual minority men? Psychol Men Masculinity. 2013;14:175–83.
20. Martins Y, Tiggemann M, Kirkbride A. Those speedos become them: the role of self-objectification in gay and heterosexual men's body image. Pers Soc Psychol Bull. 2007;33:634–47.
21. Meyer IH. Prejudice, social stress, and mental health in lesbian, gay, and bisexual populations: conceptual issues and research evidence. Psychol Bull. 2003;129:674–97.
22. Beren SE. Stigmatization and shame as determinants of subclinical eating disorder pathology: a comparison of gay and heterosexual men. [US]: ProQuest Information & Learning; 1997.
23. Torres AN. Internalized homophobia, self-esteem, gender roles, body image, and disordered eating in gay and bisexual men [Internet]. ProQuest Information & Learning. 2008. Available from: http://libproxy.sdsu.edu/login?url=http://search.ebscohost.com/login.aspx?direct=true&db=psyh&AN=2008-99100-306&login.asp&site=ehost-live&scope=site.
24. Wang SB, Borders A. Rumination mediates the associations between sexual minority stressors and disordered eating, particularly for men. Eat Weight Disord Stud Anorex Bulim Obes. 2017;22:699–706.

25. Katz-Wise SL, Scherer EA, Calzo JP, Sarda V, Jackson B, Haines J, et al. Sexual minority stressors, internalizing symptoms, and unhealthy eating behaviors in sexual minority youth. Ann Behav Med. 2015;49:839–52.
26. Siconolfi D, Halkitis PN, Allomong TW, Burton CL. Body dissatisfaction and eating disorders in a sample of gay and bisexual men. Int J Mens Health. 2009;8:254–64.
27. Wiseman MC, Moradi B. Body image and eating disorder symptoms in sexual minority men: a test and extension of objectification theory. J Couns Psychol. 2010;57:154–66.
28. Greentree S, Lewis V. Male body image and its relationship to sexual preference and homophobia. Pak J Psychol Res. 2011;26:105–26.
29. Brewster ME, Sandil R, DeBlaere C, Breslow A, Eklund A. "Do you even lift, bro?" Objectification, minority stress, and body image concerns for sexual minority men. Psychol Men Masculinity. 2017;18:87.
30. Fairburn CG, Beglin SJ. Eating disorder examination questionnaire. Cogn Behav Ther Eat Disord. New York: Guilford Press; 2008. p. 309–14.
31. Scharmer C, Donahue JM, Heiss S, Anderson DA. Factor structure of the Eating Disorder Examination – Questionnaire among heterosexual and sexual minority males. Eating Behaviors. 2020;38.
32. McCreary DR, Sasse DK, Saucier DM, Dorsch KD. Measuring the drive for muscularity: factorial validity of the Drive for Muscularity Scale in men and women. Psychol Men Masculinity. 2004;5:49–58.
33. DeBlaere C, Brewster ME. A confirmation of the Drive for Muscularity Scale with sexual minority men. Psychol Sex Orientat Gend Divers. 2017;4:227–32.
34. Nerini A, Matera C, Baroni D, Stefanile C. Drive for muscularity and sexual orientation: psychometric properties of the Italian version of the Drive for Muscularity Scale (DMS) in straight and gay men. Psychol Men Masculinity. 2016;17:137–46.
35. Tylka TL, Bergeron D, Schwartz JP. Development and psychometric evaluation of the Male Body Attitudes Scale (MBAS). Body Image. 2005;2:161–75.
36. Blashill AJ, Vander Wal JS. The Male Body Attitudes Scale: a confirmatory factor analysis with a sample of gay men. Body Image. 2009;6:322–5.
37. Hart TA, Flora DB, Palyo SA, Fresco DM, Holle C, Heimberg RG. Development and examination of the Social Appearance Anxiety Scale. Assessment. 2008;15:48–59.
38. Hart TA, Rotondi NK, Souleymanov R, Brennan DJ. Psychometric properties of the Social Appearance Anxiety Scale among Canadian gay and bisexual men of color. Psychol Sex Orientat Gend Divers. 2015;2:470–81.
39. Schaefer LM, Harriger JA, Heinberg LJ, Soderberg T, Thompson JK. Development and validation of the Sociocultural Attitudes Towards Appearance questionnaire-4-Revised (SATAQ-4R). Int J Eat Disord. 2017;50:104–17.
40. Convertino AD, Gonzales M, Malcarne VL, Blashill AJ. A psychometric investigation of the Sociocultural Attitudes Towards Appearance Questionnaire-4-Revised among sexual minority adults in the U.S. Body Image. 2019;31:96–101.
41. Becker CB, Smith LM, Ciao AC. Peer-facilitated eating disorder prevention: a randomized effectiveness trial of cognitive dissonance and media advocacy. J Couns Psychol. 2006;53:550–5.
42. Stice E, Rohde P, Gau J, Shaw H. An effectiveness trial of a dissonance-based eating disorder prevention program for high-risk adolescent girls. J Consult Clin Psychol. 2009;77:825–34.
43. Stice E, Shaw H, Burton E, Wade E. Dissonance and healthy weight eating disorder prevention programs: a randomized efficacy trial. J Consult Clin Psychol. 2006;74:263–75.
44. Festinger L. A theory of cognitive dissonance. Stanford: Stanford University Press; 1957.
45. Brown TA, Forney KJ, Pinner D, Keel PK. A randomized controlled trial of the body project: more than muscles for men with body dissatisfaction. Int J Eat Disord. 2017;50:873–83.
46. Fairburn CG. Cognitive behavior therapy and eating disorders. New York: Guilford Press; 2008.

47. Fairburn CG, Cooper Z, Doll HA, O'Connor ME, Bohn K, Hawker DM, et al. Transdiagnostic cognitive-behavioral therapy for patients with eating disorders: a two-site trial with 60-week follow-up. Am J Psychiatry. 2009;166:311–9.
48. Rieger E, Van Buren DJ, Bishop M, Tanofsky-Kraff M, Welch R, Wilfley DE. An eating disorder-specific model of interpersonal psychotherapy (IPT-ED): causal pathways and treatment implications. Clin Psychol Rev. 2010;30:400–10.
49. Couturier J, Kimber M, Szatmari P. Efficacy of family-based treatment for adolescents with eating disorders: a systematic review and meta-analysis. Int J Eat Disord. 2013;46:3–11.
50. Puckett JA, Woodward EN, Mereish EH, Pantalone DW. Parental rejection following sexual orientation disclosure: impact on internalized homophobia, social support, and mental health. LGBT Health. 2015;2:265–9.
51. Wiser S, Telch CF. Dialectical behavior therapy for binge-eating disorder. J Clin Psychol. 1999;55:755–68.
52. Pachankis JE, Hatzenbuehler ML, Rendina HJ, Safren SA, Parsons JT. LGB-affirmative cognitive-behavioral therapy for young adult gay and bisexual men: a randomized controlled trial of a transdiagnostic minority stress approach. J Consult Clin Psychol. 2015;83:875–89.
53. Blashill AJ, Safren SA, Wilhelm S, Jampel J, Taylor SW, O'Cleirigh C, et al. Cognitive behavioral therapy for body image and self-care (CBT-BISC) in sexual minority men living with HIV: a randomized controlled trial. Health Psychol. 2017;36:937–46.
54. Safren SA, Otto MW, Worth JL. Life-steps: applying cognitive behavioral therapy to HIV medication adherence. Cogn Behav Pract. 1999;6:332–41.
55. Cash T. The body image workbook: an eight-step program for learning to like your looks. 2nd ed. Oakland: New Harbinger Publications; 2008.
56. Wilhelm S, Phillips KA, Steketee G. Cognitive-behavioral therapy for body dysmorphic disorder: a treatment manual. 1st ed. New York: The Guilford Press; 2012.

Chapter 18
Eating Disorders Among Transgender and Gender Non-binary People

Allegra R. Gordon, L. B. Moore, and Carly Guss

Learning Objectives

1. Become familiar with the current literature regarding disordered eating in transgender and gender non-binary people.
2. Identify key opportunities for creating improving gender-affirming care in clinical spaces.
3. Apply these concepts to eating disorder care for transgender and gender non-binary patients.

Key Points

- Transgender and gender non-binary (T/GNB) populations experience elevated risk of disordered eating behaviors compared to their cisgender counterparts; stigma, gender dysphoria, and gendered sociocultural appearance ideals may be contributors to these health inequities although more research is needed to identify risk and resilience factors.
- Clinicians should evaluate their clinical settings to identify opportunities for increased gender-affirming practices and policies and implement changes.

A. R. Gordon (✉)
Department of Community Health Sciences, Boston University School of Public Health, Boston, MA, USA
e-mail: allegrag@bu.edu

L. B. Moore
Framingham LGBTQ+ Adolescent Social Services (Framingham GLASS), Justice Resource Institute, Health Division, Framingham, MA, USA
e-mail: lbmoore@jri.org

C. Guss
Division of Adolescent/Young Adult Medicine, Boston Children's Hospital and Department of Pediatrics, Harvard Medical School, Boston, MA, USA
e-mail: carly.guss@childrens.harvard.edu

J. M. Nagata et al. (eds.), *Eating Disorders in Boys and Men*,
https://doi.org/10.1007/978-3-030-67127-3_18

Recognize limitations of common eating disorder screening tools when evaluating T/GNB clients and patients.
- Identify personal biases and assumptions about T/GNB patients and work to mitigate the impact of these on clinical work.
- Do not delay gender-affirming treatment in order to treat an eating disorder.
- Treatment of gender dysphoria may improve disordered eating, but evaluation and involvement of a multidisciplinary team with expertise in eating disorders may be helpful.

Introduction

In the United States, an estimated 1.4 million adults and 150,000 youth aged 13–17 years identify as transgender [1, 2]. With growing visibility of diverse gender identities and communities, it is necessary for clinicians to create affirming spaces for transgender and gender non-binary (T/GNB) patients and clients—including those who are not known to the clinician as T/GNB. This chapter will synthesize the current state of the science and provide recommendations for clinicians who are just beginning to think about gender diversity in their practice as well as those who already have expertise in this area and wish to identify next steps for their clinical care, research, and/or advocacy in the field.

In this chapter, we use the term *T/GNB* to refer to people who have a gender identity different than the gender associated with their sex assigned at birth. Other key definitions can be found in Table 18.1. Language in this area is evolving rapidly, led by T/GNB communities. Although we have chosen to use terms common at the time of publication, we acknowledge that people use many different terms to describe themselves and the language people use varies widely by historical, geographic, developmental, and social context.

Table 18.1 Key terms

Term	Definition
Binding; binder	A variety of methods to flatten breast tissue. This can be employed to decrease dysphoria related to the chest. A tool that binds.
Cisgender	An umbrella term for people whose gender identity matches the gender associated with their sex assigned at birth (e.g., assigned female at birth, identify gender as a girl or woman).
Gender-affirming hormone therapy (GAHT)	Refers to when a transgender person receives hormone treatment that matches their gender identity. Gender-affirming hormones could include testosterone, estrogen, and/or anti-androgens.
Gender/sex binary	The idea that there are only two genders: female/woman and male/man.

Table 18.1 (continued)

Term	Definition
Gender dysphoria	Clinically significant distress due to an individual's experience with their primary and/or secondary sexual characteristics (e.g., genitals, body hair) and/or with the gender role assigned. In the *Diagnostic and Statistical Manual of Mental Disorders 5th Edition (DSM-5)*, this term replaced "gender identity disorder." Not all transgender people experience clinically significant gender dysphoria.
Gender expression	External manifestations of gender, such as clothing, hair, vocal inflections, mannerisms, or other characteristics.
Gender identity	A person's inner sense of gender—that is, whether they identify as a boy/man, girl/woman, both, neither, or another gender or genders. Gender identity is independent of sex assigned at birth.
Gender non-binary	An umbrella term covering gender identities that do not fit within the gender binary. Use of the label is often based on the rejection of the assumption that gender is strictly an either/or (male/men/masculine or female/woman/-feminine) based on sex assigned at birth. Words that people may use to express their non-binary gender identity include "agender," "bigender," "genderqueer," "gender-fluid," and "pangender."
Pronouns	Words used to refer to someone in the third person when not using their name. Because pronouns are gendered in English, the use of someone's correct (i.e., self-determined) pronouns is crucial to respectful interactions and culturally responsive care for T/GNB people. People may use one or multiple sets of pronouns, e.g., they/them/their, she/her/her, he/him/his, e/em/eir, or ze/zir/zir.
Sex assigned at birth	The classification of people as male, female, intersex, or another sex based on a combination of anatomy (typically genitals), chromosomes, and hormones. Sex assigned at birth is independent of gender identity.
Sexual orientation	A person's romantic or sexual attraction to other individuals, often based on gender. Components include emotional and romantic attractions, sexual behavior, self-identification, and sexual fantasies. Sexual orientation is independent of gender identity.
Transgender	An umbrella term for people whose gender identity is different than that associated with their sex assigned at birth.
Transfeminine	An umbrella term referring to gender identities of transgender and gender non-binary people who were assigned male at birth (e.g., a transfeminine patient). People may or may not identify with this term. May also refer to care provided to transfeminine people (e.g., transfeminine gender-affirming care).
Transmasculine	An umbrella term referring to gender identities of transgender and non-binary people who were assigned female at birth (e.g., a transmasculine patient). People may or may not identify with this term. May also refer to care provided to transmasculine people (e.g., transmasculine reproductive care).
Transphobia	Fear of, discrimination against, or hatred of transgender people.

Gender Diversity in Social Context

The health and clinical care of T/GNB people must be considered in relation to the social and historical context in which T/GNB people live and navigate healthcare systems. Community advocates and activists around the world have long called for more attention to mistreatment, stigmatization, and violence targeting individuals and communities perceived to violate gender norms and expectations, including T/GNB people [3–5]. Empirical research in the last two decades added to this chorus, underscoring the fact that T/GNB people of all ages are exposed to high levels of discrimination and violence. A survey of over 27,000 T/GNB adults in the United States found high prevalence of mistreatment, harassment, and violence "in every aspect of life" [6]. This includes discrimination in healthcare systems: in this study, one-third of those who saw a healthcare provider in the past year reported having a negative experience related to being transgender (e.g., refused treatment, harassed, assaulted). Over a quarter had experienced a problem in the 51
st year with their insurance (e.g., being denied coverage for routine care because they were transgender) [6]. Although research to date has predominantly been in the United States, these are global concerns [7].

Medical and mental healthcare systems have fraught histories of pathologizing gender diversity. Many excellent historical and personal accounts are worth reviewing for a better understanding of the historical context that can influence T/GNB people's interactions with healthcare systems today [8–10]. In recent years, there have been important shifts in medical and mental health practice toward approaches that seek to be less pathologizing of gender diversity, such as the removal in the DSM-5 of the diagnosis of *gender identity disorder* and its replacement with the diagnosis of *gender dysphoria* [11]. There has also been a move within healthcare systems away from a model in which mental health providers alone determine access to gender-affirming care and toward an *informed consent* model that aims to help clinicians better support personal agency of T/GNB patients [12]. Treatment paradigms are evolving and are often contested terrain [11]. The voices of T/GNB people must be central as medical and mental health systems continue to work to eliminate stigmatization and improve their capacity to provide quality care.

Gender Identity Diversity and Intersectionality

Although we use the term *T/GNB* here as an umbrella, T/GNB populations are heterogeneous. Any approach to clinical care for T/GNB people should utilize an intersectional framework, informed by Black feminist scholarship and practice [13]. From an intersectional perspective, we start this conversation by acknowledging that eating disorder risk factors, as well as eating disorder screening and treatment experiences of T/GNB people, are fundamentally shaped by interlocking systems of

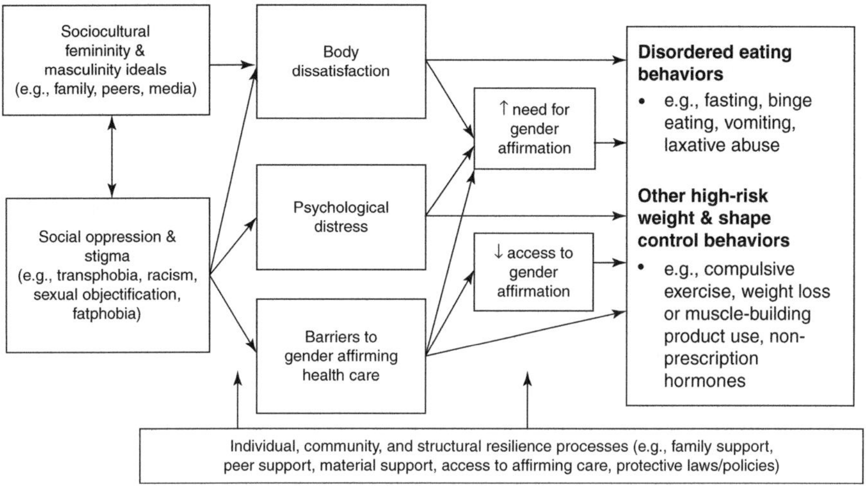

Fig. 18.1 Conceptual model of risk and protective pathways influencing high-risk weight and shape control behaviors among transgender and gender non-binary populations

power and social oppression, including transphobia, racism, sexism, heterosexism, ableism, and fatphobia [14]. These interlocking systems influence eating disorder risk through a variety of potential pathways (Fig. 18.1). However, there is an urgent need for more research on the way these pathways may vary within an individual's geographic and sociopolitical context (e.g., living in a state or nation with laws that are discriminatory or protective, effects of racism on the life opportunities of T/GNB people of color).

This chapter draws on eating disorder research and clinical experience limited to a Western/Global North context. T/GNB people and communities exist everywhere, and there is a need for more clinical and population health research in diverse global settings [7]. We are pleased to note that research and clinical interest in the field of T/GNB health, and eating disorders in particular, is growing. We look forward to increased literature in this field addressing eating disorder-related care for T/GNB people in a wide range of geographic settings.

Epidemiology and Health Inequities

In recent years, the inclusion of questions about gender identity on epidemiologic surveys has offered an unprecedented snapshot of risk for eating disorders among transgender compared to cisgender populations. These studies estimate that transgender populations are burdened by 2–4 times greater risk of eating disorder symptoms or disordered eating behaviors than their cisgender counterparts [15–17]. For example, in a study of 289,000 US college students, transgender college students reported 4.6 times greater odds of self-reported eating disorder diagnosis in the past year, and over 2 times greater odds of past-month diet pill use and purging behaviors, compared to cisgender, heterosexual women [15]. Focusing on adolescents, a probability sample of Massachusetts high school students observed no statistically significant differences in prevalence of disordered eating between transgender youth and cisgender girls; however, both groups were at significantly elevated risk of these behaviors compared to cisgender boys [16].

Most of these studies have captured self-reported eating disorder symptoms or disordered eating behaviors; few population-based studies have been able to examine prevalence or risk of clinical eating disorders among T/GNB populations. One case-control study of electronic health records of US veterans found that transgender veterans were two times more likely to have an eating disorder compared to non-transgender veterans [17]. Notably, not all studies have found the same pattern: one probability sample of students at 12 US universities found no significant differences in eating disorder symptoms between transgender students and cisgender women [18].

Few published studies have examined eating disorders specifically among gender non-binary people, who may or may not be represented within classifications of transgender participants in other studies. One study has found that non-binary people may be at even greater risk of eating disorders than binary-identified transgender peers. In this community-based sample of transgender adults, non-binary people had three times greater odds of self-reported history of anorexia nervosa or bulimia nervosa diagnosis compared to transgender men and women [19]. Two studies have reported no significant differences in risk between those on a transmasculine spectrum compared to those on a transfeminine spectrum [19, 20].

Further, few published studies have been able to take an intersectional approach to exploring differences in eating disorder risk among T/GNB people by race/ethnicity, socioeconomic position, disability status, or other dimensions of social inequality. Given the dearth of research on T/GNB people in general, and T/GNB people of color in particular, we know little about how disordered eating behaviors and eating disorders emerge across race/ethnicity for T/GNB people. Research on the intersection of race/ethnicity and sexual orientation [21] suggests T/GNB young people of color may be at particularly heightened risk of disordered eating behaviors given their experiences with multiple forms of discrimination and marginalization [22]. Given that eating disorders are underdiagnosed and undertreated among people of color, people with higher weights, and those of lower socioeconomic position [18], further work focused on T/GNB people with these experiences is urgently needed.

Risk and Protective Factors

To better understand the elevated risk of disordered eating behaviors in T/GNB populations, we propose a conceptual framework (Fig. 18.1) that draws on the extant literature on eating disorder risk and protective factors, as well as three theoretical approaches: (i) a sociocultural model of eating disorder risk, (ii) minority stress theory, and (iii) gender affirmation framework.

The *sociocultural model* is based on the premise that a society's dominant appearance ideals and norms are one key driver of eating disorders [23, 24]. More specifically, gender-related appearance ideals (e.g., the "thin ideal" for women/feminine people, the "muscular ideal" for men/masculine people) become internalized by individuals, resulting in body dissatisfaction and increasing eating disorder risk. Variants of this model posit multiple channels by which these ideals influence body dissatisfaction, including family, peer, and media influences [23]. Although this model has historically been used to describe the experiences of cisgender people (especially cisgender girls and women), sociocultural appearance ideals inevitably play a role in body satisfaction and dissatisfaction among T/GNB people as well [25]. Recent research with transgender women offers support for associations between internalization of sociocultural appearance ideals, body surveillance, body dissatisfaction, and disordered eating [26].

However, this model alone is not sufficient to fully conceptualize the disproportionate risk of disordered eating behaviors among T/GNB populations. These sociocultural processes must be considered in the context of pervasive *social stressors* targeting T/GNB people (e.g., transphobia, sexual objectification) and the intersection of these stressors with other forms of social oppression (e.g., racism, sexism, fatphobia). *Minority stress theory* [27, 28] posits that such social stressors—which manifest at multiple levels of the social environment, including structural levels such as discriminatory laws and policies and interpersonal levels such as bullying and violence—become embodied as physiologic and behavioral stress responses [29]. Experiencing such stressors can trigger a cascade of stress responses, leading to psychological distress and maladaptive coping behaviors including disordered eating behaviors [30, 31].

Growing research documents the links between social stressors and disordered eating behaviors among T/GNB people [22, 32], including a study of over 900 transgender youth in Canada that found that higher exposure to harassment and discrimination was associated with higher odds of past-year binge eating, fasting, or vomiting to lose weight [33]. In adults, there is some evidence supporting the association of anti-transgender discrimination with disordered eating among transgender women [26] and with compulsive exercise among transgender men [34].

The third framework needed to illuminate the drivers of heightened eating disorder risk among T/GNB people is the *gender affirmation framework*, which was developed to contextualize high-risk behaviors among transgender women of color [35]. Gender affirmation includes medical (e.g., access to hormones), legal (e.g., sex marker on driver's license), social (e.g., name, pronouns), and psychological (e.g., comfort with one's gender) affirmation [36]. If a T/GNB person's need for gender affirmation is high but their access is low, they may seek affirmation in higher-risk ways (e.g., disordered eating behaviors to stop menses or accessing feminizing/masculinizing hormones in non-medical settings).

Recent research has offered support for the key role of gender affirmation in exacerbating or reducing risk of disordered eating and other high-risk weight control behaviors. Nearly two-thirds (63%) of transgender youth in a clinical sample reported engaging in intentional weight manipulation for the purposes of aligning their body with their gender identity—with no statistical differences between transmasculine, transfeminine, and non-binary youth [20]. This suggests that for many T/GNB youth, attempting to manipulate weight is a key strategy for seeking needed gender affirmation. However, weight manipulation for gender affirmation was not associated with an individual's score on the Eating Disorder Examination Questionnaire; thus, although T/GNB youth may be at heightened risk for eating disorders in the future due to such weight manipulation efforts, there was no evidence that those who were manipulating their weight for gender affirmation were more likely to display eating disorder symptoms than those who were not.

Access to gender-affirming medical interventions (e.g., hormones, surgeries) may reduce risk of eating disorders [37–39]. A study of transgender adults who either desired to access or had already accessed gender-affirming medical interventions found that completing gender-affirming medical interventions was indirectly associated with lower levels of experiencing gender non-affirmation (e.g., others' use of the wrong pronouns), which in turn was associated with higher body satisfaction and lower levels of eating disorder symptoms [37]. This was a cross-sectional study and thus could not look at causality; however, it is the most specific evidence to date of gender-affirming medical care as an intervention that may reduce eating disorder risk for some T/GNB people.

Despite exposure to deeply entrenched sources of minority stress and pervasive sociocultural appearance ideals, most T/GNB people do not have eating disorders. Indeed, T/GNB people and communities have long demonstrated powerful forms of resistance and resilience in the face of social oppression. Our conceptual model proposes that resilience processes at multiple levels can intervene upon the risk pathways depicted, buffering individuals against body dissatisfaction or reducing barriers to needed gender affirmation and support.

The Basics: Gender-Affirming Healthcare Practice

Regardless of the setting in which a clinician interacts with a patient who identifies as T/GNB (e.g., outpatient, inpatient), it is crucial that the setting provides gender-affirming care to all current and potential patients. Many of the suggestions below can be implemented rapidly in a practice. It is essential that gender-affirming interactions for patients span the entire care team—including phone triage and scheduling, parking lot staff, and phlebotomy staff.

When registering as a new patient, individuals should be able to provide their pronouns and the name they want to be called recorded separately from their legal name. This can be done on an intake form or as a prompt in an electronic medical record system [40]. Patients find the routine collection of gender identity information acceptable in healthcare settings [41]. Intake paperwork can be adjusted in order to include this information, and staff must be trained to answer questions about these items in a culturally responsive way. For patients who are minors, the clinician and office staff must be careful to do this in a confidential manner in the event that the child is not "out" as T/GNB to their family.

For medical providers who may collect a review of systems on paper prior to a visit, clinicians must be careful to ensure that the forms are not "gendered" by having specific review of systems for "men" or "women." As access to gender-affirming surgeries increases for patients who require them, more and more patients may have had surgeries that may affect their relevant health screening [42, 43]; clinicians may want to consider adding a gender-neutral "*anatomy inventory*." For additional resources for assessing and strengthening the gender-affirming climate of your practice, see section "Selected Resources".

Considerations for Screening and Diagnostic Assessment

Because screening, assessment, and treatment may be provided in the same facilities—often by the same clinicians—we present here considerations for screening and diagnostic assessment in both medical and mental health settings. The following information may be implemented within all settings employing a given approach. It is important to note that clinical research on eating disorder screening and diagnostic assessment for T/GNB patients is emerging; thus, most clinical care for T/GNB patients is currently shaped by expert opinion and case studies. The information in this section is based on the limited research currently available.

Current mental health screening and diagnostic tools for the assessment of disordered eating and eating disorders are primarily normed on and validated for cisgender women (e.g., [44]); assessments validated and normed to include men are focused on cisgender men [45]. One notable exception is a recent study that gathered community norms on the Eating Disorder Examination Questionnaire (EDE-Q) in a sample of transgender men and women [46]. Though an important start, this study's authors also called for further work on the EDE-Q among gender non-binary people and in more racially and socioeconomically diverse samples.

Few if any other eating disorder screening and diagnostic tools have been examined, adapted, or validated for T/GNB populations. Because psychological properties of eating disorders feature a constellation of challenges or distortions rather than a singular fixation, many of the field's most utilized assessment instruments—such as the Eating Disorder Inventory (EDI)—are multi-scale in nature, including measurement of attitudes and behaviors across eating, body dissatisfaction, drive for thinness, ineffectiveness, and more [45]. Items on these scales may not appropriately assess disordered attitudes or risk for T/GNB patients. For example, items related to body dissatisfaction (e.g., "I feel satisfied with the shape of my body" [45]) may reflect gender dysphoria rather than disordered body image or a combination of the two. Items on the EDI's Ineffectiveness subscale (e.g., "I feel alone in the world"; "I wish I was someone else" [45]) may also unintentionally capture experiences related to transphobia and dysphoria rather than features indicative of an eating disorder. Given that assessments such as the EDI are widely validated and often recommended as part of standard best practice [47], clinicians must be attuned to the potential limitations of these measures with T/GNB patients. Further, an assessment of T/GNB patients' experiences of minority stress and dysphoria may be required for an accurate evaluation of eating disorder symptoms and risk.

Clinicians using physical measures for eating disorder screening must attend to specific physiological changes experienced by T/GNB patients accessing gender-affirming medical treatment. This may include careful consideration of growth chart use, given the fat and muscle changes affected by gender-affirming hormone therapy (GAHT) [48], and the use of medications that can suppress menses (including testosterone) [49, 50].

Considerations for Treatment

Care for T/GNB patients managing eating disorders requires some additional considerations. These considerations include review of typical tools used in the treatment of eating disorders, consideration of an individual patient's gender-related needs, and environmental-structural factors impacting the care of T/GNB clients across treatment settings.

Clinicians must consider the possible impact of "standard procedure" on T/GNB patients. A crucial part of an appointment with a medical clinician when monitoring patients with eating disorders is the assessment of vital signs. It is typical that a patient voids, changes into a hospital gown, and has a blinded weight by standing backward on a scale [51]. In providing gender-affirming care, providers must acknowledge that many tasks assumed basic for medical treatment—such as undressing into a gown—may trigger dysphoria and produce psychological distress. For example, a transgender male patient using a chest binder in the absence of gender-affirming mastectomy may experience clinically significant increases in dysphoria if required to remove the chest binder, such as for the recording of vitals. Even the act of leaving a urine sample may be distressing to patients for whom restrooms and interactions with their genitals are especially challenging. It has been suggested that a best practice would be to set clear expectations with patients about what will happen at each visit, why each portion is necessary, and what accommodations (if any) are possible [52]. It should be documented every visit whether or not vital signs are done with a binder in place and, if applicable, the reason for which no urine was obtained. If there are specific concerns for weight manipulation, it may be appropriate to have the patient remove the binder for relevant assessments only [52].

Historically, a cornerstone of recovery in anorexia nervosa among patients with uteruses has been resumption of menses [53]. However, clinicians must keep in mind that menses may be very distressing for some T/GNB patients. Additionally, patients may have been started on medication by another clinician in order to intentionally suppress menses [49]. The use of the gender-affirming hormone testosterone often results in amenorrhea as well [50, 54]. Given the importance of gender-affirming treatment to the psychological well-being of T/GNB people, clinicians should *not* discontinue GAHT as a trial to see if a patient would otherwise be menstruating. Clinicians can reference growth charts and look for other signs of improved nutritional status (such as physical exam findings and vital signs) rather than relying on menses. The use of a multidisciplinary team of a gender specialist, eating disorder specialist, and dietician can be key in order to guide therapy goals [52].

Growth charts and body mass index calculations are a mainstay of medical management of eating disorders, particularly in children [53]. Unfortunately, there are not standardized growth charts for transgender youth, including those who are being treated with gonadotropin-releasing hormone (GnRH) analogue therapy to "block" puberty [55]. It has been suggested that the use of both male and female growth charts should be incorporated, especially for youth on extreme ends of the growth chart spectrum [55]. In the context of the treatment of eating disorders, either male or female growth charts may be useful to review trends and help set weight recovery goals. A meta-analysis of ten studies of transgender individuals found that all patients, regardless of sex assigned at birth, tend to gain weight with duration of GAHT varying from 3–4 months through 54 weeks. It was noted that body fat decreases in transgender men, while it increases with transgender women; however, this paper did not specifically look at eating disorder diagnoses [48].

Treatment of gender dysphoria through therapy, supported gender identity development, and appropriate referral to gender-affirming healthcare and procedures is fundamental to responsive mental healthcare for T/GNB people [56]. Access to GAHT may also directly reduce T/GNB clients' body dissatisfaction and other risk factors for eating disorders [37–39]. When working with T/GNB patients, clinicians should collaborate with the patient and other affirming providers on the patient's team, if applicable, to identify and acknowledge the relationship between gender-related dysphoria and eating disorder symptoms. Case studies and small case series including recommendations about the treatment of eating disorders and gender dysphoria have repeatedly emphasized that these be treated in tandem [57, 58]. There can be improvement in the eating disorder pathology with treatment of gender dysphoria, but as such improvement is not always the case, T/GNB patients may still benefit from a multidisciplinary eating disorder team [58, 59].

Clinicians should also consider moving away from "body positivity" with T/GNB patients and instead focus on "body neutrality" or "body functionality" [60–62]. This concept focuses on harm reduction and acknowledges that dysphoria may present an insurmountable hurdle to body "positivity." For example, goals such as being at an adequate nutritional status for gender-affirming surgery or being able to participate in a gender sexuality alliance (GSA) activity at school represent body "neutral" approaches that center the patient's eating disorder and gender affirmation-related needs.

Finally, clinicians providing care to T/GNB patients must attend to the environmental-structural factors which impact patients in a given setting. Access to gender-aligned facilities is crucial. Inpatient and residential settings face particular facility-related challenges in this area due to typical binary sex-based segregation of treatment facilities. Lack of access to gender-aligned facilities is likely to further alienate T/GNB clients from treatment and exacerbate symptoms of body dissatisfaction and minority stress [63, 64]; this may be uniquely true for non-binary patients, for whom no truly gender-aligned inpatient facility may exist in a given setting. Increasingly, guidelines for treatment of T/GNB patients in inpatient settings recommend a collaborative process between staff and patients to acknowledge barriers and identify most affirming facility access in order to maximize rapport and efficacy of care [64]. Importantly, T/GNB patients who experience stigmatization and exclusion are less likely to complete treatment, while those who feel affirmed and included are more likely to report positive treatment experiences [65].

Conclusion: Implications and Recommendations

Despite recent growth in clinical interest in eating disorder risk factors, screening, and treatment for T/GNB people, there remains a dearth of evidence to guide clinical practice. Drawing on community advocacy and the small but growing body of epidemiologic and clinical research focused on T/GNB populations summarized above, below we highlight selected recommendations to guide mental health and medical providers who seek to offer high-quality, gender-affirming care to their patients and clients with diverse gender identities.

1. *Assess your clinical setting(s) to identify opportunities for increased gender-affirming practices and policies*. This may include visual representations of gender diversity and use of gender-inclusive language (e.g., signage), facility access (e.g., restrooms), intake forms, staff training, staff representation, and meaningful engagement with community organizations serving T/GNB communities.
2. *Standardize opportunities for self-identification for all patients*. Ensure intake forms include standardized questions about gender identity, pronouns, and chosen name (separate from name on insurance).
3. *Recognize limitations of common eating disorder screening tools when evaluating T/GNB patients*. Include assessment of gender dysphoria and minority stress experiences to capture a more complete picture of body-focused feelings. Consider using growth curve trends and other physical exam findings of malnutrition rather than binary sex-based BMI when setting goal weight.
4. *Integrate gender-affirming frameworks and T/GNB cultural responsiveness into all treatment approaches*. Acknowledge distinct body-focused experiences and treatment-related needs and barriers that may be experienced by T/GNB people. Recognize that access to or changes in gender affirmation (e.g., accessing GAHT) and eating disorder symptomatology may co-influence each other.
5. *Utilize supportive informed consent* when recommending treatment approaches that may be designed on a sex binary. Discuss possible challenges a patient or client may face (e.g., requirement to select binary sex on the phone application).

6. *Identify personal biases and assumptions about T/GNB clients and work to mitigate the impact of these on clinical work.* Access numerous existing educational and community resources to support your ongoing learning (see section "Selected Resources").
7. *Avoid terms like "body positivity" and "body acceptance."* These may be problematic or unrealistic in the context of gender dysphoria. Instead consider alternative approaches such as "body neutrality" or "body functionality."
8. *Link to supportive resources.* Connect to—or collaborate to create—T/GNB-specific eating disorder support groups and other resources.
9. *Acknowledge advocacy for T/GNB clients as a key element of eating disorder care coordination and improving long-term health outcomes.* Recognize that T/GNB patients may benefit from additional advocacy by eating disorder clinicians with primary care providers and surgeons. Clinicians are also powerful advocates beyond healthcare settings, affecting change in a range of local and national policy arenas.

Future Directions

Clinicians, researchers, and advocates interested in addressing the burden of eating disorders among T/GNB individuals and communities should consider several avenues for future research and advocacy.

- Develop evidence-based treatment guidelines specifically for T/GNB populations. These may need to be tailored with regard to gender identity, identity development, family/community support, geographic setting, and access to gender-affirming care if desired, among other factors.
- Conduct longitudinal research to better understand how puberty blockers and GAHT affect an individual's BMI and growth curve to help guide weight/recovery goals for clinicians.
- Add data collection on gender identity as well as on disordered eating behaviors and/or eating disorder symptoms to public health surveillance surveys and epidemiologic cohort studies. This is necessary in order to better track incidence, prevalence, and inequities in eating disorder risk among T/GNB populations.
- Develop research and clinical guidance on reducing weight stigma in the care of T/GNB patients, including in relation to accessing (or being prevented from accessing) gender-affirming surgeries. Research in this area remains scarce, despite growing attention to the detrimental health consequences of weight stigma, including heightened eating disorder risk.
- Conduct validation studies of existing clinical tools for screening and management of eating disorders with T/GNB populations. Create new tools that account for the potential roles of minority stress and gender dysphoria.
- Foster the next generation of clinicians, researchers, and advocates committed to improving care for T/GNB people. Create training opportunities for students

from high school to graduate levels who may be interested in pursuing a career in clinical care or research on eating disorder prevention, treatment, and policy advocacy to improve health equity for T/GNB populations. T/GNB students and trainees should be meaningfully included and mentored in these programs.

Selected Resources

National Center for Transgender Equality (NCTE): Know Your Healthcare Rights

- www.transequality.org/know-your-rights/healthcare

National LGBT Health Education Center

- www.lgbthealtheducation.org/

Trans Folx Fighting Eating Disorders (T-FFED)

- www.transfolxfightingeds.org/

Trans Students Education Resources

- www.transstudent.org/

Transgender Law Center: Identifying and Fighting Healthcare Discrimination

- transgenderlawcenter.org/issues/health/transgender-health-and-the-law-identifying-and-fighting-health-care-discrimination

UCSF Center of Excellence for Transgender Health

- https://prevention.ucsf.edu/transhealth

World Professional Association for Transgender Health Standards of Care

- https://www.wpath.org/publications/soc

References

1. Flores AR, Herman JL, Gates GJ, Brown TNT. How many adults identify as transgender in the United States? Los Angeles: The Williams Institute; 2016.
2. Herman JL, Flores AR, Brown TN, Wilson BD, Conron KJ. Age of individuals who identify as transgender in the United States. Los Angeles: The Williams Institute; 2017.
3. Feinberg L. Stone butch blues: a novel. Ithaca: Firebrand Books; 1993.
4. Mock J. Redefining realness: my path to womanhood, identity, love & so much more. In: First Atria books hardcover edition. New York: Atria Books; 2014.
5. Serano J. Whipping Girl: A Transsexual Woman on Sexism and the Scapegoating of Femininity. Seal Press. Emeryville, CA. 2007.
6. James SE, Herman JL, Rankin S, Keisling M, Mottet L, Anafi M. 2015 U.S. transgender survey. Washington, DC: National Center for Transgender Equality; 2016.

7. Reisner SL, Poteat T, Keatley J, Cabral M, Mothopeng T, Dunham E, Holland CE, Max R, Baral SD. Global health burden and needs of transgender populations: a review. Lancet. 2016;388:412–36.
8. Meyerowitz JJ. How sex changed: a history of transsexuality in the United States. Cambridge, MA: Harvard Univ. Press; 2009.
9. Daphne S, Meredith AJ. The last time I wore a dress. New York: Riverhead Books; 1998.
10. Erickson-Schroth L, editor. Trans bodies, trans selves: a resource for the transgender community. Trans bodies, trans selves: a resource for the transgender community xxi, 649–xxi, 649; 2014.
11. Turban JL, Ehrensaft D. Research review: gender identity in youth: treatment paradigms and controversies. J Child Psychol Psychiatry. 2018;59:1228–43.
12. Cavanaugh T, Hopwood R, Lambert C. Informed consent in the medical care of transgender and gender-nonconforming patients. AMA J Ethics. 2016. https://doi.org/10.1001/journalofethics.2016.18.11.sect1-1611.
13. Crenshaw K. Mapping the margins: intersectionality, identity politics, and violence against women of color. Stanford Law Rev. 1991;43:1241–99.
14. Wesp LM, Malcoe LH, Elliott A, Poteat T. Intersectionality research for transgender health justice: a theory-driven conceptual framework for structural analysis of transgender health inequities. Transgend Health. 2019;4:287–96.
15. Diemer EW, Grant JD, Munn-Chernoff MA, Patterson DA, Duncan AE. Gender identity, sexual orientation, and eating-related pathology in a national sample of college students. J Adolesc Health. 2015. https://doi.org/10.1016/j.jadohealth.2015.03.003.
16. Guss CE, Williams DN, Reisner SL, Austin SB, Katz-Wise SL. Disordered weight management behaviors, nonprescription steroid use, and weight perception in transgender youth. J Adolesc Health. 2017;60:17–22.
17. Brown GR, Jones KT. Mental health and medical health disparities in 5135 transgender veterans receiving healthcare in the veterans health administration: a case-control study. LGBT Health. 2016;3:122–31.
18. Lipson SK, Sonneville KR. Eating disorder symptoms among undergraduate and graduate students at 12 U.S. colleges and universities. Eat Behav. 2017;24:81–8.
19. Diemer EW, White Hughto JM, Gordon AR, Guss C, Austin SB, Reisner SL. Beyond the binary: differences in eating disorder prevalence by gender identity in a transgender sample. Transgend Health. 2018. https://doi.org/10.1089/trgh.2017.0043.
20. Avila JT, Golden NH, Aye T. Eating disorder screening in transgender youth. J Adolesc Health. 2019. https://doi.org/10.1016/j.jadohealth.2019.06.011.
21. Austin SB, Nelson LA, Birkett MA, Calzo JP, Everett B. Eating disorder symptoms and obesity at the intersections of gender, ethnicity, and sexual orientation in US high school students. Am J Public Health. 2013;103:e16–22.
22. Gordon AR, Austin SB, Krieger N, White Hughto JM, Reisner SL. "I have to constantly prove to myself, to people, that I fit the bill": perspectives on weight and shape control behaviors among low-income, ethnically diverse young transgender women. Soc Sci Med. 2016;165:141–9.
23. Thompson JK. Exacting beauty: theory, assessment, and treatment of body image disturbance. 1st ed. Washington, DC: American Psychological Association; 1999.
24. McCabe MP, Ricciardelli LA. Sociocultural influences on body image and body changes among adolescent boys and girls. J Soc Psychol. 2003. https://doi.org/10.1080/00224540309598428.
25. Gordon AR, Austin SB, Pantalone DW, Baker AM, Eiduson R, Rodgers R. Appearance ideals and eating disorders risk among LGBTQ college students: the being ourselves living in diverse bodies (BOLD) study. J Adolesc Health. 2019. https://doi.org/10.1016/j.jadohealth.2018.10.096.
26. Brewster ME, Velez BL, Breslow AS, Geiger EF. Unpacking body image concerns and disordered eating for transgender women: the roles of sexual objectification and minority stress. J Couns Psychol. 2019;66:131–42.

27. Meyer IH. Prejudice, social stress, and mental health in lesbian, gay, and bisexual populations: conceptual issues and research evidence. Psychol Bull. 2003;129:674–97.
28. Hendricks ML, Testa RJ. A conceptual framework for clinical work with transgender and gender nonconforming clients: an adaptation of the minority stress model. Prof Psychol Res Pract. 2012;43:460.
29. Cohen S, Janicki-Deverts D, Miller GE. Psychological stress and disease. JAMA. 2007;298:1685–7.
30. Copeland WE, Bulik CM, Zucker N, Wolke D, Lereya ST, Costello EJ. Does childhood bullying predict eating disorder symptoms? A prospective, longitudinal analysis. Int J Eat Disord. 2015. https://doi.org/10.1002/eat.22459.
31. Bucchianeri MM, Eisenberg ME, Wall MM, Piran N, Neumark-Sztainer D. Multiple types of harassment: associations with emotional well-being and unhealthy behaviors in adolescents. J Adolesc Health. 2014;54:724–9.
32. McGuire JK, Doty JL, Catalpa JM, Ola C. Body image in transgender young people: findings from a qualitative, community based study. Body Image. 2016;18:96–107.
33. Watson RJ, Veale JF, Saewyc EM. Disordered eating behaviors among transgender youth: probability profiles from risk and protective factors. Int J Eat Disord. 2017;50:515–22.
34. Velez BL, Breslow AS, Brewster ME, Cox R, Foster AB. Building a pantheoretical model of dehumanization with transgender men: integrating objectification and minority stress theories. J Couns Psychol. 2016. https://doi.org/10.1037/cou0000136.
35. Sevelius JM. Gender affirmation: a framework for conceptualizing risk behavior among transgender women of color. Sex Roles. 2013. https://doi.org/10.1007/s11199-012-0216-5.
36. Glynn TR, Gamarel KE, Kahler CW, Iwamoto M, Operario D, Nemoto T. The role of gender affirmation in psychological well-being among transgender women. Psychol Sex Orientat Gend Divers. 2016;3:336–44.
37. Testa RJ, Rider GN, Haug NA, Balsam KF. Gender confirming medical interventions and eating disorder symptoms among transgender individuals. Health Psychol. 2017;36:927–36.
38. Jones BA, Haycraft E, Bouman WP, Brewin N, Claes L, Arcelus J. Risk factors for eating disorder psychopathology within the treatment seeking transgender population: the role of cross-sex hormone treatment. Eur Eat Disord Rev. 2018. https://doi.org/10.1002/erv.2576.
39. Van De Grift TC, Elaut E, Cerwenka SC, Cohen-Kettenis PT, De Cuypere G, Richter-Appelt H, Kreukels BPC. Effects of medical interventions on gender dysphoria and body image: a follow-up study. Psychosom Med. 2017. https://doi.org/10.1097/PSY.0000000000000465.
40. Vance SR, Mesheriakova VV. Documentation of gender identity in an adolescent and young adult clinic. J Adolesc Health. 2017. https://doi.org/10.1016/j.jadohealth.2016.10.018.
41. Rullo JE, Foxen JL, Griffin JM, Geske JR, Gonzalez CA, Faubion SS, van Ryn M Patient acceptance of sexual orientation and gender identity questions on intake forms in outpatient clinics: a pragmatic randomized multisite trial. Health Serv Res. 2018. https://doi.org/10.1111/1475-6773.12843.
42. Deutsch MB, Green J, Keatley JA, Mayer G, Hastings J, Hall AM. Electronic medical records and the transgender patient: recommendations from the world professional association for transgender health EMR working group. J Am Med Inform Assoc. 2013. https://doi.org/10.1136/amiajnl-2012-001472.
43. Rosendale N, Goldman S, Ortiz GM, Haber LA. Acute clinical care for transgender patients: a review. JAMA Intern Med. 2018. https://doi.org/10.1001/jamainternmed.2018.4179.
44. Aardoom JJ, Dingemans AE, Slof Op't Landt MCT, Van Furth EF. Norms and discriminative validity of the eating disorder examination questionnaire (EDE-Q). Eat Behav. 2012. https://doi.org/10.1016/j.eatbeh.2012.09.002.
45. Garner DM, Olmstead MP, Polivy J. Development and validation of a multidimensional eating disorder inventory for anorexia nervosa and bulimia. Int J Eat Disord. 1983. https://doi.org/10.1002/1098-108X(198321)2:2<15::AID-EAT2260020203>3.0.CO;2-6.
46. Nagata JM, Murray SB, Compte EJ, Pak EH, Schauer R, Flentje A, Capriotti MR, Lubensky ME, Lunn MR, Obedin-Maliver J. Community norms for the Eating Disorder Examination Questionnaire (EDE-Q) among transgender men and women. Eat Behav. 2020;37:101381.

47. Lock J, La Via MC. Practice parameter for the assessment and treatment of children and adolescents with eating disorders. J Am Acad Child Adolesc Psychiatry. 2015. https://doi.org/10.1016/j.jaac.2015.01.018.
48. Klaver M, Dekker MJHJ, de Mutsert R, Twisk JWR, den Heijer M. Cross-sex hormone therapy in transgender persons affects total body weight, body fat and lean body mass: a meta-analysis. Andrologia. 2017. https://doi.org/10.1111/and.12660.
49. Carswell JM, Roberts SA. Induction and maintenance of amenorrhea in transmasculine and nonbinary adolescents. Transgender Health. 2017. https://doi.org/10.1089/trgh.2017.0021.
50. Hembree WC, Cohen-Kettenis PT, Gooren L, Hannema SE, Meyer WJ, Murad MH, Rosenthal SM, Safer JD, Tangpricha V, T'Sjoen GG. Endocrine treatment of gender-dysphoric/gender-incongruent persons: an endocrine society clinical practice guideline. J Clin Endocrinol Metab. 2017;102:3869–903.
51. Katzman DK, Golden NH. Feeding and eating disorders. In: Neinstein LS, Katzman DK, Callahan ST, Gordon CM, Joffe A, Rickert VI, editors. Adolescent and young adult health care: a practical guide. 6th ed. Wolters Kluwer; Philadelphia, PA. 2017. p. 301–310.
52. Donaldson AA, Hall A, Neukirch J, Kasper V, Simones S, Gagnon S, Reich S, Forcier M. Multidisciplinary care considerations for gender nonconforming adolescents with eating disorders: a case series. Int J Eat Disord. 2018;51:475–9.
53. Golden NH, Katzman DK, Sawyer SM, Ornstein RM. Position paper of the society for adolescent health and medicine: medical management of restrictive eating disorders in adolescents and young adults references. J Adolesc Health. 2015. https://doi.org/10.1016/j.jadohealth.2014.10.259.
54. Carswell JM, Roberts SA. Induction and maintenance of amenorrhea in transmasculine and nonbinary adolescents. Transgend Health. 2017. https://doi.org/10.1089/trgh.2017.0021.
55. Kidd KM, Sequeira GM, Dhar CP, Montano GT, Witchel SF, Rofey D. Gendered body mass index percentile charts and transgender youth: making the case to change charts. Transgend Health. 2019. https://doi.org/10.1089/trgh.2019.0016.
56. Coleman E, Bockting W, Botzer M, et al. Standards of care for the health of transsexual, transgender, and gender-nonconforming people, version 7. Int J Transgend. 2012. https://doi.org/10.1080/15532739.2011.700873.
57. Ewan LA, Middleman AB, Feldmann J. Treatment of anorexia nervosa in the context of transsexuality: a case report. Int J Eat Disord. 2014. https://doi.org/10.1002/eat.22209.
58. Strandjord SE, Ng H, Rome ES. Effects of treating gender dysphoria and anorexia nervosa in a transgender adolescent: lessons learned. Int J Eat Disord. 2015. https://doi.org/10.1002/eat.22438.
59. Ålgars M, Alanko K, Santtila P, Sandnabba NK. Disordered eating and gender identity disorder: a qualitative study. Eat Disord. 2012. https://doi.org/10.1080/10640266.2012.668482.
60. Martha P, Inwards-Breland DJ, Watson L, Lara H. Bodies beyond the binary: developing a collaborative gender affirming approach to eating disorder management in gender nonconforming youth (conference presentation). Society for Adolescent Health and Medicine; 2019.
61. Bushell J. How current eating disorder discourse fails the LGBTQ community. And how we can change that. In: Huffington Post (blog). 2017. https://www.huffingtonpost.com/entry/how-current-eating-disorder-discourse-fails-the-lgbtq_us_5975e0fce4b0f1feb89b44e7.
62. Perry M, Watson L, Hayden L, Inwards-Breland D. Using body neutrality to inform eating disorder management in a gender diverse world. Lancet Child Adolesc Health. 2019;3:597–8.
63. Duffy ME, Henkel KE, Earnshaw VA. Transgender clients' experiences of eating disorder treatment. J LGBT Issues Couns. 2016;10:136–49.
64. Walton HM, Baker SL. Treating transgender individuals in inpatient and residential mental health settings. Cogn Behav Pract. 2019. https://doi.org/10.1016/j.cbpra.2017.09.006.
65. Lyons T, Shannon K, Pierre L, Small W, Krüsi A, Kerr T. A qualitative study of transgender individuals' experiences in residential addiction treatment settings: stigma and inclusivity. Subst Abuse Treat Prev Policy. 2015. https://doi.org/10.1186/s13011-015-0015-4.

Chapter 19
Eating Disorders in Boys and Men: Considerations in Sport and Exercise

Eva Pila and Sasha Gorrell

Learning Objectives

1. Examine the prevalence and unique presentations of eating pathology as it relates to dysfunctional exercise in at-risk and clinical samples of boys and men, as well as athletes.
2. Explore conceptualizations, theoretical frameworks, and models that can be applied to eating disorders in boys and men as contextualized to sport and exercise.
3. Overview athlete-specific assessment tools and intervention strategies aimed at prevention and treatment among boys and men.
4. Critically consider the contexts in which exercise and sport may exacerbate and protect against eating pathology.

Key Points

- Exercise is often central to the presentation of eating pathology in boys and men, thereby conferring critical diagnostic and treatment considerations.
- Knowledge of the role of sport and exercise in the context of eating pathology in boys and men is predominantly based on clinical observation and empirical evidence from samples of girls and women and may not capture the experiences of men.
- Tailored assessment and intervention strategies that consider unique sex- and gender-specific characteristics of eating pathology are needed for male and men-identifying athletes.

E. Pila (✉)
School of Kinesiology, Western University, London, ON, Canada
e-mail: epila@uwo.ca

S. Gorrell
Department of Psychiatry, Weill Institute for Neurosciences, University of California San Francisco, San Francisco, CA, USA
e-mail: sasha.gorrell@ucsf.edu

J. M. Nagata et al. (eds.), *Eating Disorders in Boys and Men*,
https://doi.org/10.1007/978-3-030-67127-3_19

Exercise in the Presentation of Eating Pathology

Exercise has enumerable benefits, but in the context of eating pathology, some individuals develop a problematic relationship with exercise as a central or tertiary symptom of an eating disorder [1]. Across boys and men that are non-treatment-seeking [2] or in treatment for an eating disorder [3], exercise may supersede other symptoms, such as dietary restriction or purging, as a primary method of weight control and/or affect regulation. There is evidence that engagement in exercise may serve to reduce body dissatisfaction and related eating pathology [4], with further evidence indicating that weight-bearing exercise may have protective effects on bone density [5–7], as well as improve strength and power [8]. Despite this potential for exercise to be protective, sport-specific pressures related to performance or body ideals in sport and exercise contexts may initiate or perpetuate disordered behaviors [9]. Taken together, knowledge of factors that confer increased risk for, or protection from, concurrent maladaptive eating and exercise pathology among men relies almost exclusively on theoretical underpinnings and empirical evidence from samples of women. As such, this chapter will discuss how commonly used assessment methods may not appropriately capture the unique prevalence, characteristics, and consequences of eating disorders among men, including men athletes. Further, efforts to prevent and treat the co-occurrence of exercise and eating pathology have focused almost exclusively on samples of women. As such, this chapter will summarize and critically consider empirical gaps in prevalence rates, presentation, theoretical considerations, and interventions related to sport and exercise in the context of eating disorders in boys and men.

Characterizations and Prevalence of Problematic Exercise in Boys and Men

Non-treatment-Seeking Samples As a symptom, compulsive exercise has an early onset [10] and demonstrates prevalence rates that are similar across sex in adolescent community samples (5.3% vs. 5.4%, for boys and girls, respectively) [11]. Rates appear to be slightly lower in adult samples. Specifically, German and Australian population surveys of 20–44-year-olds found that 3.5% [12] and 3.2% [13] of adult men report engaging in compulsive exercise in the past month. Aligned with documented trends in younger cohorts, these studies did not evidence sex differences in the proportion of individuals reporting these behaviors. Among adolescent boys, exercise may serve affective regulatory functions [14], a feature that has also been evidenced in adulthood. For example, in a community sample of US adults, men and women were equally likely to engage in problematic exercise; in this sample, men were more likely than women to engage in exercise that serves to reduce negative affect [15]. In a study of non-treatment-seeking undergraduate men in the United States, over 30% endorsed engaging in compulsive exercise in the prior month [16]. In another sample of US men college athletes, while the frequency of disordered eating behaviors was low overall, 37% reported using exercise as the primary means for weight control [2]. Considering this phenomenon internationally, 48% of Australian college men reported that exercise was important to their self-esteem, 34% were distressed when they could not exercise as much as they wanted, 27% followed rules about exercising, and 14% worried about the amount of exercise they were doing [17].

Clinical Samples Prevalence estimates identify that up to 80% of girls and women with anorexia nervosa and 40% of those with bulimia nervosa report problematic exercise behaviors [18]. The very limited research that has specifically examined the presentation of exercise behavior in clinical samples of boys and men suggests that as a symptom, it may be central to the presentation of anorexia nervosa [3]. A recent study using aggregate data from several adolescent family-based treatment trials for anorexia and bulimia nervosa did not find significant differences in baseline or end-of-treatment report of compulsive exercise, across sex (Gorrell et al., *under review*). In the whole sample, 58% of adolescent boys reported at least one episode of compulsive exercise in the month prior to treatment; prevalence rates were 54% and 71% in anorexia and bulimia nervosa, respectively.

Athletes The study of eating and exercise pathology in the sporting context has increased over the past three decades, but investigation of athletes has largely focused on samples of women, resulting in a comparative void of samples of men in the extant literature [19]. Studies that have focused on men athletes suggest that they may be at unique risk for sport-specific leanness and muscularity concerns [9], as pressure to achieve and maintain a lean physique may be particularly salient in sports that emphasize a specific body ideal (e.g., figure skating) [20]. A recent review established that prevalence of eating disorders is lower among men athletes compared to the women athletes [21]; however, one study found that eating disorders appear more frequently in men athletes compared to men non-athletes and a similar frequency of men elite athletes and women controls met criteria for eating disorders [22].

While findings related to vulnerability for eating pathology among athletes are mixed, increased risk for eating disorders has consistently been identified among men athletes who participate in weight class sports (e.g., wrestling, boxing, jockeys, rowers) [21] or aesthetic sports [23]. Vulnerability for eating pathology in these specific sport categories may be linked with sport-specific body dissatisfaction [24]. Risk for eating disorders and higher levels of maladaptive physical activity have also been identified among athletes who use performance- or image-enhancing drugs [25].

Vulnerability for cognitive vs. behavioral eating disorder symptoms may differ, relative to other types of sport categories. For example, a study comparing athletes participating in lean (e.g., distance running, wrestling) vs. non-lean sports (e.g., football, golf) across sex found that men athletes in non-lean sports had the highest overall scores in *attitudinal* eating disorder symptoms, while men in lean sports had the lowest scores [26]. However, men in lean sports reported significantly higher scores on reported eating disorder *behaviors* than men in non-lean sports. A recent study of collegiate men athletes compared eating and exercise pathology across 19 different sport categories; across both cognitive and behavioral domains, this study identified overall greatest risk in baseball players, cyclists, wrestlers, and rowers [27]. In team sports such as rugby, eating pathology may also differ as a function of the players' position, whereby players in forward positions (i.e., those necessitating greater body mass for engagement in scrums) endorse greater eating pathology than back-positioned team players [28]. In support of these findings, a recent meta-analysis of literature on eating disorders in men athletes underscores the notion that eating pathology and compulsive exercise behavior in men should be investigated separately and within specific sport environments [29].

In summary, among boys and men across the lifespan (i.e., among adolescents and adults) and in non-treatment-seeking, collegiate, clinical, and athlete samples, exercise may be more central to the presentation of eating pathology. Further, results suggest that men present with symptoms that are as severe as those observed in women. While evidence consistently supports increased risk for eating and exercise pathology among men participating in weight class sports, classification of sport categories across the literature has varied tremendously, precluding generalizability across samples. It is also noteworthy that disordered eating attitudes, and, to an extent, behaviors, may also occur in sports that do not emphasize weight or leanness [29], although this is less commonly recognized and may therefore be more likely overlooked. Further, commentary on maladaptive exercise behavior among treatment-seeking men with eating disorders is cautionary, given the paucity of research directly probing this symptom. Overall, given that a clear majority of all research, particularly in clinical samples, has focused on the presence of eating and exercise pathology among women, there is a critical need for increased awareness and early identification of maladaptive exercise behavior among men, including those who regularly participate in athletics.

Delineating Disordered Eating Practices from Committed Elite Athletic Performance

Identifying and characterizing disordered eating in high-level elite athletes may be particularly challenging, given that certain personality traits that are desirable for athletic achievement (e.g., perseverance in training, perfectionism, rigidity in exercise and dietary routines) can also characterize individuals with eating disorders [30] and are central to conceptualizations of problematic exercise (e.g., compulsive exercise; [1]). This presents a particular challenge of delineating disordered eating from normative and even necessary behavior patterns in the context of highly committed elite athletic training. Further, discerning medical consequences secondary to eating pathology in this population becomes particularly difficult given that conditions that result from physiological demands of the sport (e.g., bradycardia, endocrine dysregulation, and secondary amenorrhea) overlap with complications arising from relative energy deficiency. As such, the National Athletic Trainers' Association Position Statement [31] outlines recommendations, including the serial monitoring and recording of cardiovascular indicators (e.g., pulse rate and quality, blood pressure, orthostatic measurements, body temperature) and body composition with reference to gradual changes in fat and fat-free mass, while de-emphasizing ideal metrics of body composition. Relevant to men athletes, it is recommended that bradycardia is no longer considered a benign physiological adaptation in highly conditioned athletes when resting heart rate is less than 50 beats/minute during the day and less than 45 beats/min at night. This indicator suggests physiological instability in athletes and may be used to identify eating pathology. More recently, clinical assessment and management guidelines for eating disorders in athletes [32] suggest that screening for disordered behaviors ought to be a standard component of athletic care in order to distinguish disordered behaviors in athletes where extreme diet and exercise rigidity are contextually normative. Routine recommendations include screening questions, comprehensive physical examinations, and adopting a high index of suspicion for medical consequences of relative energy deficiency among all high-performance athletes. Assessment of an athlete's day-to-day function and eating and exercise/training behaviors are also recommended.

Conceptualizations and Frameworks Identifying Factors Related to Sport and Exercise

Conceptualizations of Compulsive Exercise Researchers have widely debated the definition, conceptualization, and assessment of maladaptive or disordered exercise behavior [33], thereby leading to challenges with the study of the phenomena [34]. To date, compulsive exercise is the most supported term for conceptualizing maladaptive exercise cognitions, emotions, and behaviors in clinical and nonclinical populations of women and men [34, 35]. There has been a limited focus on athlete populations, potentially due to the difficulty in characterizing compulsive exercise among those who engage in highly committed and rigorous training schedules for performance reasons [30]. Despite this, researchers have reported a higher risk of compulsive exercise in elite and competitive athletes (ranging from 7% to 42% prevalence) vs. leisure or recreational exercisers [36]. Further, given that higher levels of exercise are more aligned with the pursuit of muscularity, compulsive exercise may be a critical component of eating pathology for men [27]. Nevertheless, there are considerable challenges in assessing this phenomenon in the athlete population, given that athletes with high training needs may inherently experience a conflict with other life demands and negative affect as a result of missing important training sessions with performance implications. Further, there has been robust evidence to suggest that compulsive exercise is problematic when it is confounded with eating pathology and may not present considerable health risk in the absence of disordered eating symptoms [37]. Notably, research on compulsive exercise has not focused exclusively on men, at the expense of developing gender-specific conceptualizations.

Maintenance Model of Compulsive Exercise Embedded within an addiction framework, compulsive exercise has been recognized as a critical factor in the development and maintenance of eating disorders. Indeed, compulsive exercise is one of the most difficult and treatment resistance symptoms [38, 39]. The maintenance model of compulsive exercise [1] posits that exercise functions as an affect regulation strategy via positive reinforcement (e.g., mitigating affective withdrawal when not exercising) and negative reinforcement (e.g., alleviating/avoiding internal discomfort). Additionally, weight and shape concerns, compulsivity, perfectionism, and rigidity are all functional components that maintain compulsive exercise. This model was derived from research that was almost exclusively conducted in young samples of girls and women, with very limited investigations focusing on men or athletes. One of the main investigations of the multidimensional model of compulsive exercise in athletes [40] found that weight control and avoidance of negative affect were critical components associated with compulsive exercise, beyond other dimensions which were more relevant in non-athlete-specific samples (e.g., exercise rigidity, lack of exercise enjoyment). By nature of the rigid and habitual exercise routines inherent to training programs, these features are likely not predictive of compulsive exercise. Some evidence suggests that athletic identity, the extent to which one identifies with their role as an athlete, may be an important factor to consider in the maintenance of compulsive exercise. Specifically, individuals with a high athletic identity may ascribe upmost importance to sport in their life, with their self-worth being highly contingent on their performance, and a high willingness to sacrifice other life domains. Indeed, athletic identity tends to be higher among athletes who are at risk of compulsive exercise – yet no discernable differences have been reported between women and men athletes [41–43]. It is plausible to suggest that men may be particularly prone to compulsive exercise as a predictor of eating pathology, given that in some nonclinical undergraduate samples, men engage in higher frequencies of compulsive exercise compared to women [44]. Further, exercise is more aligned with reaching masculine physique ideals (compared to feminine ideals), and compulsive exercise is a critical component of the drive for muscularity and muscle dysmorphia [45] – two conditions that are disproportionately observed in men.

Objectification Theory (and Embodiment) Grounded in feminist frameworks, objectification theory was originally developed to understand how sexual objectification of women's bodies is associated with a range of conditions that disproportionately impact women, including eating disorders [46]. Since then, researchers have extended this framework to men, given that men are similarly subject to gendered sociocultural ideals around masculine physique, and men's bodies are sexually objectified [47–49]. Indeed, pervasive body ideals center around a highly mesomorphic (i.e., muscular) body as the masculine physique ideal [50]. There is a growing body of research that has demonstrated replication of the proposed pathways in men [51, 52], whereby self-objectification has been associated with disordered eating, via body surveillance and body shame. Notably, Calogero [52] noted that self-objectification experiences in men may be more robustly linked with disordered exercise given the use of exercise as an appearance management strategy in men. Strelan and Hargreaves [53] found that among men, self-objectification and appearance motives for exercise were linked with lower body esteem. A small cross-sectional study of university-aged men reported that high self-objectification was associated with greater drive for muscularity and higher levels of muscle dysmorphia symptoms [54]. Further research integrated the internalization of body ideals and drive for muscularity [55], finding support for the mediating role of body surveillance in the association between internalization of cultural standards of attractiveness and body shame, and that internalization of cultural standards may be associated with tendencies to use anabolic-androgenic steroids. Given that traditional sport and exercise contexts are often highly social, evaluative, and physique-focused, there is ample opportunity for self-objectification. Based on tenets of objectification theory, those participating in physique-salient activities (e.g., bodybuilding) will endorse higher levels of self-objectification, compared to more functional activities (e.g., weightlifting), a hypothesis that has been supported in previous work [56].

However, it has also been postulated that sport and exercise contexts can promote embodying opportunities that may mitigate the impact of objectifying experiences within and beyond sport [4]. Specifically, physical activity contexts can support features of embodiment by enhancing mind-body integration, increasing body awareness and responsiveness, physical empowerment, and providing a sense of physical competence. This internal orientation toward the physical self in sport and exercise recognizes the body as instrumental and expressive, thereby fundamentally embodied [57]. Menzel and Levine [4] state that all sport contexts, regardless of their physique-oriented nature, endorse the devotion of time and attention to the development of physical skills that promote an internal orientation of one's body function, skills, and capabilities. According to this framework, caring for the body, being aware of its needs, and preventing injury are critical to peak athletic performance. As such, by participating in a context that lends itself to development of embodiment, men may be protected against self-objectification and thereby at lower risk of disordered eating. Overall, there are important considerations for the role of objectification in athletic contexts, whereby sport and exercise are highly evaluative and often ascribe to specific physique ideals that are associated with performance – and, yet, can also empower individuals to experience and appreciate the body's functional capabilities. It is noteworthy that embodiment frameworks have had limited applications in men, and it is unclear how embodied experiences via physical activity may reduce men's objectification experiences and therefore risk for eating disorders. There is substantial conceptual support for applying objectification frameworks to men and moderate empirical support for the utility of objectification theory. However, to date, there have been very limited applications of protective features (e.g., embodiment) in understanding risk factors contributing to men's eating disorders in sport and exercise contexts.

Sociocultural Model of Eating Disorders in Sport Drawing on Petrie and Greenleaf's [2, 58] conceptual model, athletes are exposed to pressures to change their body weight, shape, and size which are communicated through traditional (e.g., friends, family, friends, media) and sport sources (e.g., coaches, teammates, officials). Pervasive exposure to these sociocultural pressures, along with exposure to the physique-salient and evaluative sport context, can lead athletes to internalize a given observer's perspective of their bodies. As a result, athletes may engage in disordered eating and exercise behaviors to alleviate these internalized evaluations by managing their body appearance. Competitive sport environments in particular may perpetuate sociocultural pressures relating to appearance, function, eating, and performance, thereby uniquely contributing to eating pathology risk. Notably, competitive and elite athletes who are highly embedded in the sport context are considerably exposed to these sociocultural messages from sport sources, which may exert negative effects, regardless of degree of internalization. More recently, researchers [59] have proposed initial conceptual and empirical support for extension of the model to include factors that are specific to men athletes, including evaluations of body fat, training regimens, and sport competitive levels. Indeed, men athletes face unique vulnerability due to commonly perpetuated notions that optimal performance is weight-contingent (e.g., wrestlers need to meet weight limits to compete at specific levels; rowers at lower weights may have a performance advantage). Indeed, sociocultural pressures and influences for men communicate that highly muscular bodies demonstrate social capital, strength, competence, and power. Despite this promising conceptual framework, longitudinal research is needed to test the causal nature of the proposed pathways [60].

Biopsychosocial Model in Adolescent Boys Ricciardelli and McCabe's [18] conceptual model summarized the empirical similarities of biopsychosocial risk factors associated with both eating disorders and the pursuit of muscularity in adolescent boys. Although this model was not specific to exercise and sport contexts, it did identify that participation in aesthetic sports is an important risk factor for boys during this pubertal period and that exercise engaged in for the pursuit of muscularity may be a core component of disordered eating practices in boys.

Transdiagnostic Cognitive-Behavioral Model of Eating Disorders Fairburn and colleagues [61] proposed that anorexia nervosa, bulimia nervosa, and eating disorders not otherwise specified share foundational psychopathological underpinnings (i.e., perfectionism, low self-esteem, mood intolerance, and interpersonal difficulties) which function to interact and maintain disordered eating cognitions and behaviors. Empirical evidence has supported the applicability of the model to a wide range of girl and women athletes (e.g., individual, team, recreational, elite sport), although the model was not supported in men athletes [62]. Notably, interpersonal difficulties with the coaching relationship were not involved in the eating pathology for men compared to women athletes. Considering the substantial level of empirical support for the underpinnings of this model [63], further research is needed on the applicability of this model in men athletes.

Relative Energy Deficiency in Sports (RED-S) Consensus statements released by the International Olympic Committee (IOC) [64, 65] identified relative energy deficiency in sport (RED-S) as a syndrome which may include metabolic, menstrual, bone health, immune, protein, and cardiovascular complications that interrelate to compromise physiological function, psychological health, and athletic performance. Despite original definition as the female athlete triad, a syndrome exclusive to female athletes, recent clinical and empirical evidence has drawn parallels to male athletes [66]. This emergent evidence has found that low energy availability is similarly experienced in male athletes, as identified by a discrepancy between energy intake via nutrition and energy expenditure via exercise in the sport context. Male athletes, particularly those engaged in sports that endorse leanness and weight restrictions (e.g., runners, cyclists, rowers, athletes in weight-limiting sports), are at risk of presenting with interrelated issues around inadequate nutrition, impaired bone health, and endocrine dysfunction. Indeed, eating pathology and biomarkers indicative of RED-S (e.g., reduced testosterone) have been reported among male athletes competing in intense endurance sport; however, there has been a predominant focus on physiological markers at the expense of understanding presentations of eating pathology in men [67]. And unlike the well-documented clinical consequences of RED-S in female athletes, there is substantially limited research for the consequences in men. Although current guidelines parallel those for female athletes, considerable caution is recommended when applying prevention, screening, treatment, and return-to-play guidelines that were developed for female athletes to men athletes, given the lack of gender-specific empirical support. As such, the IOC [65] calls for further identification of risk factors and development of screening tools, evidence-based prevention and treatment programs, continued development in RED-S among male athletes, and further development of associated health and performance consequences [65].

Assessment and Measures of Exercise Behavior in the Context of Eating Disorders in Boys and Men

Included in the earliest descriptions of anorexia nervosa [68], problematic exercise was initially conceptualized as *excessive* and subsequently evaluated for its duration, frequency, or intensity [69]. More recent evidence suggests that *motivation* to exercise (e.g., for weight control) is more salient than the amount of exercise per se in predicting eating disorder pathology [1, 70–72]. Over the past three decades, the assessment of exercise has burgeoned and includes measures that describe exercise as compulsive [1, 18, 73, 74], addictive [75], dependent [76–79], and obligatory [80], among other terms. Driven exercise has also been considered a primary disorder (i.e., exercise that is more addictive in nature and serves to reduce negative affect) or secondary to an eating disorder (i.e., exercise that is more compulsive in nature and serves to control body weight and shape) [15, 76].

There is considerable overlap in this panoply of conceptualizations, as well as the possibility that the sheer number of terms used to describe exercise in the context of eating pathology has diluted the conclusions that may be drawn across the broader literature. Arguably more problematic is the questionable validity of certain measures among men samples, as a consequence of their original development in women samples, or with items that imply that exercise is aimed exclusively at weight loss. Referring to eating disorder symptom evaluation more broadly, a majority of gold standard assessments reveal lower scores among men, likely due to a lack of validity and sensitivity within specific items [81]. Despite these potential reliability issues, efforts to assess exercise behavior and related eating pathology in mixed-gender samples have burgeoned.

Measures Used to Assess Exercise and Eating Pathology in Boys and Men

Some measures of exercise that demonstrate potential utility in assessing exercise behavior in the context of eating pathology among men include the *Obligatory Exercise Questionnaire* (OEQ; [80]). A 20-item self-report questionnaire, the OEQ assesses the frequency of exercise-related situations and has demonstrated good internal consistency and 2-week test-retest reliability in men [80]. Limited investigation of OEQ outcomes specific to men has been published, but in one sample of university students, no significant differences were evidenced in OEQ scores, across gender [82]. The OEQ has three subscales, *Exercise Fixation*, *Exercise Frequency*, and *Exercise Commitment*. In one study that reported predictors of two of these subscales specifically among men, only perceived pressure from a dating partner significantly predicted exercise commitment, with no significant findings relevant to exercise fixation [83].

A different measure that has been validated in men samples is the *Compulsive Exercise Test* (CET), a self-report 24-item assessment of cognitive, behavioral, and emotional characteristics of exercise with 5 subscales: *Avoidance and Rule-Driven Behavior*, *Weight Control Exercise*, *Mood Improvement*, *Exercise Rigidity*, and *Lack of Exercise Enjoyment* [1, 84]. The CET has demonstrated strong psychometric properties in both adolescents and adult men [84, 85]. The CET uniquely captures multidimensional aspects of exercise (i.e., cognitive, behavioral, and emotional features). In a study of young adult men and women with anorexia nervosa using the CET, findings indicated that men reported significantly greater overall exercise pathology, compared to women [3]. Subscale analysis showed that men were more likely to report engaging in compulsive exercise to avoid negative affect and increase positive affect and endorsed more rigidity in their exercise habits than women. This study suggests that compulsive exercise in anorexia nervosa among men serves both physiological and psychological purposes and appears more functionally linked to affect regulation than in women [3].

The CET is predicated upon the idea that exercise may be undertaken to avoid or escape the experience of negative affect (e.g., guilt, anxiety) [1]. In contrast, exercise has also been conceptualized as approach-oriented and reward-driven rather than avoidant, akin to engagement in substance use [79]. Accordingly, the *Exercise Dependence Scale* (EDS) is a 21-item measure that was designed to assess exercise dependence, based on criteria for substance dependence [79]. One study which evaluated associations between EDS scores and body image concerns in university students found that for men, exercise behavior was the strongest negative predictor of body dissatisfaction and social physique anxiety [86]. For men, but not for women, the amount of time spent on activities necessary to obtain exercise as well as the experience of engaging in activity for longer than was intended was associated with improved body image.

The *Exercise Addiction Inventory* (EAI) shares the theoretical basis as the EDS, in that the etiology and maintenance of exercise are considered to align with a model of behavioral addiction [87]. This six-item measure assesses for six domains related to reasons for engagement in or consequences of exercise behavior: salience, mood modification, tolerance, withdrawal symptoms, conflict, and relapse. Gender invariance in the EAI was evaluated in cross-cultural secondary analyses of studies using the EAI across five countries (i.e., Denmark, Hungary, Spain, the United Kingdom, and the United States) [88]. Findings suggest that men and women may use the starting points on the scales differently, and therefore, comparison of means directly across gender may be misleading. Further, the authors suggest that different cutoffs should be calculated for men and women. An adolescent adaptation of the EAI has recently been validated in a mixed-gender sample of adolescents, but while analyses controlled for gender, outcomes were not delineated specifically to men [89].

Notably, despite the preponderance of measures that have been developed in samples of women, a majority of the literature indicates that men are equally or even more likely to endorse problematic exercise, compared to women (e.g., [3, 15]). A recent study identified item-level gender bias in the *Female Athlete Screening Tool* (FAST; [90], a measure designed to assess eating and exercise behavior in women athletes [91]. Specifically, in this study that assessed both men and women athletes, men-derived item bias was demonstrated in items that queried attributing weight loss attempts to weight class requirements, restricting food, and frequent weighing. Further, while women athletes were more likely to score above the median on cognitive symptoms, men athletes are more likely to score above the median on behavioral symptoms. In efforts to improve assessment efforts in a sporting context, a new multidimensional measure, the *Athletes' Relationships with Training* scale, was recently developed for use specifically among athletes, to capture self-report of unhealthy training behaviors associated with eating disorders [92]. Scores from this scale have thus far demonstrated validity evidence among women athletes, with current research efforts underway for validation among men.

Body Image and Exercise in Boys and Men

With the aim of better capturing the experience of men who are compelled to engage in problematic exercise, some work has investigated relations between muscle dysmorphia, exercise behavior, and eating pathology. A single case study describing a young adult man diagnosed with eating disorder not otherwise specified and muscle dysmorphia identified similar psychological function between compulsive muscle-building and binge eating/purging episodes [93]. For this individual, compulsive exercise was directly related to interpersonal stressors, and binge eating/purging was tied with mood regulation. This emotional and behavioral link was echoed in another study where the functional utility and features of compulsive exercise were equivalent in both men diagnosed with muscle dysmorphia or with anorexia nervosa [93]. Specifically, both clinical groups reported exercise for mood regulation and rigid and rule-driven exercise patterns.

Given the considerable overlap in exercise symptom presentation in muscle dysmorphia and eating disorders, the importance of muscularity has been highlighted in its diagnostic relevance to eating pathology, particularly among men [94, 95]. Scores from the recently developed *Muscularity-Oriented Eating Test* have shown initial validity evidence in collegiate men [96], with current research efforts underway to test score validity among men athletes. To date, only one scale has been developed to directly probed body satisfaction in men athletes, the *Weight Pressures in Sport Scale for Male Athletes* (WPS-M; [58]). The WPS-M is a 14- item self-report questionnaire with two subscales, one reflecting pressure to maintain a weight seen as desirable by coaches or teammates and the other reflecting pressure to maintain a desirable weight and appearance for individuals outside of sport (i.e., family, friends, spectators). Scores from the WPS-M have demonstrated good reliability and validity evidence in a sample of collegiate men athletes [9]. Some studies have used a wider variety of body image domains in their assessment protocol. For example, in a sample of men who were either non-regular exercisers or those participating in one of two different types of sports (runners/aerobic exercisers, weightlifting/bodybuilding), men were queried about facets of body image including partner preference, ideals, and overall dissatisfaction [97]. In this study, the authors noted that it was somewhat surprising that little differences in body image dissatisfaction or eating pathology were identified, relative to both sport status and sexual orientation [97].

Overall, research querying the unique experience of men's body image, related eating pathology, and maladaptive exercise is considerably limited. Given the role that sport-specific body dissatisfaction may play in exacerbating risk for eating disorders among men athletes [24], further research specific to men's experience of the body is warranted. When at all possible, efforts should be made to stratify samples according to not only the type of exercise (e.g., weightlifting, distance running) but also to consider that idealized body types may differ within sport, according to position of play (e.g., defensive vs. offensive football).

The limited research base to date indicates that measures that have directly assessed problematic exercise in the context of eating pathology among men have generally identified rates that are comparable to, or exceed, those in women. Further, the motivation for exercise among men appears to be predominantly for mood regulation purposes (i.e., reducing negative affect or increasing positive affect) or, when relevant, to achieve a sport-specific body ideal. While men report less exercise for reasons of weight control on measures that directly probe internalization of a thin ideal, they do report significantly more rigid and rule-based exercise behavior than women [3]. There are few sport-specific, athlete-specific, or multidimensional instruments with which to measure a problematic relationship with exercise specifically among men. The development and testing of exercise assessment tools specifically among men, and men athletes, is unequivocally essential to future assessment, diagnostic, and treatment endeavors.

Interventions in Prevention and Treatment

Athlete-Specific Eating Disorder Prevention Despite a large body of literature on eating disorder prevention focused on non-athlete samples of women, there are some documented efforts aimed at reducing symptoms of disordered eating or eating disorder incidence in athletes [98–100]. Not surprisingly, most of these prevention efforts have focused on women athletes, thereby precluding an understanding of the need for gender-specific intervention. A universal primary prevention intervention – ATHENA (Athletes Targeting Healthy Exercise and Nutrition Alternatives) – targeted high school athletes [101, 102]. This peer-led, team-based program consisted of eight sessions embedded within athlete training activities and targeted adolescent girls. Outcomes from a randomized trial revealed reductions in diet pill use and eating pathology that were sustained 1 year and 3 years post-intervention. A parallel gender-specific team-based intervention has also been developed for adolescent boys in sport and applied in young men non-athletes [103] – ATLAS (Athletes Training and Learning to Avoid Steroids) – reporting success in reduced use of anabolic steroids and other illicit substances, as well as some indices of eating behavior [102, 104]. Further, Martinsen and colleagues [99] developed and tested an intervention aimed at primary prevention among adolescent girl and boy athletes. Utilizing a social-cognitive framework, the intervention aimed to enhance self-esteem, self-efficacy, intrinsic motivation, and mastery goals. The multimodal school-based program consisted of delivering educational content (e.g., lectures, assignments) and targeted elite student athletes, coaches, and parents for a period of 1 year. Results from the randomized controlled trial demonstrated effective prevention of new cases of eating disorders, but only for women athletes. The lack of significant effects among men was hypothesized to be due to the utilization of women-centric assessments (e.g., drive for thinness, body dissatisfaction subscale of the EDI). Other eating disorder prevention programs in athletes have focused exclusively on women (i.e., [105]) and include programs such as Bodies in Motion [23], the Female Athlete Body Project [106], BodySense [107], and Nutrition for Optimal Performance [108]. Overall, the limited literature on eating disorder prevention suggests that primary interventions with multiple targets (e.g., athletes, coaches) and multimodal approaches show effectiveness at reducing eating disorder symptoms in higher-risk women athletes. Due to the high risk of eating disorders in elite men athletes, the development of prevention interventions targeting this subsample is critical.

Treatment Guidelines Despite several calls for athlete-specific interventions in prevention and treatment of eating disorders (e.g., International Olympic Committee, American College of Sports Medicine, National Collegiate Athletic Association, National Athletic Trainers' Association), there is a paucity of research and practice for athletes more generally, and there are no known recommendations or interventions specific to men athletes. Indeed, eating disorders are more likely to be undetected and untreated in men athletes, in that this subset of individuals faces cumulative gender and mental health stigma and convoluted perceptions of risk in athletic domains. Collectively, these factors contribute to worsened health risk and outcomes for men athletes with eating disorders [109]. Practitioners have called for the reduction of barriers, enhanced stigma, and bias education in sport contexts, which will promote early detection and intervention among men athletes [110]. Athlete-tailored treatment has the capacity to appropriately address sport-related performance needs and athlete's unique presentations of the condition and may be ideally suited to promote eating disorder prevention, recovery, and return-to-play among athletes. Treatment guidelines and protocols for athletes are limited, and especially so for men athletes, precluding the availability of evidence-based recommendations for optimal treatment efficacy in this population.

Treatment Recommendations Despite several calls for athlete-specific interventions in prevention and treatment of eating disorders (e.g., International Olympic Committee, American College of Sports Medicine, National Collegiate Athletic Association, National Athletic Trainers Association), there is a paucity of research and practice for athletes more generally, and there are no known recommendations or interventions specific to men athletes. Indeed, eating disorders are more likely to be undetected and untreated in men athletes, in that this subset of individuals faces cumulative stigmas directed toward men more generally and the convoluted perceptions of risk in the athletic domains – thereby increasing the health risk and outcomes for men athletes with eating disorders [109]. Practitioners have called for the reduction of barriers, enhanced stigma, and bias education in sport contexts, which will promote early detection and intervention among men athletes [110]. Athlete-tailored treatment has the capacity to appropriately address sport-related performance needs and athlete's unique presentations of the condition and may be ideally suited to promote eating disorder prevention, recovery, and return-to-play among

Table 19.1 Summary of treatment recommendations for athletes with eating disorders

	Summary of treatment guidelines
Multidisciplinary team	Coordinated multidisciplinary team with specialized training for athletes with eating disorders. Personnel include athletic supports such as coaches, strength and conditioning specialists, primary care physician, psychiatrist, psychotherapist, and registered dietician. Consultation with sport psychiatrist is valuable
Psychoeducation	Psychoeducation for athletes, families, coaches, and trainers will help to reduce stigma and reduce normalization of disordered practices in athletic setting (e.g., decouple body fat and weight from performance in the coaching practice)
Medical care	Primary care physicians are integral in the evaluation and management of medical complications (e.g., cardiovascular, gastrointestinal, orthopedic, psychiatric, and endocrinological). Psychiatric care is highly recommended for pharmacological management and monitoring. Support pharmacological care that is sensitive to the athlete's competitive environment
Comorbidities	Common comorbidities include anxiety, depression, obsessive-compulsive disorder, posttraumatic stress, substance abuse, and/or self-injury. Screening and management are recommended
Weight restoration and monitoring	Restoring weight and metabolic balance are primary goals, with regular weight monitoring and assessment of body composition. Special considerations of weight history, hormonal functioning, energy balance, and athletic demands on the body. Care is recommended in de-emphasizing weight and reducing athlete's exposure to weight metrics
Nutritional support	Working closely with dietician to calculate energy expenditure and matching energy intake. Consulting evidence on energy availability hypothesis when treating athletes is recommended
Psychotherapy	Evidence-based psychotherapy is integral to treatment (e.g., cognitive-behavior therapy, enhanced cognitive-behavior therapy, dialectical behavior therapy, acceptance and commitment therapy, and family-based treatment). Psychological care that integrates key stakeholders in the athlete's sporting environment (e.g., teammates, coaches, family) and considers the role of the athletic environment is most effective. Consideration of the athlete's involvement in sport, the level of competition, and the type of sport needs to be assessed in a compassionate manner that recognizes and respects the importance of one's athletic identity
Evaluation of sport involvement	Cautiously consider and continuously adjust frequency and intensity of training, according to weight restoration and medical status Maintaining appropriate levels of sport participation in medically stable athletes is important. Using an athlete-centered approach to treatment is of critical importance during treatment and in considering return-to-play. In cases where sport involvement is detrimental to athlete's health, re-consider involvement in competitive sport or consider alternate sports

athletes. Recommendations for athlete-focused treatment guidelines [19, 111, 112] are summarized in Table 19.1.

Integrating Exercise in Eating Disorder Treatment There is some debate regarding the inclusion of exercise in the treatment of eating disorders, and limited empirical data and clinical guidelines further stymie efforts [113]. Advocates for the inclusion of exercise in the treatment of eating disorders posit that exercise intervention can be safe and beneficial if nutritionally supported and appropriately monitored [114]. In a review of literature, Cook and colleagues [114] report several core strategies for appropriate therapeutic integration of exercise in eating disorder treatment:

(i) Assimilation of multidisciplinary team of experts in the treatment context.
(ii) Management of medical contraindications.
(iii) Screening for exercise-related psychopathology.
(iv) Development of a collaborative written contract between team members and patient regrading exercise plan.
(v) Including psychoeducation.
(vi) Exercise is available as positive reinforcement.
(vii) Develop an incremental exercise program.
(viii) Limit intensity of activity and build gradually.
(ix) Tailor mode of exercise to individual needs.
(x) Enroll dietetics and nutritional expertise in weight restoration.
(xi) Probe the emotions and cognitions associated with each exercise session.

These evidence-based strategies comprise a set of clinical guidelines for incorporating exercise in the treatment of eating disorders; however, they do not focus on men samples specifically. As such, further evaluation is needed to determine the extent to which these guidelines apply in samples of men with eating disorders, given common exercise-related intricacies in male-oriented presentations of illness. To date, there is preliminary support targeting exercise pathology among individuals with eating disorders in "sport therapy" educational programs [115] and cognitive behavioral programs [116]; however, this is limited by small sample sizes and predominantly female samples.

Treatment Interventions in Clinical Samples The existing limited reports of athlete-specific intensive treatment programs feature either female- or women-only samples (e.g., [110]) or predominantly female or women samples (e.g., [117]). Drawing upon a collaborative multidisciplinary team of clinicians [118], the Victory Program is a clinical initiative designed to treat eating disorders in elite men and women athletes. Despite the lack of robust randomized clinical trial data, preliminary outcomes from the Victory Program have demonstrated enhanced strength and power among a small sample of athletes (predominantly diagnosed with anorexia nervosa) in residential and partial hospitalization programs [117]. Similarly, the Walden GOALS program is an intensive outpatient treatment program formulated using the IOC guidelines to treat competitive athletes and has demonstrated promise in improving outcomes among women athletes predominantly diagnosed with other specified feeding and eating disorders [110]. The evidence of treatment strategies does not consider the clinical considerations that may be important to men athletes, which carries critical implications given that men are diagnosed at more developed stages of illness [21].

Implications

Considerations of the role of sport and exercise as applied to eating disorders have been overwhelmingly reliant on empirical evidence in women. In light of clinical observations and emerging empirical literature among males and men, sex- and gender-specific considerations in the conceptualization, assessment, and treatment of eating disorders as related to sport and exercise warrant further attention. Considering that exercise pathology is more salient in the presentation of eating disorders in men, it becomes critical to seek robust and psychometrically supported assessment tools that are specific to men's experience of body image, sport characteristics, and function of exercise. Indeed, the convoluted characterization of eating and exercise pathology in clinical samples of men precludes a nosological understanding about diagnostic criteria in boys and men. Relatedly and likely consequentially to the gaps in assessment, current interventions lack appropriate male representation and do not appropriately consider unique components that may be relevant for boys and men. Focusing on athletes in higher-risk sports that inextricably link appearance features (e.g., weight, muscularity) with performance outcomes is of critical importance. Considering the unique characteristics (e.g., drive for muscularity) and disordered behaviors (e.g., anabolic steroid use) that are inherently linked with sport and exercise contexts are also imperative in advancing the understanding of eating disorders in boys and men. The limited evidence does converge to suggest that in the clinical treatment of athletes, there is a need to integrate the athletic community and emphasize a multidisciplinary approach to care that recognizes the salience of athletic identity. Collectively, these advances will support sex- and gender-specific approaches that will promote the prevention and treatment of eating disorders among boys and men, in the context of sport and exercise.

References

1. Meyer C, Taranis L, Goodwin H, Haycraft E. Compulsive exercise and eating disorders. Eur Eat Disord Rev. 2011;19:174–89.
2. Petrie TA, Greenleaf C, Reel J, Carter J. Prevalence of eating disorders and disordered eating behaviors among male collegiate athletes. Psychol Men Masculinity. 2008;9:267–77.
3. Murray SB, Griffiths S, Rieger E, Touyz S. A comparison of compulsive exercise in male and female presentations of anorexia nervosa: what is the difference? Adv Eat Disord. 2014;2:65–70.
4. Menzel JE, Levine MP. Embodying experiences and the promotion of positive body image: the example of competitive athletics. In: Self-objectification in women: causes, consequences, and counteractions. Washington DC: American Psychological Association; 2010.
5. Seeman E, Szmukler GI, Formica C, Tsalamandris C, Mestrovic R. Osteoporosis in anorexia nervosa: the influence of peak bone density, bone loss, oral contraceptive use, and exercise. J Bone Miner Res. 1992;7:1467–74.
6. Gordon CM, Goodman E, Emans SJ, Grace E, Becker KA, Rosen CJ, et al. Physiologic regulators of bone turnover in young women with anorexia nervosa. J Pediatr. 2002;141:64–70.

7. Waugh EJ, Woodside DB, Beaton DE, CotI P, Hawker GA. Effects of exercise on bone mass in young women with anorexia nervosa. Med Sci Sports Exerc. 2011;43:755–63.
8. Fewell LK, Nickols R, Schlitzer Tierney A, Levinson CA. Strength and power improvements in athlete and non-athletes during intensive eating disorder treatment. J Clin Sport Psychol. 2018;12:1–28.
9. Galli N, Petrie TA, Chatterton JM, Baghurst TM, Reel JJ. Assessing the validity of the weight pressures in sport scale for male athletes. Psychol Men Masculinity. 2014;15:170–81.
10. Allen KL, Byrne SM, Oddy WH, Crosby RD. Early onset binge eating and purging eating disorders: course and outcome in a population-based study of adolescents. J Abnorm Child Psychol. 2013;41:1083–96.
11. Mond J, Hall A, Bentley C, Harrison C, Gratwick-Sarll K, Lewis V. Eating-disordered behavior in adolescent boys: eating disorder examination questionnaire norms. Int J Eat Disord. 2014;47:335–41.
12. Hilbert A, de Zwaan M, Braehler E. How frequent are eating disturbances in the population? Norms of the eating disorder examination-questionnaire. PLoS One. 2012;7:e29125.
13. Bentley C, Mond J, Rodgers B. Sex differences in psychosocial impairment associated with eating-disordered behavior: what if there aren't any? Eat Behav. 2014;15:609–14.
14. Goodwin H, Haycraft E, Meyer C. The relationship between compulsive exercise and emotion regulation in adolescents. Br J Health Psychol. 2012;17:699–710.
15. Cunningham HE, Pearman S, Brewerton TD. Conceptualizing primary and secondary pathological exercise using available measures of excessive exercise. Int J Eat Disord. 2016;49:778–92.
16. Lavender JM, De Young KP, Anderson DA. Eating disorder examination questionnaire (EDE-Q): norms for undergraduate men. Eat Behav. 2010;11:119–21.
17. O'Dea JA, Abraham S. Eating and exercise disorders in young college men. J Am Coll Health Assoc. 2002;50:273–8.
18. Dalle Grave R, Calugi S, Marchesini G. Compulsive exercise to control shape or weight in eating disorders: prevalence, associated features, and treatment outcome. Compr Psychiatry. 2008;49:346–52.
19. Baum A. Eating disorders in the male athlete. Sports Med. 2006;36:1–6.
20. Voelker DK, Reel JJ. An inductive thematic analysis of male competitive figure skaters' experiences of weight pressure in sport. J Clin Sport Psychol. 2018;12:1–28.
21. Bratland-Sanda S, Sundgot-Borgen J. Eating disorders in athletes: overview of prevalence, risk factors and recommendations for prevention and treatment. Eur J Sport Sci. 2013;13:499–508.
22. Sundgot-Borgen J, Torstveit MK. Prevalence of eating disorders in elite athletes is higher than in the general population. Clin J Sport Med. 2004;14:25–32.
23. Voelker DK, Petrie TA, Reel JJ, Gould D. Frequency and psychosocial correlates of eating disorder symptomatology in male figure skaters. J Appl Sport Psychol. 2018;30;119–26.
24. Goltz FR, Stenzel LM, Schneider CD. Disordered eating behaviors and body image in male athletes. Rev Bras Psiquiatr. 2013;35:237–42.
25. Piacentino D, Longo L, Pavan A, Ferracuti S, Brugnoli R, Girardi P, et al. Body image and eating disorders are common in professional and amateur athletes using performance and image-enhancing drugs (pieds). A cross-sectional study. Eur Psychiatry. 2017;49:373–84.
26. McDonald AH, Pritchard M, McGuire MK. Self-reported eating disorder risk in lean and non-lean NCAA Collegiate Athletes. Eat Weight Disord. 2020;25:745–50.
27. Gorrell S, Nagata JM, Hill KB, Carlson JL, Shain AF, Wilson J, et al. Eating behavior and reasons for exercise among competitive collegiate male athletes. Eat Weight Disord [Internet]. 2019;(0123456789). Available from: http://www.ncbi.nlm.nih.gov/pubmed/31782028.
28. Compte EJ, Murray SB, Sepúlveda AR, Schweiger S, Bressan M, Torrente F. What position do you play? Eating disorder pathology among rugby players, and the understudied role of player position. Int J Eat Disord. 2018;51:1015–9.

29. Chapman J, Woodman T. Disordered eating in male athletes: a meta-analysis. J Sports Sci. 2016;34:101–9.
30. Thompson RA, Sherman R. Reflections on athletes and eating disorders. Psychol Sport Exerc. 2014;15:729–34.
31. Bonci CM, Bonci LJ, Granger LR, Johnson CL, Malina RM, Milne LW, et al. National athletic trainers' association position statement: preventing, detecting, and managing disordered eating in athletes. J Athl Train. 2008;43:80–108.
32. Joy E, Kussman A, Nattiv A. 2016 update on eating disorders in athletes: a comprehensive narrative review with a focus on clinical assessment and management. Br J Sports Med. 2016;50:154–62.
33. Allegre B, Souville M, Therme P, Griffiths M. Definitions and measures of exercise dependence. Addict Res Theory. 2006;14:631–46.
34. Davies RR. The treatment of compulsive physical activity in anorexia nervosa lacks a conceptual base. Adv Eat Disord. 2015;3:103–12.
35. Touyz S, Hay P, Noetel M. Is the neglect of exercise in anorexia nervosa research a case of "running out" of ideas or do we need to take a "LEAP" of faith into the future? J Eat Disord. 2017;35:1–3.
36. Szabo A, Griffiths MD, de La Vega Marcos R, Mervó B, Demetrovics Z. Methodological and conceptual limitations in exercise addiction research. Yale J Biol Med. 2015;88:303–8.
37. Mond JM, Hay PJ, Rodgers B, Owen C. Eating disorder examination questionnaire (EDE-Q): norms for young adult women. Behav Res Ther. 2006;44:53–62.
38. Solenberger SE. Exercise and eating disorders. Eat Behav. 2001;2:151–68.
39. Carter JC, Blackmore E, Sutandar-Pinnock K, Woodside DB. Relapse in anorexia nervosa: a survival analysis. Psychol Med. 2004;34:671–9.
40. Plateau CR, Shanmugam V, Duckham RL, Goodwin H, Jowett S, Brooke-Wavell KSF, et al. Use of the compulsive exercise test with athletes: norms and links with eating psychopathology. J Appl Sport Psychol. 2014;26:287–301.
41. Cabrita T, Rosado A, De La Vega R, Serpa S. Athletic identity and athlete characteristics as predictor of exercise dependence. Rev Psicol del Deport. 2017;27:99–106.
42. Gapin JI, Petruzzello SJ. Athletic identity and disordered eating in obligatory and non-obligatory runners. J Sports Sci. 2011;29:1001–10.
43. Turton R, Goodwin H, Meyer C. Athletic identity, compulsive exercise and eating psychopathology in long-distance runners. Eat Behav. 2017;26:129–32.
44. Guidi J, Pender M, Hollon SD, Zisook S, Schwartz FH, Pedrelli P, et al. The prevalence of compulsive eating and exercise among college students: an exploratory study. Psychiatry Res. 2009;165:154–62.
45. Murray SB, Rieger E, Touyz SW. Muscle dysmorphia symptomatology during a period of religious fasting: a case report. Eur Eat Disord Rev. 2011;19:162–8.
46. Fredrickson BL, Roberts TA. Toward understanding women's lived experiences and mental health risks. Psychol Women Q. 1997;21:173–206.
47. Pope HG, Olivardia R, Borowiecki JJ, Cohane GH. The growing commercial value of the male body: a longitudinal survey of advertising in women's magazines. Psychother Psychosom. 2001;70:189–92.
48. Martins Y, Tiggemann M, Kirkbride A. Those speedos become them: the role of self-objectification in gay and heterosexual men's body image. Pers Soc Psychol Bull. 2007;33:634–47.
49. Morry MM, Staska SL. Magazine exposure: internalization, self-objectification, eating attitudes, and body satisfaction in male and female university students. Can J Behav Sci. 2001;33:269–79.
50. Thompson JK, Cafri G. The muscular ideal: Psychological, social, and medical perspectives. Washington, DC: Springer. 2007.

51. Tiggemann M, Kuring JK. The role of body objectification in disordered eating and depressed mood. Br J Clin Psychol. 2004;43:299–311.
52. Calogero RM. Objectification processes and disordered eating in british women and men. J Health Psychol. 2009;14(3):394–402.
53. Strelan P, Hargreaves D. Reasons for exercise and body esteem: men's responses to self-objectification. Sex Roles. 2005;53:495–503.
54. Grieve R, Helmick A. The influence of men's self-objectification on the drive for muscularity: self-esteem, body satisfaction and muscle dysmorphia. Int J Mens Health. 2008;7:288–98.
55. Parent MC, Moradi B. An abbreviated tool for assessing conformity to masculine norms: psychometric properties of the conformity to masculine norms inventory-46. Psychol Men Masculinity. 2011;12:339–53.
56. Hallsworth L, Wade T, Tiggemann M. Individual differences in male body-image: an examination of self-objectification in recreational body builders. Br J Health Psychol. 2005;10:453–65.
57. Piran N, Teall T. The developmental theory of embodiment. In: Preventing eating-related and weight-related disorders: collaborative research, advocacy, and policy change. Waterloo: Wilfred Laurier Press; 2012.
58. Galli N, Reel J, Petrie T, Greenleaf C, Carter J. Preliminary development of the weight pressures in sport scale for male athletes. J Sport Behav. 2011;34:47–68.
59. de Sousa Fortes L, Ferreira MEC, de Oliveira SMF, Cyrino ES, Almeida SS. A socio-sports model of disordered eating among Brazilian male athletes. Appetite. 2015;92:29–35.
60. Stoyel H, Slee A, Meyer C, Serpell L. Systematic review of risk factors for eating psychopathology in athletes: a critique of an etiological model. Eur Eat Disord Rev [Internet]. 2019;(May):3–25. Available from: http://www.ncbi.nlm.nih.gov/pubmed/31793151.
61. Fairburn CG, Cooper Z, Shafran R. Cognitive behaviour therapy for eating disorders: a "transdiagnostic" theory and treatment. Behav Res Ther. 2003;41:509–28.
62. Shanmugam V, Jowett S, Meyer C. Eating psychopathology amongst athletes: links to current attachment styles. Eat Behav. 2012;13:5–12.
63. Pennesi JL, Wade TD. A systematic review of the existing models of disordered eating: do they inform the development of effective interventions? Clin Psychol Rev. 2016;43:175–92.
64. Mountjoy M, Sundgot-Borgen J, Burke L, Carter S, Constantini N, Lebrun C, et al. The IOC consensus statement: beyond the Female Athlete Triad-Relative Energy Deficiency in Sport (RED-S). Br J Sports Med. 2014;48(7):491–7.
65. Mountjoy M, Sundgot-Borgen JK, Burke LM, Ackerman KE, Blauwet C, Constantini N, et al. IOC consensus statement on relative energy deficiency in sport (RED-S): 2018 update. Br J Sports Med. 2018;52(11):687–97.
66. Tenforde AS, Barrack MT, Nattiv A, Fredericson M. Parallels with the female athlete triad in male athletes. Sports Med. 2016;46:171–82.
67. Torstveit MK, Fahrenholtz IL, Lichtenstein MB, Stenqvist TB, Melin AK. Exercise dependence, eating disorder symptoms and biomarkers of Relative Energy Deficiency in Sports (RED-S) among male endurance athletes. BMJ Open Sport Exerc Med. 2019;5:1–8.
68. Gull WW. Anorexia nervosa (apepsia hysterica, anorexia hysterica). 1868. Obes Res. 1997;5:498–502.
69. Davis C, Fox J. Excessive exercise and weight preoccupation in women. Addict Behav. 1993;18:201–11.
70. Adkins EC, Keel PK. Does "excessive" or "compulsive" best describe exercise as a symptom of bulimia nervosa? Int J Eat Disord. 2005;38:24–9.
71. Mond JM, Calogero RM. Excessive exercise in eating disorder patients and in healthy women. Aust N Z J Psychiatry. 2009;43:227–34.
72. Seigel K, Hetta J. Exercise and eating disorder symptoms among young females. Eat Weight Disord. 2001;6:32–9.
73. Cook B, Hausenblas H, Freimuth M. Exercise addiction and compulsive exercising: relationship to eating disorders, substance use disorders, and addictive disorders. In: Eating disor-

ders, addictions and substance use disorders: research, clinical and treatment perspectives. New York: Springer; 2014.
74. Dittmer N, Voderholzer U, von der Mühlen M, Marwitz M, Fumi M, Mönch C, et al. Specialized group intervention for compulsive exercise in inpatients with eating disorders: feasibility and preliminary outcomes. J Eat Disord. 2018;6:27.
75. Adams J, Kirkby RJ. Excessive exercise as an addiction: a review. Addict Res Theory. 2002;10:415–37.
76. Bamber DJ, Cockerill IM, Rodgers S, Carroll D. Diagnostic criteria for exercise dependence in women. Br J Sports Med. 2003;37:393–400.
77. Bratland-Sanda S, Martinsen EW, Rosenvinge JH, Rã Ã, Hoffart A, Sundgot-Borgen J. Exercise dependence score in patients with longstanding eating disorders and controls: the importance of affect regulation and physical activity intensity. Eur Eat Disord Rev. 2011;19:249–55.
78. Cook B, Hausenblas H, Tuccitto D, Giacobbi PR. Eating disorders and exercise: a structural equation modelling analysis of a conceptual model. Eur Eat Disord Rev. 2011;19:216–25.
79. Hausenblas HA, Downs DS. Exercise dependence: a systematic review. Psychol Sport Exerc. 2002;3:89–123.
80. Pasman L, Thompson JK. Body image and eating disturbance in obligatory runners, obligatory weightlifters, and sedentary individuals. Int J Eat Disord. 1988;7:P759–69.
81. Darcy AM, Doyle AC, Lock J, Peebles R, Doyle P, Le Grange D. The eating disorders examination in adolescent males with anorexia nervosa: how does it compare to adolescent females? Int J Eat Disord. 2012;45:110–4.
82. Matheson H, Crawford-Wright A. An examination of eating disorder profiles in student obligatory and non-obligatory exercisers. J Sport Behav. 2000;23:42–50.
83. Chalk HM, Miller SE, Roach ME, Schultheis KS. Predictors of obligatory exercise among undergraduates: differential implications for counseling college men and women. J Coll Couns. 2013;16:102–14.
84. Taranis L, Touyz S, Meyer C. Disordered eating and exercise: development and preliminary validation of the compulsive exercise test (CET). Eur Eat Disord Rev. 2011;19:256–68.
85. Goodwin H, Haycraft E, Taranis L, Meyer C. Psychometric evaluation of the compulsive exercise test (CET) in an adolescent population: links with eating psychopathology. Eur Eat Disord Rev. 2011;19:269–79.
86. Hausenblas HA, Fallon EA. Relationship among body image, exercise behavior, and exercise dependence symptoms. Int J Eat Disord. 2002;32:179–85.
87. Terry A, Szabo A, Griffiths M. The exercise addiction inventory: a new brief screening tool. Addict Res Theory. 2004;12:489–99.
88. Griffiths MD, Urbán R, Demetrovics Z, Lichtenstein MB, de la Vega R, Kun B, et al. A cross-cultural re-evaluation of the Exercise Addiction Inventory (EAI) in five countries. Sport Med Open. 2015;1:5.
89. Lichtenstein MB, Griffiths MD, Hemmingsen SD, Støving RK. Exercise addiction in adolescents and emerging adults - validation of a youth version of the Exercise Addiction Inventory. J Behav Addict. 2018;7:117–25.
90. McNulty KY, Adams CH, Anderson JM, Affenito SG. Development and validation of a screening tool to identify eating disorders in female athletes. J Am Diet Assoc. 2001;101:886–92.
91. Gallagher KA, Sonneville KR, Hazzard VM, Carson TL, Needham BL. Evaluating gender bias in an eating disorder risk assessment questionnaire for athletes. Eat Disord. 2019;29:29–41.
92. Chapa DAN, Hagan KE, Forbush KT, Perko VL, Sorokina DA, Alasmar AY, et al. The Athletes' Relationships with Training scale (ART): a self-report measure of unhealthy training behaviors associated with eating disorders. Int J Eat Disord. 2018;51:1080–9.
93. Murray SB, Maguire S, Russell J, Touyz SW. The emotional regulatory features of bulimic episodes and compulsive exercise in muscle dysmorphia: a case report. Eur Eat Disord Rev. 2012;20:68–73.

94. Lavender JM, Brown TA, Murray SB. Men, muscles, and eating disorders: an overview of traditional and muscularity-oriented disordered eating. Curr Psychiatry Rep. 2017;19:32.
95. Murray SB, Rieger E, Touyz SW, García YDLG. Muscle dysmorphia and the DSM-V conundrum: where does it belong? A review paper. Int J Eat Disord. 2010;43:483–91.
96. Murray SB, Brown TA, Blashill AJ, Compte EJ, Lavender JM, Mitchison D, et al. The development and validation of the muscularity-oriented eating test: a novel measure of muscularity-oriented disordered eating. Int J Eat Disord. 2019;52:1389–98.
97. Boroughs M, Thompson JK. Exercise status and sexual orientation as moderators of body image disturbance and eating disorders in males. Int J Eat Disord. 2002;31:307–11.
98. Bar RJ, Cassin SE, Dionne MM. Eating disorder prevention initiatives for athletes: a review. Eur J Sport Sci. 2016;16:325–35.
99. Martinsen M, Bahr R, BØrresen R, Holme I, Pensgaard AM, Sundgot-Borgen J. Preventing eating disorders among young elite athletes: a randomized controlled trial. Med Sci Sports Exerc. 2014;46:435–47.
100. Torres-McGehee TM, Pritchett KL, Zippel D, Minton DM, Cellamare A, Sibilia M. Sports nutrition knowledge among collegiate athletes, coaches, athletic trainers, and strength and conditioning specialists. J Athl Train. 2012;47:205–11.
101. Elliot DL, Goldberg L, Moe EL, DeFrancesco CA, Durham MB, McGinnis W, Lockwood C. Long-term outcomes of the ATHENA program for female high school athletes. J Alcohol Drug Educ. 2008;52:73–92.
102. Elliot DL, Goldberg L, Moe EL, Defrancesco CA, Durham MB, Hix-Small H. Preventing substance use and disordered eating: initial outcomes of the ATHENA (Athletes Targeting Healthy Exercise and Nutrition Alternatives) program. Arch Pediatr Adolesc Med. 2004;158:1043–9.
103. Yager Z, McLean SA, Li X. Body image outcomes in a replication of the ATLAS program in Australia. Psychol Men Masculinity. 2019;20:418–28.
104. Goldberg L, Elliot D, Clarke GN, MacKinnon DP, Moe E, Zoref L, et al. Effects of a multidimensional anabolic steroid prevention intervention: the adolescents training and learning to avoid steroids (ATLAS) program. JAMA. 1996;276:1555–62.
105. Smith A, Petrie T. Reducing the risk of disordered eating among female athletes: a test of alternative interventions. J Appl Sport Psychol. 2008;20:392–407.
106. Becker CB, McDaniel L, Bull S, Powell M, McIntyre K. Can we reduce eating disorder risk factors in female college athletes? A randomized exploratory investigation of two peer-led interventions. Body Image. 2012;9:31–42.
107. Buchholz A, Mack H, McVey G, Feder S, Barrowman N. BodySense: an evaluation of a positive body image intervention on sport climate for female athletes. Eat Disord. 2008;16:308–21.
108. Doyle-Lucas AF, Davy BM. Development and evaluation of an educational intervention program for pre-professional adolescent ballet dancers: nutrition for optimal performance. J Dance Med Sci. 2011;15:65–75.
109. Mond J, Mitchison D, Hay P. Eating disordered behavior in men: prevalence, impairment in quality of life, and implications for prevention and health promotion. In: Current findings on males with eating disorders. New York: Routledge/Taylor & Francis Group; 2013.
110. Stranberg M, Slager E, Spital D, Coia C, Quatromoni PA. Athlete-specific treatment for eating disorders: initial findings from the Walden GOALS program. J Acad Nutr Diet. 2020;120:183–92.
111. Conviser JH, Tierney AS, Nickols R. Assessment of athletes with eating disorders: essentials for best practice. J Clin Sport Psychol. 2018;12:1–26.
112. Glazer JL. Eating disorders among male athletes. Curr Sports Med Rep. 2008;7:332–7.
113. Hausenblas HA, Cook BJ, Chittester NI. Can exercise treat eating disorders? Exerc Sport Sci Rev. 2008;36:43–7.
114. Cook BJ, Wonderlich SA, Mitchell JE, Thompson R, Sherman R, McCallum K. Exercise in eating disorders treatment: systematic review and proposal of guidelines. Med Sci Sports Exerc. 2016;48:1408–14.

115. Schlegel S, Hartmann A, Fuchs R, Zeeck A. The Freiburg sport therapy program for eating disordered outpatients: a pilot study. Eat Weight Disord. 2015;20:319–27.
116. Hay P, Touyz S, Arcelus J, Pike K, Attia E, Crosby RD, et al. A randomized controlled trial of the compuLsive Exercise Activity TheraPy (LEAP): a new approach to compulsive exercise in anorexia nervosa. Int J Eat Disord. 2018;51(8):999–1004.
117. Fewell LK, Nickols R, Schlitzer Tierney A, Levinson CA. Eating disorders in sport: comparing eating disorder symptomatology in athletes and non-athletes during intensive eating disorder treatment. J Clin Sport Psychol. 2018;12:1–28.
118. Conviser JH, Schlitzer Tierney A, Nickols R. Essentials for best practice: treatment approaches for athletes with eating disorders. J Clin Sport Psychol. 2018;12:1–23.

Chapter 20
Social Media and Eating and Body Image Concerns Among Men and Boys

Alexandra Rhodes Lonergan, Deborah Mitchison, Kay Bussey, and Jasmine Fardouly

Learning Objectives

1. Identify differences in social networking sites (SNS) appearance-based behaviors among boys and men compared to girls and women.
2. Identify relationships between SNS, body image, and eating disorders among boys and men, including which platforms and/or behaviors may be more damaging.
3. Discuss the role of social comparison in mediating the relationship between SNS, body image, and eating disorders among boys and men.
4. Identify avenues for future research, clinical implications, and eating disorder/SNS interventions for men and boys.

Key Points

- Studies examining the relationship between social networking sites (SNS) and eating and body image concerns in boys and men are limited. Existing research has extended findings from populations of girls and women to identify both common and distinct features of maladaptive SNS use among boys and men. Evidence suggests that across age and cultural groups, boys and men participate in appearance-based SNS behaviors, such as posting "selfies."

A. R. Lonergan · K. Bussey · J. Fardouly
Centre for Emotional Health, Department of Psychology, Macquarie University, Sydney, NSW, Australia
e-mail: alexandra.lonergan@mq.edu.au; kay.bussey@mq.edu.au; jasmine.fardouly@mq.edu.au

D. Mitchison (✉)
Centre for Emotional Health, Department of Psychology, Macquarie University, Sydney, NSW, Australia

Translational Health Research Institute, School of Medicine, Western Sydney University, Sydney, NSW, Australia
e-mail: deborah.mitchison@westernsydney.edu.au

J. M. Nagata et al. (eds.), *Eating Disorders in Boys and Men*,
https://doi.org/10.1007/978-3-030-67127-3_20

- Maladaptive gendered stereotypes that promote a lean and muscular physique are widespread on photo-based SNS, such as Instagram. Boys and men who internalize "masculine" bodily ideals may be vulnerable to the pressures to adapt images shared on photo-based SNS.
- Photo-based SNS provide ample opportunity for social comparison. Outcomes of appearance comparisons to others' selfies may motivate exercise and dietary behaviors that contribute to eating disorders.
- Social media literacy interventions are required to educate boys and men about hypermasculine appearance norms that may be expressed in pro-muscularity selfies and related online content. Practitioners may consider how SNS behaviors may reflect markers of eating disorders and muscle dysmorphia among boys and men.

Social Media Use Among Men and Boys

Social networking sites (SNS), such as YouTube, Facebook, Instagram, and TikTok, are globally popular forms of contemporary online communication [1]. SNS enables users to create, share, and directly participate in online content with individuals and organizations within their networks. These may include celebrities, peers, family members, businesses, and other organizations. Applications, such as Tinder, Grindr, and Bumble, are SNS with the primary purpose of connecting users that are interested in romantic relationships, casual sex, or friendship. As opposed to traditional forms of media, participation in SNS is immediate, highly interactive, targeted toward individual users, and able to be accessed on a frequent basis, particularly via smartphones. Frequency statistics from the United States indicates that adolescents are the most active SNS users, particularly regarding "photo-based" platforms, such as Instagram and Snapchat [2]. The primary function of photo-based SNS is for users to post and share videos and images, often in the form of "selfies" (photos of oneself taken by oneself). Selfies are inherently "active," appearance-focused SNS behaviors, as taking, editing, and posting selfies, as well as scrutinizing responses to such images, require greater cognitive effort toward one's appearance than passively browsing a newsfeed or user profile [3]. Across genders, men are more likely to use YouTube and Twitter, while women are more likely to use photo-based SNS, including Facebook and Instagram [4]. While adults of all ages use SNS, engagement appears to decrease across older generations. Nine out of ten young adults, aged 23–38 years, use some form of SNS, while 76% and 59% of adults aged 39–54 and 55–73 years, respectively, use SNS [4]. SNS have positive functions, such as sharing and increasing information, communication, and technological skills across social groups otherwise separated by geographic location. However, it may also be a risk factor for negative outcomes, such as eating psychopathology for men and women [5–7].

Gendered SNS behaviors have been investigated in relation to motivations underlying SNS use. Men tend to take and post fewer selfies than women [8], suggesting that it may be less gender-normative for men to post selfies on SNS. Rather, men appear to be motivated to gain general knowledge and information, such as through YouTube videos, possibly to enhance their position within online and "offline" networks [9]. Table 20.1 provides an overview of the five most popular SNS among men in the United States at the time of writing. As shown in Table 20.1, most studies that have examined the relationship between SNS and eating and body image concerns have focused on photo-based SNS (e.g., Instgram and Facebook). Research attention toward photo-based SNS reflects an extension of studies traditionally conducted with populations of girls and women, whereby active, photo-based SNS behaviors have been related to eating and body image concerns (e.g., [10, 11, 12, 13, 14, 15]). Among men who post selfies, content analyses suggested that men post full-body photos, while women use portrait photos [16]. Men's physiques may therefore be an important aspect of self-presentation on social media. This is consistent with findings that suggest men edit and post selfies to SNS to cultivate their "best" appearance for external validation [17]. Moreover, personality traits such as narcissism have been more strongly related to frequency of posting selfies among men compared to women [18].

Gendered preferences in SNS use and distinct forms of self-presentation may be conceptualized via a self-construction model [38], whereby innate differences, in conjunction with socialized gender-normative views and expectations, contribute to different self-construal behaviors for men and women. In investigating SNS behaviors in men and boys, celebrities and peers may provide a "blueprint" for appropriate SNS etiquette and self-presentation. While men may not strive for thinness in the same way that women do [39], they are concerned with muscularity enhancement and experience body image and eating disturbances related to this preoccupation [31]. Gender stereotypes that promote a lean and muscular physique are widespread on photo-based SNS [34]. Incidental browsing, sharing images, and searching for and/or using specific hashtag terms (e.g., "#bulking") ultimately increase engagement with such stereotypes due to algorithmic targeting across social media platforms [32]. Accordingly, men who explore stereotypical male bodily ideals and eating behaviors required to attain such an ideal may

Table 20.1 Studies across the popular social networking sites used by men

Social media site	Primary media used	List of citations
YouTube	Videos	[19, 20, 21, 22]
Facebook	Photos, videos, messaging, news, advertising	[5, 6, 7, 15, 16, 17, 18, 20, 21, 22, 23, 24, 25, 26, 27, 28, 29]
Snapchat	Photos	[5, 7, 15, 17, 18, 20, 23, 24, 26, 27, 28, 30]
Twitter	Short text messages limited to a number of characters	[21, 22, 26, 31, 32, 33]
Instagram	Photos, videos	[5, 6, 7, 8, 12, 15, 17, 18, 20, 22, 23, 24, 26, 27, 28, 29, 34, 35, 36, 37]

Note: The five most popular social networking sites are listed in descending order according to percentage of men who endorsed using them in the United States in 2018 [1]

be exposed to ever increasingly similar content across multiple SNS. Given the pervasive use of SNS among men of different ages and nationalities, it is important to determine which specific social media behaviors, as well as which mediating factors, pose the greatest risk for eating psychopathology. As with eating disorder literature in general, investigation into the relationship between SNS and eating psychopathology among men is limited. This may be attributed to female-focused conceptualizations of eating disorders, research attention toward the thin ideal as opposed to muscularity concerns, and sampling bias toward women [40]. Exploring the nuanced relationships between SNS and eating disorders among men is therefore important to elucidate the role of potentially damaging online behaviors.

Social Networking Sites and Eating Disorder/Body Image Outcomes Within a Sociocultural Theoretical Context

From a sociocultural framework, exposure to physical bodily ideals via the media is a key precipitant in the development of body dissatisfaction among men and women [19, 41]. As outlined in Chap. 2, the "tripartite" dual pathway model of body image and disordered eating has been revised to account for men's engagement in muscularity enhancement and disordered eating [42]. Specifically, men who experience high internalization of contemporary "masculine" body ideals and are dissatisfied with their muscularity and body fat may be more vulnerable to the pressures of media images. SNS may have stronger associations with body dissatisfaction than traditional media, as it is more interactive and self-exposing, allows for greater peer-to-peer scrutiny, and can be accessed on a frequent basis, particularly via smartphones [15]. However, a meta-analysis of correlational research has suggested that the effect of SNS use on body image is similar to traditional media [23]. Given the pervasive use of smartphones, SNS may provide ample opportunities for comparison of men's bodies against the lean and muscular ideal, which may result in muscularity and body fat dissatisfaction in relation to unrealistic sociocultural norms.

Research on pro-muscularity websites show evidence of SNS-endorsed maladaptive eating behaviors and drive for muscularity, which may contribute to eating disorders in men [31]. These include rigid dietary and exercise practices, emphasis on muscularity and body size, and minimization of health risks associated with muscularity enhancement [31]. Examination of maladaptive pro-muscularity behaviors on SNS with the hashtag "#cheatmeal" (i.e., a single meal that deviates from dietary rules) suggested that more than one half of images promoted energy-dense food to be eaten in large quantities, which may promote objective binge episodes [6]. Moreover, images that contained individuals often portrayed highly muscular bodies and intentional body exposure, suggesting both promotion of unrealistic bodily ideals and overeating and/or binge behaviors [6].

Appearance-Based Social Networking Site Behaviors

More explicit photo-based behaviors on SNS, rather than overall time spent on SNS, has been related to body dissatisfaction among men and women and boys and girls [5, 24, 25, 43]. SNS that are associated with eating disorder behaviors also include those that are primarily photo-based [5, 6]. Photo-based SNS behaviors include the use of appearance-related features, such as posting selfies and editing selfies to improve bodily appearance prior to posting images on social media, such as reshaping legs [14], and investment in selfies, that is, effort expended in choosing selfies and monitoring comments and Likes to posted images [15]. Beyond posting selfies, photo-based SNS may also include engagement with others' selfies, such as scrutinizing images posted by peers and monitoring comments and Likes on others' selfies. Accordingly, even if users do not take or post selfies, engagement with others' selfies may be related to features of eating psychopathology, such as appearance comparison. Emerging research supports this notion, as young women who reported greater engagement with others' selfies also reported greater social comparison [13]. Similar research is yet to be conducted with young men, although a similar pattern would be expected.

In correlational studies (i.e., examination of the relationship between SNS use and eating behaviors at one point in time), which included both men and women, SNS use in general has been related to eating disorder concerns and symptomology across genders for Western [20], Lebanese [33], and Singaporean-Chinese [35] samples. This relationship between photo-based SNS and eating disorder symptoms has been identified among sexual minority men [35]. There also appears to be increasing prevalence of muscularity-oriented selfies among men [6]. Smartphone photo-editing applications such as "Manly" have been developed specifically for men, whereby users may alter their appearance, such as increasing muscle mass (e.g., enhancing a "six-pack"). Such applications emphasize hypermasculine appearance norms, such as physical strength, which may contribute to body image concerns and disordered eating in boys and men. While limited research has examined social media use and body dissatisfaction in male cohorts [44], men appear to be similarly susceptible to the effects of photo-based SNS on body dissatisfaction [25, 26, 29]. In terms of the directionality of the relationship between body dissatisfaction and SNS, longitudinal findings with boys suggest that frequent SNS use predicts body dissatisfaction [25]. Further, editing but not posting selfies to SNS has been found to predict higher levels of face and body appearance concerns over a 6-month period among Chinese boys [27]. Such longitudinal findings are critical in establishing the causal relationships between SNS use and eating psychopathology.

In terms of disordered eating, in the only study examining SNS use in boys with an eating disorder to date, it was found that compared to healthy peers, adolescent boys who meet criteria for an eating disorder have been found to report greater avoidance of posting selfies, photo investment, photo manipulation, and investment in others' selfies [28]. The same study found that adolescent boys who reported greater avoidance of posting selfies were more likely than adolescent girls to meet criteria for clinical and subclinical anorexia nervosa [28]. Avoidance of posting selfies may reflect "offline" body avoidance typically observed in eating disorders [45, 46]. Boys who meet criteria for clinical and subclinical anorexia nervosa may purposefully avoid presenting themselves on SNS, possibly due to the inconsistency between pervasive muscularity ideals and their own muscularity.

The Role of Social Comparison in the Relationship Between Social Networking Sites and Eating Psychopathology

Festinger's [47] model of social comparison proposed that individuals have an innate drive to determine their progress and standing on different aspects of their lives and evaluate themselves against others when more objective points of comparison are unavailable. SNS are a pivotal environment for social comparison as users can compare their appearance to celebrities, peers, and other users within their networks and make comparisons on the basis of the image posted. Users may also compare number of "Likes" and comments that others receive [24, 48]. Upward social comparisons, whereby individuals compare themselves to others who are perceived to be better than themselves, are relevant to the experience and expression of eating disorders in a SNS context. Specifically, users may may compare themselves to others' posted images perceived to be superior according to certain criteria, such as physical attractiveness, weight and shape, and adherence to dietary rules. Research with women has found that upward appearance comparisons through social media were associated with greater body dissatisfaction and more thoughts of dieting and exercising to lose weight than when no comparisons were made [11]. Of the limited research pertaining to men, men who viewed more fitspiration content on social media reported greater internalization of muscular bodily ideals and appearance comparison, which, in turn, was associated with lower body satisfaction and exercise motivation based on appearance as opposed to health [34]. Further highlighting the role of appearance comparison, experimental research with men showed that upward social comparisons with attractive models on social media strengthened motivation for self-improvement in terms of physical activity [36].

Specific to eating disorders, pro-anorexia nervosa and pro-bulimia nervosa Instagram SNS accounts have been identified as "inspiration" for those striving to lose weight, where (mostly girls/women) users post idealized images of thin bodies and their own "progress" selfies [12]. Instagram has banned search terms such as "thinspiration" to limit access to pro-eating disorder accounts [37]. On the other hand, terms such as "fitspiration" and "clean eating," which reflect bodily ideals for a lean and toned physique, as well as dietary rules required to achieve such a physique [21], have become normalized on photo-based SNS. Terms such as "fitspiration" may be more relevant to the male experience of drive for muscularity, muscle dysphoria, and eating psychopathology. However, such terms and accounts have not been monitored to the same extent as their "thinspiration" counterparts. This may be due to "fitspiration" accounts purporting to encourage a "healthy" lifestyle. Research among populations of girls and women has identified a relationship between exposure to fitspiration content and body dissatisfaction [49, 50, 51] and that appearance comparison mediated the relationship between fitspiration and symptom severity in eating disorder samples [29]. However, over one third of fitspiration content on Instagram features images of just men [22], and men are exposed to a greater amount of fitspiration than thinspiration content [30]. Fewer studies have examined the relationship between exposure to "fitspiration" and "clean eating" content and disordered eating in samples of boys or men. This is a notable omission, as exposure to "fitspiration" content may provide an avenue for social and/or appearance comparison and increased body dissatisfaction that may contribute to body image disorders among men and boys.

Future Directions

Primarily, greater research attention toward the male experience of eating and body image concerns in an online setting is required. Experimental and longitudinal studies are particularly required to confirm causality and inform evidence-based treatment and intervention programs. Photo-based SNS literacy interventions that have been successfully applied to girls and women, for example, to reduce dietary restraint in adolescents [52] may be adapted for boys and men. Such interventions may involve having adolescent boys critique the use of apps, such as "Manly," that are designed specifically for male users. As with samples of girls or women [10], identification of problematic behaviors, such as particular interest in taking and editing selfies, and excessive monitoring of Likes/comments may be addressed in relation to body image concerns relevant to male users, such as muscularity enhancement. Other relevant targets may include high levels of social comparison to muscular and lean bodily ideals seen on SNS and following and/or seeking fitspiration and related content.

From a clinical perspective, the role of social media may be considered in the current transdiagnostic model of eating disorders, whereby SNS behaviors may reflect "offline" indicators of eating disorders and muscle dysmorphia. Body checking (i.e., compulsive scrutiny of perceived appearance flaws or areas of overvaluation) and avoidance (e.g., avoiding one's reflection) are prominent eating disorder maintaining factors [45] that may extend in online contexts through obsessive monitoring and selection of selfies or avoidance of posting selfies (and "un-tagging"). Further, monitoring of "Likes"/comments on uploaded selfies may be an online manifestation of reassurance-seeking [10]. Finally, compulsive appearance-fixing and camouflaging are also maintaining factors in the drive for muscularity and associated muscularity-driven behaviors. This approach would assist assessment of the role of social media in maintaining eating disordered behaviors among boys and men. Both social and clinical interventions may target mental health literacy in general to distinguish "healthy" and maladaptive eating behaviors related to drive for muscularity (e.g., overconsumption accompanied by driven exercise).

Conclusion

Across cultures and age groups, boys and men are as at risk as girls and women in developing body image concerns and eating disorder symptoms through SNS use. Photo-based SNS, such as Instagram, and appearance-based behaviors, including editing and posting selfies, are relevant avenues for the development and/or maintenance of eating disorders among men and boys. Those who engage in social comparison may be particularly at risk, as exposure to muscularity-related content, such as "fitspiration," may increase body dissatisfaction that leads to eating psychopathology. Maladaptive SNS behaviors relevant to boys and men have received less focus compared to SNS content that promotes anorexia- and bulimia nervosa-type behavior in girls and women. Current interventions may therefore be adapted to better target eating and body image concerns as they more typically present in boys and men. In eating disorder settings, clinicians may also assess and intervene with how men and boys engage with SNS, particularly in relation to appearance-based behaviors that maintain symptomology.

References

1. Perrin A, Anderson M. Share of U.S. adults using social media, including Facebook, is mostly unchanged since 2018 Pew Research Centre Pew Research Centre 2019. Available from: https://www.pewresearch.org/fact-tank/2019/04/10/share-of-u-s-adults-using-social-media-including-facebook-is-mostly-unchanged-since-2018/.
2. Smith A, Anderson M. Social media use in 2018: A majority of Americans use Facebook and YouTube, but young adults are especially heavy users of Snapchat and Instagram Pew Research Centre Pew Research Centre 2018. Available from: https://www.pewresearch.org/internet/2018/03/01/social-media-use-in-2018/.
3. de Vries DA, Vossen HGM, van der Kolk-van der Boom P. Social media and body dissatisfaction: investigating the attenuating role of positive parent-adolescent relationships. J Youth Adolesc. 2019;48(3):527–36.
4. Vogels EA. Pew Research Centre Pew Research Centre 2019. Available from: https://www.pewresearch.org/internet/2018/03/01/social-media-use-in-2018/.
5. Cohen R, Newton-John T, Slater A. 'Selfie'-objectification: the role of selfies in self-objectification and disordered eating in young women. Comput Hum Behav. 2018;79:68–74.
6. Pila E, Mond JM, Griffiths S, Mitchison D, Murray SB. A thematic content analysis of #cheatmeal images on social media: characterizing an emerging dietary trend. Int J Eat Disord. 2017;50(6):698–706.
7. Smith AR, Hames JL, Joiner TE Jr. Status update: maladaptive Facebook usage predicts increases in body dissatisfaction and bulimic symptoms. J Affect Disord. 2013;149(1–3):235–40.
8. Wagner C, Aguirre E, Sumner EM. The relationship between Instagram selfies and body image in young adult women. First Monday. 2016;21(9). https://doi.org/10.5210/fm.v21i9.6390.
9. Krasnova H, Veltri NF, Eling N, Buxmann P. Why men and women continue to use social networking sites: the role of gender differences. J Strateg Inf Syst. 2017;26(4):261–84.
10. Chua THH, Chang L. Follow me and like my beautiful selfies: Singapore teenage girls' engagement in self-presentation and peer comparison on social media. Comput Hum Behav. 2016;55:190–7.

11. Fardouly J, Pinkus RT, Vartanian LR. The impact of appearance comparisons made through social media, traditional media, and in person in women's everyday lives. Body Image. 2017;20:31–9.
12. Ging D, Garvey S. 'Written in these scars are the stories I can't explain': a content analysis of pro-ana and thinspiration image sharing on Instagram. New Media Soc. 2017;20(3):1181–200.
13. Hogue JV, Mills JS. The effects of active social media engagement with peers on body image in young women. Body Image. 2019;28:1–5.
14. Kleemans M, Daalmans S, Carbaat I, Anschütz D. Picture perfect: the direct effect of manipulated instagram photos on body image in adolescent girls. Media Psychol. 2018;21(1):93–110.
15. McLean SA, Paxton SJ, Wertheim EH, Masters J. Photoshopping the selfie: self photo editing and photo investment are associated with body dissatisfaction in adolescent girls. Int J Eat Disord. 2015;48(8):1132–40.
16. Haferkamp N, Eimler SC, Papadakis AM, Kruck JV. Men are from Mars, women are from Venus? Examining gender differences in self-presentation on social networking sites. Cyberpsychol Behav Soc Netw. 2012;15(2):91–8.
17. Fox J, Vendemia MA. Selective self-presentation and social comparison through photographs on social networking sites. Cyberpsychol Behav Soc Netw. 2016;19(10):593–600.
18. Sorokowski P, Sorokowska A, Oleszkiewicz A, Frackowiak T, Huk A, Pisanski K. Selfie posting behaviors are associated with narcissism among men. Personal Individ Differ. 2015;85:123–7.
19. Ferguson CJ. In the eye of the beholder: thin-ideal media affects some, but not most, viewers in a meta-analytic review of body dissatisfaction in women and men. Psychol Pop Media Cult. 2013;2(1):20–37.
20. Sidani JE, Shensa A, Hoffman B, Hanmer J, Primack BA. The association between social media use and eating concerns among US young adults. J Acad Nutr Diet. 2016;116(9):1465–72.
21. Griffiths S, Murray SB, Krug I, McLean SA. The contribution of social media to body dissatisfaction, eating disorder symptoms, and anabolic steroid use among sexual minority men. Cyberpsychol Behav Soc Netw. 2018;21(3):149–56.
22. Carrotte ER, Prichard I, Lim MS. "Fitspiration" on social media: a content analysis of gendered images. J Med Internet Res. 2017;19(3):e95.
23. Saiphoo AN, Vahedi Z. A meta-analytic review of the relationship between social media use and body image disturbance. Comput Hum Behav. 2019;101:259–75.
24. Lonergan AR, Bussey K, Mond J, Brown O, Griffiths S, Murray SB, et al. Me, my selfie, and I: the relationship between editing and posting selfies and body dissatisfaction in men and women. Body Image. 2019;28:39–43.
25. de Vries DA, Peter J, de Graaf H, Nikken P. Adolescents' social network site use, peer appearance-related feedback, and body dissatisfaction: testing a mediation model. J Youth Adolesc. 2016;45(1):211–24.
26. Holland G, Tiggemann M. A systematic review of the impact of the use of social networking sites on body image and disordered eating outcomes. Body Image. 2016;17:100–10.
27. Wang Y, Xie X, Fardouly J, Vartanian LR, Lei L. The longitudinal and reciprocal relationships between selfie-related behaviors and self-objectification and appearance concerns among adolescents. New Media Soc. 2019;23(1):56–77.
28. Lonergan AR, Bussey K, Fardouly J, Griffiths S, Murray SB, Hay P, et al. Protect me from my selfie: examining the association between photo-based social media behaviors and self-reported eating disorders in adolescence. Int J Eat Disord. 2020;53(5):485–96.
29. Griffiths S, Castle D, Cunningham M, Murray SB, Bastian B, Barlow FK. How does exposure to thinspiration and fitspiration relate to symptom severity among individuals with eating disorders? Evaluation of a proposed model. Body Image. 2018;27:187–95.
30. Griffiths S, Stefanovski A. Thinspiration and fitspiration in everyday life: an experience sampling study. Body Image. 2019;30:135–44.
31. Murray SB, Griffiths S, Hazery L, Shen T, Wooldridge T, Mond JM. Go big or go home: a thematic content analysis of pro-muscularity websites. Body Image. 2016;16:17–20.
32. Aruguete N, Calvo E. Time to #protest: selective exposure, cascading activation, and framing in social media. J Commun. 2018;68(3):480–502.

33. Zeeni N, Doumit R, Abi Kharma J, Sanchez-Ruiz MJ. Media, technology use, and attitudes: associations with physical and mental well-being in youth with implications for evidence-based practice. Worldviews Evid-Based Nurs. 2018;15(4):304–12.
34. Fatt S, Fardouly J, Rapee R. #malefitspo: Links between viewing fitspiration posts, muscular-ideal internalisation, appearance comparisons, body satisfaction, and exercise motivation in men. New Media & Soc. 2019;21(6):1311–25.
35. Teo NSY, Collinson SL. Instagram and risk of rumination and eating disorders: an Asian perspective. Psychol Pop Media Cult. 2019;8(4):491–508.
36. Peng C-T, Wu T-Y, Chen Y, Atkin DJ. Comparing and modeling via social media: the social influences of fitspiration on male instagram users' work out intention. Comput Hum Behav. 2019;99:156–67.
37. Chancellor S, Pater JA, Clear T, Gilbert E, Choudhury MD. #thyghgapp: Instagram Content Moderation and Lexical Variation in Pro-Eating Disorder Communities. Proceedings of the 19th ACM Conference on Computer-Supported Cooperative Work & Social Computing. San Francisco: Association for Computing Machinery; 2016. p. 1201–13.
38. Cross SE, Madson L. Models of the self: self-construals and gender. Psychol Bull. 1997;122(1):5–37.
39. Strother E, Lemberg R, Stanford SC, Turberville D. Eating disorders in men: underdiagnosed, undertreated, and misunderstood. Eat Disord. 2012;20(5):346–55.
40. Murray SB, Nagata JM, Griffiths S, Calzo JP, Brown TA, Mitchison D, et al. The enigma of male eating disorders: a critical review and synthesis. Clin Psychol Rev. 2017;57:1–11.
41. Barlett CP, Vowels CL, Saucier DA. Meta-Analyses of the effects of media images on men's body-image concerns. J Soc Clin Psychol. 2008;27(3):279–310.
42. Tylka TL. Refinement of the tripartite influence model for men: dual body image pathways to body change behaviors. Body Image. 2011;8(3):199–207.
43. Mingoia J, Hutchinson AD, Wilson C, Gleaves DH. The relationship between social networking site use and the internalization of a thin ideal in females: a meta-analytic review. Front Psychol. 2017;8:1351.
44. Perloff RM. Social media effects on young Women's body image concerns: theoretical perspectives and an agenda for research. Sex Roles. 2014;71(11):363–77.
45. Fairburn CG, Cooper Z, Shafran R. Enhanced cognitive behavior therapy for eating disorders ("CBT-E"): an overview. Cognitive behavior therapy and eating disorders. New York: Guilford Press; 2008. p. 23–34.
46. Mitchison D, Crino R, Hay P. The presence, predictive utility, and clinical significance of body dysmorphic symptoms in women with eating disorders. J Eat Disord. 2013;1(1):20.
47. Festinger L. A theory of social comparison processes. Hum Relat. 1954;7(2):117–40.
48. Tiggemann M, Hayden S, Brown Z, Veldhuis J. The effect of Instagram "likes" on women's social comparison and body dissatisfaction. Body Image. 2018;26:90–7.
49. Prichard I, McLachlan AC, Lavis T, Tiggemann M. The impact of different forms of #fitspiration imagery on body image, mood, and self-objectification among young women. Sex Roles. 2017;78(11–12):789–98.
50. Robinson L, Prichard I, Nikolaidis A, Drummond C, Drummond M, Tiggemann M. Idealised media images: the effect of fitspiration imagery on body satisfaction and exercise behaviour. Body Image. 2017;22:65–71.
51. Tiggemann M, Zaccardo M. "Exercise to be fit, not skinny": the effect of fitspiration imagery on women's body image. Body Image. 2015;15:61–7.
52. McLean SA, Wertheim EH, Masters J, Paxton SJ. A pilot evaluation of a social media literacy intervention to reduce risk factors for eating disorders. Int J Eat Disord. 2017;50(7):847–51.

Chapter 21
Eating Disorders and Body Image Across the Lifespan: A Focus on Boys and Men in Midlife and Beyond

Tiffany A. Brown and Jason M. Lavender

Learning Objectives

1. Discuss body image attitudes and dissatisfaction among preadolescent and adolescent boys.
2. Describe the nature and prevalence of disordered eating and clinical eating disorders in preadolescent and adolescent boys.
3. Identify age-related changes in body image among men in midlife and beyond.
4. Explain the nature and prevalence of disordered eating and clinical eating disorders among men in midlife and beyond.

Key Points

- Attitudes about body sizes and body image begin to develop in early childhood, and boys exhibit positive perceptions about muscularity and socioculturally prescribed ideal body sizes.
- Attitudes and behaviors consistent with traditional eating disorders or those associated with muscularity and/or leanness concerns can emerge in younger boys, and adolescence is a time of elevated risk for symptom onset or exacerbation.

T. A. Brown (✉)
Department of Psychiatry, University of California, San Diego, San Diego, CA, USA

San Diego State University Research Foundation, San Diego, CA, USA
e-mail: tiffanybrown@ucsd.edu

J. M. Lavender (✉)
Department of Medicine, Military Cardiovascular Outcomes Research (MiCOR) Program, Uniformed Services University of the Health Sciences, Bethesda, MD, USA

The Metis Foundation, San Antonio, TX, USA
e-mail: jason.lavender.ctr@usuhs.edu

J. M. Nagata et al. (eds.), *Eating Disorders in Boys and Men*,
https://doi.org/10.1007/978-3-030-67127-3_21

- Men continue to experience body image concerns into midlife, including concerns regarding age-related weight gain and muscle loss.
- Midlife men also exhibit disordered eating/clinical eating disorders, and gender differences observed in young adulthood may diminish later in life.

Introduction

The literature on eating disorders in men remains small compared to the corresponding literature in women, and much of the research focused on eating pathology and related body image concerns in men has been conducted in young adult, college-aged samples. However, these concerns can affect boys and men across the lifespan, from childhood through older adulthood [1–8]. Importantly, there are unique developmental and life course considerations for boys and for older adult men that are salient to understanding the form and trajectory of body dissatisfaction and eating disorder symptoms in these younger and older age groups. As such, this chapter will offer a concise overview of the nature and prevalence of body image concerns, disordered eating, and eating disorders among boys (age < 18) and among men in midlife and beyond (age ~40+).

Childhood and adolescence represent developmental periods of particular relevance to the onset of body image concerns and eating pathology, including among boys [2–5, 9–13]. In particular, as boys move from childhood into early and later adolescence, numerous factors may be important to consider in relation to body dissatisfaction and disordered eating, including pubertal onset and development (e.g., hormonal changes, physical growth, shifting caloric requirements), psychological development (e.g., overall sexuality, gender and sexual identity), neurodevelopment, and social and familial changes (e.g., increased autonomy around food access and intake, greater salience of peer influences), among others. Within the section focused on boys, we consider research on body image, disordered eating, and full threshold eating disorders in boys from childhood (preadolescence) through adolescence. Table 21.1 presents a summary of major findings from selected empirical or review papers of particular relevance that are focused on boys.

Table 21.1 Summary of major findings from selected papers on boys

Citation	Article title	Summary of major findings
Pearson et al. (2010) [49]	A risk model for disordered eating in late elementary school boys	In 5th grade boys (M_{age} = 10.9 years): 10% endorsed objective binge eating and 4.2% endorsed purging during the past 2 weeks Found empirical support for a risk model involving pubertal development, negative urgency, thinness expectancies, and eating expectancies

Table 21.1 (continued)

Citation	Article title	Summary of major findings
Wang et al. (2019) [40]	Fifteen-year prevalence, trajectories, and predictors of body dissatisfaction from adolescence to middle adulthood	Prospective study from Project EAT that included data from adolescent boys (at baseline) with follow-up through middle adulthood Body dissatisfaction increased slightly but significantly overall over 15 years; classified participants into groups based on trajectory of body dissatisfaction Vast majority showed predominantly consistent levels of body dissatisfaction, either low (71.4%) or high (18.9%)
Ricciardelli and McCabe (2004) [5]	A biopsychosocial model of disordered eating and the pursuit of muscularity in adolescent boys	Offers a biopsychosocial model for traditional disordered eating behaviors and those associated with the drive for muscularity, as well as a review of the literature Example social factors: Pressure from parents, peers, and media (both), weight-focused/leanness sports (disordered eating) vs strength/power-focused sports (pursuit of muscularity) Example biological factors: BMI (both), pubertal growth, and timing (both) Example psychological factors: Body dissatisfaction (both), self-esteem (both), perfectionism (both)
Calzo et al. (2016) [54]	Male eating disorder symptom patterns and health correlates from 13 to 26 years of age	Prospective study using Growing Up Today Study (GUTS) data from adolescent boys (baseline) with follow-up through young adulthood Prevalence during adolescence: At age 13–15 years: 3.1% high leanness concern, 4.2% high muscularity concern, 0.4% recurrent (≥ monthly) purging, 0.5% recurrent (at least monthly) binge eating At age 16–18 years: 2.2% high leanness concern, 5.0% high muscularity concern, 0.4% recurrent (≥ monthly) purging, 0.8% recurrent (≥ monthly) binge eating Latent class analyses identified groups across ages with distinct characteristics and health correlates: Asymptomatic (largest class), mostly asymptomatic, body image disturbance, binge eating/purging, muscularity concerns

(continued)

Table 21.1 (continued)

Citation	Article title	Summary of major findings
Rozzell et al. (2019) [57]	Prevalence of eating disorders among US children aged 9 to 10 years: data from the Adolescent Brain Cognitive Development (ABCD) Study	In a US nationally representative study of 9–10-year-olds that applied DSM-5 criteria for EDs, population-level prevalence estimates for boys were: 1.6% any ED; 0% for BN, 0.2% AN, 0.7% BED, 0.7% OSFED No differences found in ED prevalence across boys and girls
Allen et al. (2013) [59]	DSM-IV-TR and DSM-5 eating disorders in adolescents: prevalence, stability, and psychosocial correlates in a population-based sample of male and female adolescents	Prospective, population-based study of Australian adolescents that applied both DSM-IV and DSM-5 criteria Age 14 prevalence in boys: 1.2% for any DSM-IV ED; 0% AN, 0.1% BN, 1% EDNOS 1.2% for any DSM-5 ED; 0% AN, 0.4% BN, 0% BED, 0.7% OSFED Age 17 prevalence in boys 1.2% for any DSM-IV ED; 0% AN, 0.3% BN, 0.9% EDNOS 2.6% for any DSM-5 ED; 0% AN, 0.7% BN, 1.2% BED, 0.9% OSFED

Further, the relative inattention to men in general within the eating disorder literature is even more notable for research specifically focused on body dissatisfaction and eating disorder symptoms among older adult men in midlife and beyond. Similar to women, as men age, they experience several physical and life course changes that may impact body image and disordered eating, including age-related weight gain, andropause (reductions in testosterone in midlife), marriage, divorce, parenting, medical issues, career growth, and retirement [2, 8, 14]. Within the section focused on men in midlife and beyond, we address research on body image, disordered eating, and clinical eating disorders in this older age group of men. Table 21.2 presents a summary of major findings from selected empirical or review papers of particular relevance that are focused on older adult men.

Boys in Preadolescence and Adolescence

Body Dissatisfaction

Body image is a complex and multidimensional construct comprising attitudinal, affective, perceptual, cognitive, and behavioral components [15, 16]. Within the field of eating disorders, body satisfaction and dissatisfaction historically were

Table 21.2 Summary of major findings from selected papers on men in midlife and beyond

Citation	Article title	Summary of major findings
Lodge and Umberson (2013) [62]	Midlife gay and heterosexual men talk about their bodies	In a qualitative study, midlife men identified the following age-related body image concerns: "Functional deterioration" (lower athleticism, physical functioning) Perceived loss of masculinity (lower libido, less muscularity)
Keel et al. (2007) [14]	A 20-year longitudinal study of body weight, dieting, and eating disorder symptoms	In a longitudinal study of men from their 20s to 40s: Increase in percentage of men wanting to lose weight: 37% at age 20, 71% at age 40 Decrease in percentage of men wanting to gain weight: 24% at age 20 to 2% at age 40
Mangweth-Matzek et al. (2016) [69]	Eating disorder symptoms in middle-aged and older men	6.8% of men aged 40–75 years reported eating disorder symptoms 0.9% had a BMI < 18.5, 2.3% reported binge eating only, 1.5% reported binge eating and purging, and 2.1% reported purging only
Kummer et al. (2019) [70]	Aging male symptomatology and eating behavior	Midlife men reporting greater symptoms of andropause had significantly higher BMI, greater eating disorder symptoms, and more negative body image than men with lower andropause symptoms
Brown et al. (2020) [61]	A 30-year longitudinal study of body weight, dieting, and eating pathology across women and men from late adolescence to later midlife	In a longitudinal sample, from age 20 to 50, the proportion of OSFED cases increased in men through midlife: Age 20 = 20.0%, age 30 = 42.9%, age 40 = 75.0%, age 50 = 71.4% Point prevalence of DSM-5 EDs at age 50: AN, 0%; BN, 0%; BED, 1.1%; atypical AN, 1.1%; purging disorder, 1.7%
Hudson et al. (2007) [72]	The prevalence and correlates of eating disorders in the National Comorbidity Survey Replication	In a US nationally representative cross-sectional sample, gender differences in ED point prevalence in younger age groups were not evident in midlife: Ages 18–29: women = 3.6% versus men = 0.7% Over age 45: women = 2.3% versus men = 2.5%

conceptualized in relation to the traditional thin ideal. This is reflected in the content or format of older body image measures, such as the body dissatisfaction scale of the Eating Disorder Inventory (i.e., concern about large thighs) [17] or silhouette/figure rating scales reflecting a single dimension of body weight/body fat [18, 19]. These measures were based on conceptualizations emphasizing the drive for thinness or fear of weight gain, such that body dissatisfaction was most commonly equated with a desire to be thinner or less heavy than one's current body shape or weight. Given what is now understood about the more complex nature of body image and body ideals in boys and men (i.e., the emphasis on muscularity and leanness [20–23]), some early research based on the more "gendered" unidimensional approach to assessment inadvertently arrived at the inaccurate conclusion that boys and men had few body image concerns.

Evidence suggests that body dissatisfaction can emerge in early childhood [2–4, 24–26] and that boys as young as 4 demonstrate preferences for socioculturally prescribed ideal body sizes [27]. Results from qualitative research studies have provided some insights into the experience of body image during preadolescence. For example, young preadolescent boys have been found to endorse the perceptions that greater body size is associated with better physical performance (e.g., athletics) and independence [28] and that masculinity is equated with muscularity and strength [29]. Similarly, older preadolescent boys have been found to ascribe to a fit body ideal that reflects a dislike of fatness, the salience of physical performance and ability, and preferences for muscularity [30]. Consistent with this notion, a majority of boys aged 8–11 years have been found to rate both their weight and muscles as important, and a substantial proportion reported engaging in body change strategies to increase muscles or lose weight [31]. Further, boys aged 6 years have been found to show both muscularity- and thinness-oriented body dissatisfaction, with muscularity being perceived as more rewarding versus thinness [32]. There also is evidence indicating that among preadolescent boys who are dissatisfied with their bodies, some exhibit a desire for a larger body shape, and others exhibit a desire for a smaller body shape [2, 24, 25]. Overall, there has been inconsistent measurement across studies of preadolescent boys and a focus on general body size in some investigations, leading to mixed findings on the specific nature, degree, and prevalence of body dissatisfaction in this age group. In particular, while the desire for larger body shapes among some younger boys may reflect a specific desire for greater muscularity, it may also reflect a conflation of larger body sizes with perceptions of greater height, age, or physical capabilities [28, 29]. Notably, research has also addressed factors that may contribute to body dissatisfaction in young boys, including communication about and exposure to body ideals, as well as other psychological and sociocultural influences [4, 24, 33, 34].

Adolescence is a time of particular relevance to the experience of body image among boys, given the shifting physical, psychological, and social factors during this period (e.g., pubertal development, increased peer influences) [5, 10, 11, 35, 36]. Evidence suggests that body dissatisfaction is common among adolescent boys and, similar to findings among preadolescents, can take the form of a desire to be smaller/thinner, a desire to be larger/bigger, and/or specific concerns about muscularity [37–41]. Further, findings from longitudinal research suggest that overall, adolescent boys experience a decrease in body satisfaction corresponding to the typical period of pubertal development [42], which is consistent with evidence that advanced pubertal status may be associated with greater risk for body dissatisfaction and weight/shape concerns in this population [11]. However, highlighting the complexity of body image concerns in boys, longitudinal changes in body satisfaction have been found to differ based on changes in weight, with increased satisfaction for boys decreasing weight from overweight categories versus decreased satisfaction for boys decreasing weight from average to underweight [42]. Similarly, other research has found a curvilinear relationship between body mass index (BMI) and body dissatisfaction in boys, such that either underweight or overweight/obesity weight status may elevate risk for body image concerns among adolescent boys [43, 44].

Disordered Eating

Although the overall prevalence of specific full threshold eating disorders among boys in school and community settings is relatively low, evidence clearly indicates that disordered eating behaviors are more common. Specific forms of disordered eating that have received the most attention include disinhibited eating behaviors, such as loss of control eating and binge eating, as well as unhealthy weight control/body change strategies (i.e., compensatory behaviors). In addition to disordered eating behaviors consistent with traditional eating disorder diagnoses, more recent research has also begun to examine muscularity-oriented attitudes and behaviors.

Evidence suggests that disordered eating behaviors can emerge among some boys even in preadolescence [25], although prevalence rates differ based on a number of study-related factors (e.g., measures, sample age range). For example, in a population-based study of elementary school children aged 6–11 years, 5% of boys met the criteria for disordered eating (indicated by two out of five endorsed items on the SCOFF [45]), with rates higher among boys with overweight (11.5%) or obesity (18.6%) versus normal weight (3.6%) [46]. Further, in a large cohort study with a mixed-gender (approximately equal) sample of 11- and 12-year-old boys and girls, 7% of the sample reported recurrent disordered eating behavior (i.e., engaging in fasting, purging, or binge eating at least monthly for the past year), and no gender differences were found [47]. Additionally, in a large community sample of youth aged 8–11 years, approximately one in five boys reported engaging in loss of control eating during the past month [48], whereas a large study of 5th grade boys found that 10% endorsed objective binge eating in the past 2 weeks, as well as 4.2% endorsing purging behavior [49].

In general, adolescent boys have received more attention in the literature on disordered eating than younger boys. In particular, a number of larger-scale epidemiological studies have provided relevant data. For example, data collected from nearly 40,000 9th and 12th grade boys as part of the Minnesota Student Survey found that

29.1% reported any form of disordered eating behavior, such as binge eating (12.5%), fasting/skipping meals (14.0%), vomiting (1.6%), and laxative use (1.7%) [50]. Further, a study of nearly one thousand German adolescent boys aged 11–17 years selected from a nationally representative sample found that 14.4% of boys met the criteria for disordered eating (indicated by 2 out of 5 endorsed items on the SCOFF [45]), with rates notably higher among boys with overweight (24.7%) or obesity (51.6%) [51]. In a study of 3270 Australian adolescents aged 14–15 years using data from the Longitudinal Study of Australian Children, estimated population prevalence rates for anorexia nervosa (AN) symptoms in boys were found to be 7.58% for behaviors interfering with/fear of weight gain, 15.95% for overvaluation/disturbance in experience of body weight, and 3.41% for both; rates for bulimia nervosa (BN) symptoms in boys were found to be 0.38% for binge eating, 10.84% for overvaluation of weight, 3.88% for compensatory behaviors, and 0% for all three [52]. Consistent with other studies, prevalence rates were generally higher in those boys with higher weight. Notably, a Project EAT-III study that included 10-year follow-up data on boys who were originally recruited during adolescence reported rates of disordered eating in early and middle adolescence, including 27.9–34.8% for unhealthy weight control behaviors (e.g., fasting, skipping meals, food substitute use), 2.1–2.2% for extreme weight control behaviors (e.g., vomiting, laxatives, diet pills), and 3.0–3.5% for binge eating; findings also revealed that in general, the prevalence of disordered eating behaviors either remained stable or increased from adolescence through young adulthood [53]. Taken together, although specific rates vary, evidence generally suggests that various traditional disordered eating attitudes and behaviors become more prevalent from childhood through adolescence in boys, with greater rates commonly found among those with overweight or obesity.

More recently, large-scale studies have also assessed disordered eating attitudes and behaviors that more directly reflect the sociocultural body ideals for boys and men (e.g., muscularity and leanness). For example, a prospective study that used Growing Up Today Study (GUTS) data from participants who were adolescents at baseline (with follow-up data through young adulthood) reported prevalence rates for boys: high leanness concern (age 13–15, 3.1%; age 16–18, 2.2%), high muscularity concern (age 13–15, 4.2%; age 16–18, 5.0%), recurrent purging (age 13–15, 0.4%; age 16–18, 0.4%), and recurrent binge eating (age 13–15, 0.5%; age 16–18, 0.8%); a latent class analysis identifying subgroups based on symptoms found multiple classes, with the asymptomatic class largest for all age groups [54]. Additionally, data from Wave I of the National Longitudinal Study of Adolescent to Adult Health (Add Health) showed that among boys aged 11–18 years, 29.2% reported trying to gain weight/bulk up and 25.2% reported any muscle-enhancing behavior, including dieting to gain weight/bulk up (3.8%), exercising to gain weight/bulk up (15.4%), lifting weights to gain weight/bulk up (17.5%), and taking food supplements to gain weight/bulk up (3.3%) [55].

Eating Disorders

Nationally representative studies of eating disorders in preadolescent boys have reported a range of prevalence rates, likely due in part to differing assessment methods, diagnostic frameworks, and other factors. For example, based on data from the National Health and Nutrition Examination Survey (NHANES) study that applied DSM-IV criteria, 12-month prevalence rates for any eating disorder were found to be 0.1% for boys aged 8–15 years, with the same rate found in the combined sample of boys and girls aged 8–11 years [56]. In a more recent nationally representative study of youth aged 9–10 years that applied DSM-5 criteria, the population-level prevalence estimate for any eating disorder was 1.6% for boys, and prevalence estimates of specific diagnoses ranged from 0% for BN to 0.7% for binge eating disorder (BED) and for other specified feeding or eating disorder (OSFED) [57]. Consistent with other research, these studies indicate small or nonsignificant differences in prevalence between preadolescent boys and girls, suggesting that the differences that are apparent in older age groups likely emerge during adolescence, perhaps related to pubertal onset or other aspects of development.

In adolescent boys, various epidemiological studies have reported prevalence rates for full threshold eating disorders, typically within the approximate range of 0–1% for each core eating disorder diagnosis [see 1]. For example, in a nationally representative sample of adolescents aged 13–18 years that applied DSM-IV criteria, the lifetime rates for full threshold eating disorders in boys were 0.3% for AN, 0.5% for BN, and 0.8% for BED, with rates of 0.1% and 2.6% for subthreshold AN and subthreshold BED, respectively; prevalence was lower in boys than girls for BN, BED, and subthreshold AN [58]. Further, in a prospective, population-based sample of Australian adolescents that applied both DSM-IV and DSM-5 criteria, prevalence rates for boys were as follows: (a) at age 14, 1.2% for any DSM-IV eating disorder (0% AN, 0.1% BN, 1% eating disorder not otherwise specified [EDNOS]) versus 1.2% for any DSM-5 eating disorder (0% AN, 0.4% BN, 0% BED, 0.7% OSFED) and (b), at age 17, 1.2% for any DSM-IV eating disorder (0% AN, 0.3% BN, 0.9% EDNOS) versus 2.6% for any DSM-5 eating disorder (0% AN, 0.7% BN, 1.2% BED, 0.9% OSFED) [59]. Notably, other studies have reported greater prevalence rates. For instance, in a recent population-based study of Australian adolescents aged 11–19 years recruited from school settings that applied DSM-5 criteria, the 1-month prevalence rate among boys for any eating disorder was 12.8%, with 2.1% meeting criteria for a full-syndrome eating disorder (0% AN, 1.8% probable BN, 0.2% probable BED) and 8.5% for other specific feeding or eating disorder [60]. However, this study assessed symptoms over only a 1-month period, and along with other methodological considerations and in the context of prior research, findings from the study may reflect an overestimation of the true prevalence.

Men in Midlife and Beyond

Body Dissatisfaction

As men age, natural changes in body shape, increases in body fat, and a decrease in muscularity may exacerbate body image concerns and disordered eating [14, 61]. As such, aging may confer increased concerns regarding losing a "masculine" physique. Many studies have examined body weight dissatisfaction in men or body image concerns more broadly, with few studies exploring muscularity concerns in older ages. Qualitative research supports that changes in body functionality and appearance may impact body dissatisfaction in midlife men. Indeed, men aged 40–60 years reported distress regarding the "functional deterioration" of their bodies (lower athleticism, physical functioning) and concerns regarding perceived loss of masculinity (lower libido, less muscularity) as they aged [62]. Interestingly, a study of men aged 65–85 years found that while midlife and beyond men reported becoming increasingly dissatisfied with their physical appearance as they age, particularly in regard to bodily functioning, they were still less likely than women to engage in appearance-enhancing activities [63]. These results suggest a potentially important role regarding the impact of body functionality on body image in midlife and beyond men.

One major body image concern for midlife men is age-related weight gain. Consistent with this, a longitudinal study of men from their 20s to 40s demonstrated that the percentage of men who wanted to lose weight increased from 37% at age 20 to 71% at age 40 [14]. Conversely, the percentage of men wanting to gain weight decreased from 24% at age 20 to 2% at age 40. Notably, this study did not ask about the desire to gain muscle and lose body fat, which may have influenced results. Beyond weight and shape concerns specifically, a cross-sectional survey of men in 1997 revealed that appearance dissatisfaction may persist through midlife. Indeed, 38–41% of young men aged 13–29 years, 48% of men aged 30–39 years, 43% of men aged 40–49 years, and 48% of men aged 50–59 years reported dissatisfaction with their appearance [64]. Body image and appearance-related concerns may be maintained via negative conversations about one's body and the body of others (sometimes termed "fat talk" or "negative body talk"). While this construct has been investigated predominantly in samples of girls and young women, research supports that men engage in negative body talk across the lifespan and that this behavior is associated with disordered eating in midlife men [65]. While several studies support that body image concerns may increase as men age, other studies have found no associations between aging and body image for midlife men, suggesting that men may become more accepting of their bodies as they age [66]. Consistent with this, a cross-sectional study reported that men aged 46–55 years had lower drive for muscularity attitudes and muscle dysmorphia physique protection (i.e., behaviors to avoid one's body being seen by others) compared to younger men aged 19–25 years [67]. Given the limited research on this topic, future research should continue to explore how aging may affect body image in men beyond young adulthood.

Disordered Eating

With regard to dieting behaviors, data from the Netherlands Twin Registry indicate that women aged 35–65 years and men aged 45–65 years report the highest rates (31.7–31.9% and 56.6–63.0%, respectively) compared to all other age categories [68]. These results are comparable to those from Keel and colleagues who found that dieting frequency prospectively increased in men as they aged from 20 to 40, with 25% reporting sometimes or often dieting at age 40 [14]. However, while dieting appears to increase into midlife for men, recent research supports that dieting may confer less risk for disordered eating across ages. Indeed, in a longitudinal cohort study of men from their 20s to 50s, the impact of dieting as a risk factor on drive for thinness decreased prospectively as men aged, to the point that there was no longer a significant association between dieting and drive for thinness at 50, while this relationship remained significant and stable across time for women [61]. This may suggest that dieting may be motivated less by disordered eating and more by health-focused behaviors among midlife versus younger men. However, more research on this topic is needed.

In addition to dieting, midlife men are also at risk for symptoms of eating disorders including binge eating, purging (e.g., self-induced vomiting, laxative and diuretic misuse), and pathological exercise. For example, in a sample of Austrian men aged 40–75 years, 6.8% reported eating disorder symptoms, 0.9% had a BMI < 18.5, 2.3% reported binge eating, 1.5% reported binge eating and purging, and 2.1% reported purging without binge eating [69]. Midlife and beyond men reporting these symptoms demonstrated significantly greater eating pathology, exercise addiction, and lower body satisfaction compared to those that did not report symptoms. Notably, the cutoff score on the measure of eating pathology used identified only 9% of the men, suggesting that existing measures of eating pathology may lead to under-recognition of disordered eating in midlife and beyond men [69]. Supporting that age-related changes may lead to increased disordered eating in midlife men, in the same sample of Austrian men aged 40–75 years, those with greater symptoms of andropause had significantly higher BMI, greater eating disorder symptoms, greater risk of exercise addiction, and more negative body image than men with lower andropause symptoms [70]. Although the research on disordered eating in older men has largely been cross-sectional in nature, data has also examined cross-sectional trends over time in midlife men. While purging is typically less often endorsed by men versus women, evidence indicates that purging behavior has increased in men and women aged 45 years or older from 1998 to 2008 [71].

Research has also examined dimensional measures of eating pathology in midlife men, most notably the Eating Disorder Inventory Drive for Thinness and Bulimia subscales. For example, in a 30-year longitudinal study of women and men from their 20s to their 50s, women demonstrated higher drive for thinness and bulimia scores across time compared to men [14, 61]. Importantly, there were also gender differences in the trajectory of eating pathology over time; drive for thinness decreased over time for women and increased over time for midlife men, while bulimic symptoms decreased over time for both genders [14, 61].

Eating Disorders

Few studies have examined the current or lifetime prevalence of eating disorders in men in midlife and beyond. The limited research on this topic suggests that prevalence rates range from 0% to 0.3% for AN, 0% to 2.8% for BN, 0.9% to 2.7% for BED, and 1.1 to 2.8% for OSFED [61, 72, 73].

While a preponderance of evidence suggests that eating disorders are more prevalent in women compared to men during adolescence and young adulthood [72], recent research suggests that these gender differences may diminish in midlife [61, 72, 73]. Cross-sectional research from the US National Comorbidity Survey supports that women demonstrate higher lifetime eating disorder point prevalence compared to men between ages 18 and 29 (women = 3.6%, men = 0.7%), but gender differences in point prevalence disappear in those over age 45 (women = 2.3%, men = 2.5%; [72]. Notably, few studies have examined OSFED in midlife men. Keel and colleagues [74] examined prospective changes in DSM-III-R diagnoses of BN and related EDNOS cross-sectionally at ages 20, 30, and 40 in women and men. Bulimic syndrome point prevalence declined significantly in women but remained stable in men from late adolescence to early midlife. However, at approximately 40 years of age, women were still significantly more likely to have a current eating disorder compared to men [74]. In a more recent study using DSM-5 criteria in the same cohort, Brown and colleagues [61] examined eating disorder point prevalence in men through age 50. The percentage of men meeting criteria for any ED diagnosis did not change significantly from age 20 to 50. Over time, the proportion of OSFED cases increased for men (age 20 = 20.0%, age 30 = 42.9%, age 40 = 75.0%, age 50 = 71.4%). At age 50, no men met criteria for AN or BN, while 1.1% met criteria for BED, 1.1% met criteria for atypical AN, and 1.7% met criteria for purging disorder. Of the individuals who had an eating disorder at age 50, 50.0% of men represented new-onset cases, and the majority of these were diagnosed with OSFED (new onset, 66.7%). Thus, OSFED may better capture eating disorders in men, particularly in midlife.

Conclusions

Evidence suggests that body image and disordered eating behaviors can occur even in young children, with adolescence appearing to be a period of particular risk for development or exacerbation of eating disorder symptoms and body dissatisfaction. Although the prevalence of full threshold eating disorders is relatively low among boys in school and community settings, disordered eating symptoms and elevated body dissatisfaction are more common and may reflect risk for future development of clinical eating disorders. Unfortunately, appropriate diagnosis and treatment seeking among boys with eating disorders remain low, perhaps due in part to stigma/shame given the still "gendered" views of eating disorders that are common, particularly for boys in adolescence [75–77]. Additional research using prospective, longitudinal designs and measures that account for the unique manifestations of body image concerns and eating pathology in boys (e.g., concerns about leanness and muscularity and associated behaviors) is needed. Further research examining the impact of body weight on these attitudes and behaviors, as well as the interactions of body weight in associations with other clinical and functional correlates, is warranted. From a measurement perspective, there is a need for more research to validate measures with boys, particularly with regard to content validity (e.g., assessing multiple body dissatisfaction dimensions such as body fat, muscularity, and height); broader adoption of validated measures in future research will also be important. Lastly, more research on subgroups of boys, particularly those who may be at elevated risk for body dissatisfaction and eating pathology (e.g., racial and ethnic minorities, sexual and gender minorities), is suggested.

With regard to men in midlife and beyond, there has been an encouraging increase in research on body image and eating disorders within this population in recent years. However, there is still a relative dearth of information on this older age group of men. Additional research will be critical to better help identify, prevent, and treat appearance and eating-related concerns in this group. Future studies would benefit from the use of longitudinal designs to confirm that cross-sectional findings across age groups are not due to cohort effects. Further, to better understand the associations between changes in testosterone and changes in eating pathology across the lifespan, future studies would benefit from multimethod approaches to assessment that include endocrinological measures (e.g., testosterone levels). Importantly, few studies have examined muscularity concerns in midlife men using validated measurements, which may be masking an important area of relevant concern for this age group. Finally, studies of midlife men could benefit from examining how risk may change across the lifespan for different subgroups of men (e.g., sexual and gender minorities, racial and ethnic minorities, etc.) to help better identify subgroups of midlife men that may be at greater risk.

Disclaimer The opinions and assertions expressed herein are those of the author and do not necessarily reflect the official policy or position of the Uniformed Services University or the Department of Defense.

References

1. Mitchison D, Mond J. Epidemiology of eating disorders, eating disordered behaviour, and body image disturbance in males: a narrative review. J Eat Disord. 2015;3:20.
2. McCabe MP, Ricciardelli LA. Body image dissatisfaction among males across the lifespan: a review of past literature. J Psychosom Res. 2004;56:675–85.

3. Cohane GH, Pope HG Jr. Body image in boys: a review of the literature. Int J Eat Disord. 2001;29:373–9.
4. Littleton HL, Ollendick T. Negative body image and disordered eating behavior in children and adolescents: what places youth at risk and how can these problems be prevented? Clin Child Fam Psychol Rev. 2003;6:51–66.
5. Ricciardelli LA, McCabe MP. A biopsychosocial model of disordered eating and the pursuit of muscularity in adolescent boys. Psychol Bull. 2004;130:179–205.
6. Tiggemann M. Body image across the adult life span: stability and change. Body Image. 2004;1:29–41.
7. Mangweth-Matzek B, Hoek HW. Epidemiology and treatment of eating disorders in men and women of middle and older age. Curr Opin Psychiatry. 2017;30:446–51.
8. Reas DL, Stedal K. Eating disorders in men aged midlife and beyond. Maturitas. 2015;81:248–55.
9. Muise AM, Stein DG, Arbess G. Eating disorders in adolescent boys: a review of the adolescent and young adult literature. J Adolesc Health. 2003;33:427–35.
10. Markey CN. Invited commentary: why body image is important to adolescent development. J Youth Adolesc. 2010;39:1387–91.
11. Klump KL. Puberty as a critical risk period for eating disorders: a review of human and animal studies. Horm Behav. 2013;64:399–410.
12. Limbers CA, Cohen LA, Gray BA. Eating disorders in adolescent and young adult males: prevalence, diagnosis, and treatment strategies. Adolesc Health Med Ther. 2018;9:111–6.
13. Nagata JM, Ganson KT, Murray SB. Eating disorders in adolescent boys and young men: an update. Curr Opin Pediatr. 2020;32:476–81.
14. Keel PK, Baxter MG, Heatherton TF, Joiner TE Jr. A 20-year longitudinal study of body weight, dieting, and eating disorder symptoms. J Abnorm Psychol. 2007;116:422.
15. Banfield SS, McCabe MP. An evaluation of the construct of body image. Adolescence. 2002;37:373–93.
16. Thompson JK. The (mis)measurement of body image: ten strategies to improve assessment for applied and research purposes. Body Image. 2004;1:7–14.
17. Garner DM, Olmstead MP, Polivy J. Development and validation of a multidimensional eating disorder inventory for anorexia nervosa and bulimia. Int J Eat Disord. 1983;2:15–34.
18. Gardner RM, Brown DL. Body image assessment: a review of figural drawing scales. Pers Individ Dif. 2010;18:107–11.
19. Cafri G, Thompson JK. Measuring male body image: a review of the current methodology. Psychol Men Masc. 2004;5:18–29.
20. Pope HG, Phillips KA, Olivardia R. The Adonis complex: the secret crisis of male body obsession. New York: The Free Press; 2000.
21. Murray SB, Griffiths S, Mond JM. Evolving eating disorder psychopathology: conceptualizing muscularity-oriented disordered eating. Br J Psychiatry. 2016;208:414–5.
22. Murray SB, Nagata JM, Griffiths S, Calzo JP, Brown TA, Mitchison D, Blashill AJ, Mond JM. The enigma of male eating disorders: a critical review and synthesis. Clin Psychol Rev. 2017;57:1–11.
23. Lavender JM, Brown TA, Murray SB. Men, muscles, and eating disorders: an overview of traditional and muscularity-oriented disordered eating. Curr Psychiatry Rep. 2017;19:32.
24. Tatangelo G, McCabe M, Mellor D, Mealey A. A systematic review of body dissatisfaction and sociocultural messages related to the body among preschool children. Body Image. 2016;18:86–95.
25. Ricciardelli LA, McCabe MP. Children's body image concerns and eating disturbance: a review of the literature. Clin Psychol Rev. 2001;21:325–44.
26. Dion J, Hains J, Vachon P, Plouffe J, Laberge L, Perron M, McDuff P, Kalinova E, Leone M. Correlates of body dissatisfaction in children. J Pediatr. 2016;171:202–7.
27. Damiano SR, Gregg KJ, Spiel EC, McLean SA, Wertheim EH, Paxton SJ. Relationships between body size attitudes and body image of 4-year-old boys and girls, and attitudes of their fathers and mothers. J Eat Disord. 2015;3:16.

28. Birbeck D, Drummond M. Understanding boys' bodies and masculinity in early childhood. Int J Mens Health. 2006;5:238–50.
29. Drummond MJ. Boys' bodies in early childhood. Aust J Early Childhood. 2012;37:107–14.
30. Tatangelo GL, Ricciardelli LA. A qualitative study of preadolescent boys' and girls' body image: gendered ideals and sociocultural influences. Body Image. 2013;10:591–8.
31. Ricciardelli LA, McCabe MP, Holt KE, Finemore J. A biopsychosocial model for understanding body image and body change strategies among children. J Appl Dev Psychol. 2003;24:475–95.
32. McLean SA, Wertheim EH, Paxton SJ. Preferences for being muscular and thin in 6-year-old boys. Body Image. 2018;26:98–102.
33. Nichols TE, Damiano SR, Gregg K, Wertheim EH, Paxton SJ. Psychological predictors of body image attitudes and concerns in young children. Body Image. 2018;27:10–20.
34. Pope HG Jr, Olivardia R, Gruber A, Borowiecki J. Evolving ideals of male body image as seen through action toys. Int J Eat Disord. 1999;26:65–72.
35. Smolak L, Murnen SK, Thompson JK. Sociocultural influences and muscle building in adolescent boys. Psychol Men Masc. 2005;6:227–39.
36. Smolak L, Stein JA. The relationship of drive for muscularity to sociocultural factors, self-esteem, physical attributes gender role, and social comparison in middle school boys. Body Image. 2006;3:121–9.
37. Baker JH, Higgins Neyland MK, Thornton LM, Runfola CD, Larsson H, Lichtenstein P, Bulik C. Body dissatisfaction in adolescent boys. Dev Psychol. 2019;55:1566–78.
38. Carlson JD. Body image among adolescent girls and boys: a longitudinal study. Dev Psychol. 2004;40:823–35.
39. Jones DC, Bain N, King S. Weight and muscularity concerns as longitudinal predictors of body image among early adolescent boys: a test of the dual pathways model. Body Image. 2008;5:195–204.
40. Wang SB, Haynos AF, Wall MM, Chen C, Eisenberg ME, Neumark-Sztainer D. Fifteen-year prevalence, trajectories, and predictors of body dissatisfaction from adolescence to middle adulthood. Clin Psychol Sci. 2019;7:1403–15.
41. Dion J, Blackburn ME, Auclair J, Laberge L, Veillette S, Gaudreault M, Vachon P, Perron M, Touchette É. Development and aetiology of body dissatisfaction in adolescent boys and girls. Int J Adolesc Youth. 2015;20:151–66.
42. Eisenberg ME, Neumark-Sztainer D, Paxton SJ. Five-year change in body satisfaction among adolescents. J Psychosom Res. 2006;61:521–7.
43. Austin SB, Haines J, Veugelers PJ. Body satisfaction and body weight: gender differences and sociodemographic determinants. BMC Public Health. 2009;9:313.
44. Calzo JP, Sonneville KR, Haines J, Blood EA, Field AE, Austin SB. The development of associations among body mass index, body dissatisfaction, and weight and shape concern in adolescent boys and girls. J Adolesc Health. 2012;51:517–23.
45. Morgan JF, Reid F, Lacey JH. The SCOFF questionnaire: assessment of a new screening tool for eating disorders. BMJ. 1999;319:1467–8.
46. Jendrzyca A, Warschburger P. Weight stigma and eating behaviours in elementary school children: a prospective population-based study. Appetite. 2016;102:51–9.
47. Stemann Larsen P, Nybo Andersen AM, Olsen EM, Kragh Andersen P, Micali N, Strandberg-Larsen K. Weight trajectories and disordered eating behaviours in 11- to 12-year-olds: a longitudinal study within the Danish National Birth Cohort. Eur Eat Disord Rev. 2019;27:436–44.
48. Goossens L, Braet C, Bosmans G, Decaluwé V. Loss of control over eating in pre-adolescent youth: the role of attachment and self-esteem. Eat Behav. 2011;12:289–95.
49. Pearson CM, Combs JL, Smith GT. A risk model for disordered eating in late elementary school boys. Psychol Addict Behav. 2010;24:696–704.
50. Croll J, Neumark-Sztainer D, Story M, Ireland M. Prevalence and risk and protective factors related to disordered eating behaviors among adolescents: relationship to gender and ethnicity. J Adolesc Health. 2002;31:166–75.

51. Herpertz-Dahlmann B, Wille N, Hölling H, Vloet TD, Ravens-Sieberer U; BELLA study group. Disordered eating behaviour and attitudes, associated psychopathology and health-related quality of life: results of the BELLA study. Eur Child Adolesc Psychiatry. 2008;17 Suppl 1:82–91.
52. Hughes EK, Kerr JA, Patton GC, Sawyer SM, Wake M, Le Grange D, Azzopardi P. Eating disorder symptoms across the weight spectrum in Australian adolescents. Int J Eat Disord. 2019;52:885–94.
53. Neumark-Sztainer D, Wall M, Larson NI, Eisenberg ME, Loth K. Dieting and disordered eating behaviors from adolescence to young adulthood: findings from a 10-year longitudinal study. J Am Diet Assoc. 2011;111:1004–11.
54. Calzo JP, Horton NJ, Sonneville KR, Swanson SA, Crosby RD, Micali N, Eddy KT, Field AE. Male eating disorder symptom patterns and health correlates from 13 to 26 years of age. J Am Acad Child Adolesc Psychiatry. 2016;55:693–700.
55. Nagata JM, Ganson KT, Griffiths S, Mitchison D, Garber AK, Vittinghoff E, Bibbins-Domingo K, Murray SB. Prevalence and correlates of muscle-enhancing behaviors among adolescents and young adults in the United States. Int J Adolesc Med Health. 2020. https://doi.org/10.1515/ijamh-2020-0001
56. Merikangas KR, He JP, Brody D, Fisher PW, Bourdon K, Koretz DS. Prevalence and treatment of mental disorders among US children in the 2001–2004 NHANES. Pediatrics. 2010;125:75–81.
57. Rozzell K, Moon DY, Klimek P, Brown T, Blashill AJ. Prevalence of eating disorders among US children aged 9 to 10 years: data from the Adolescent Brain Cognitive Development (ABCD) study. JAMA Pediatr. 2019;173:100–1.
58. Swanson SA, Crow SJ, Le Grange D, Swendsen J, Merikangas KR. Prevalence and correlates of eating disorders in adolescents. Results from the national comorbidity survey replication adolescent supplement. Arch Gen Psychiatry. 2011;68:714–23.
59. Allen KL, Byrne SM, Oddy WH, Crosby RD. DSM–IV–TR and DSM-5 eating disorders in adolescents: prevalence, stability, and psychosocial correlates in a population-based sample of male and female adolescents. J Abnorm Psychol. 2013;122:720–32.
60. Mitchison D, Mond J, Bussey K, Griffiths S, Trompeter N, Lonergan A, Pike KM, Murray SB, Hay P. DSM-5 full syndrome, other specified, and unspecified eating disorders in Australian adolescents: prevalence and clinical significance. Psychol Med. 2020;50:981–90.
61. Brown TA, Forney KJ, Klein KM, Grillot C, Keel PK. A 30-year longitudinal study of body weight, dieting, and eating pathology across women and men from late adolescence to later midlife. J Abnorm Psychol. 2020;129:376.
62. Lodge AC, Umberson D. Age and embodied masculinities: midlife gay and heterosexual men talk about their bodies. J Aging Stud. 2013;27:225–32.
63. Baker L, Gringart E. Body image and self-esteem in older adulthood. Ageing Soc. 2009;29:977–95.
64. Garner D. Body image survey results. Psychology Today-New York. 1997;30:30–45.
65. Tzoneva M, Forney KJ, Keel PK. The influence of gender and age on the association between "fat-talk" and disordered eating: an examination in men and women from their 20s to their 50s. Eat Disord. 2015;23:439–54.
66. Forrester-Knauss C, Stutz EZ. Gender differences in disordered eating and weight dissatisfaction in Swiss adults: which factors matter? BMC Public Health. 2012;12:809.
67. Hughes EK, Dean C, Allen JS. Measures of eating disorder symptoms, drive for muscularity, and muscle dysmorphia: norms and typologies of Australian men. Aust J Psychol. 2016;68:270–80.
68. Slof-Op't Landt MC, van Furth EF, van Beijsterveldt CE, Bartels M, Willemsen G, de Geus EJ, et al. Prevalence of dieting and fear of weight gain across ages: a community sample from adolescents to the elderly. Int J Public Health. 2017;62:911–9.
69. Mangweth-Matzek B, Kummer KK, Pope HG. Eating disorder symptoms in middle-aged and older men. Int J Eat Disord. 2016;49:953–7.

70. Kummer KK, Pope HG, Hudson JI, Kemmler G, Pinggera G-M, Mangweth-Matzek B. Aging male symptomatology and eating behavior. Aging Male. 2019;22:55–61.
71. Mitchison D, Hay P, Slewa-Younan S, Mond J. The changing demographic profile of eating disorder behaviors in the community. BMC Public Health. 2014;14:943.
72. Hudson JI, Hiripi E, Pope HG Jr, Kessler RC. The prevalence and correlates of eating disorders in the National Comorbidity Survey Replication. Biol Psychiatry. 2007;61:348–58.
73. Mitchell KS, Wolf EJ. PTSD, food addiction, and disordered eating in a sample of primarily older veterans: the mediating role of emotion regulation. Psychiatry Res. 2016;243:23–9.
74. Keel PK, Gravener JA, Joiner TE Jr, Haedt AA. Twenty-year follow-up of bulimia nervosa and related eating disorders not otherwise specified. Int J Eat Disord. 2010;43:492–7.
75. Forrest LN, Smith AR, Swanson SA. Characteristics of seeking treatment among U.S. adolescents with eating disorders. Int J Eat Disord. 2017;50:826–33.
76. Griffiths S, Mond JM, Li Z, Gunatilake S, Murray SB, Sheffield J, Touyz S. Self-stigma of seeking treatment and being male predict an increased likelihood of having an undiagnosed eating disorder. Int J Eat Disord. 2015;48:775–8.
77. Griffiths S, Mond JM, Murray SB, Touyz S. The prevalence and adverse associations of stigmatization in people with eating disorders. Int J Eat Disord. 2015;48:767–74.

Chapter 22
Eating Disorders in Boys and Men: Conclusions and Future Research Directions

Jason M. Nagata, Tiffany A. Brown, Stuart B. Murray, and Jason M. Lavender

Despite progress within recent years, boys and men with eating disorders continue to be under-recognized and underserved within both research and clinical contexts. The overarching aim of this book was to provide a comprehensive and empirically informed overview of the most up-to-date information on wide-ranging and clinically relevant topics related to the presentation, assessment, medical and nutritional considerations, prevention, treatment, and sociocultural considerations of eating disorders among boys and men. Key takeaways for this book are reflected in the "Nine truths about eating disorders in boys and men" presented in Table 22.1 [1]; the subsequent sections of this concluding chapter, organized by the primary sections of the book, highlight core gaps in the existing literature and knowledge base, along with recommendations for future research to expand our collective knowledge base on the nature, assessment, prevention, and treatment of these serious psychiatric disorders in boys and men from diverse backgrounds.

J. M. Nagata (✉)
Division of Adolescent and Young Adult Medicine, Department of Pediatrics, University of California, San Francisco, San Francisco, CA, USA
e-mail: jason.nagata@ucsf.edu

T. A. Brown
Department of Psychiatry, University of California, San Diego, San Diego, CA, USA

San Diego State University Research Foundation, San Diego, CA, USA

S. B. Murray
Department of Psychiatry and the Behavioral Sciences, USC Keck School of Medicine, University of Southern California, Los Angeles, CA, USA

J. M. Lavender
Department of Medicine, Military Cardiovascular Outcomes Research (MiCOR) Program, Uniformed Services University of the Health Sciences, Bethesda, MD, USA

The Metis Foundation, San Antonio, TX, USA

J. M. Nagata et al. (eds.), *Eating Disorders in Boys and Men*,
https://doi.org/10.1007/978-3-030-67127-3_22

Table 22.1 Nine truths about eating disorders in boys and men

1	The eating disorder field historically developed through a female-centric lens
2	Boys and men with eating disorders remain under-recognized and underserved
3	Eating disorders can, but do not necessarily, present differently in boys and men
4	Medical complications of eating disorders in boys and men can be severe, and mortality is elevated
5	Seeking treatment for an eating disorder can be especially challenging for boys and men
6	Boys and men can face additional eating disorder treatment barriers
7	Eating disorders can affect boys and men across the lifespan
8	Eating disorders can affect cisgender and transgender boys and men of all sexual orientations, race/ethnicities, cultures, socioeconomic backgrounds, and body shapes and weights
9	Body ideals in boys and men are diverse and can be influenced by many factors

Overview and Perspectives

Continued research is imperative in order to expand our collective knowledge regarding the onset, conceptualization, and prevalence of eating disorders in boys and men. From an epidemiological perspective, the development of more sensitive methods to screen for eating disorders in boys and men is crucial to developing a more accurate understanding of prevalence and onset timing, as well as facilitating early intervention. Moreover, additional studies are needed to generate better understanding of the extent to which theoretical models of body image and eating disorder psychopathology are applicable to boys and men. Further, and in recognition of the complexity of disordered eating symptoms among boys and men, it is important for future research to develop robust methods to more fully differentiate the drive for muscularity, which is ubiquitous among boys and men, from the pathological pursuit of muscularity and muscularity-disordered eating.

Diagnosis and Assessment

There are multiple areas in which additional research related to the diagnosis and assessment of eating disorders and related symptomology in boys and men is recommended. Broadly, there is a need for more research to better understand the extent to which existing eating disorder diagnostic frameworks and criteria adequately capture the full spectrum of symptoms in boys and men. Relatedly, it is important to understand how behaviors or other symptoms may present uniquely in boys and men (e.g., perception of loss of control over eating, muscularity-oriented concerns). For avoidant/restrictive food intake disorder in particular, given the novelty of the diagnosis and evidence that boys and men may be overrepresented compared to other restrictive eating disorders (e.g., anorexia nervosa), there is a need for more research in boys and men. Further, it is important for more research to investigate the factors that contribute to under-recognition of symptoms and barriers to eating disorder treatment for boys and men and, particularly, strategies for overcoming these difficulties. With regard to measurement, there is a general need for ongoing research to address the degree to which existing assessments of eating disorder symptoms and related constructs (e.g., body image), particularly those originally developed and tested with female-centric conceptualizations and samples, are reliable and valid in samples of boys and men. Finally, additional empirical work is needed to understand how muscle dysmorphia is best conceptualized in relation to eating disorder psychopathology in boys and men, as well as the extent to which symptoms may overlap concurrently or show a pattern diagnostic shifting over time.

Medical

The chapters of the medical section identified several important gaps to be addressed by future research. For example, the nature and extent of medical complications of specific eating disorder diagnoses in boys and men, particularly atypical anorexia nervosa and avoidant/restrictive food intake disorder, should be examined. Additionally, short- and long-term medical consequences of muscularity-oriented disordered eating behaviors and use of appearance- and performance-enhancing substances need to be investigated. Future research in clinical samples is particularly essential to inform medical standards and guidelines for eating disorders in boys and men focused on monitoring bone health, testosterone testing, determining goal weights in treatment, and protocols for refeeding. In particular, randomized controlled trials would have substantial utility in establishing appropriate refeeding guidelines as well as micronutrient and macronutrient needs for boys and men with eating disorders. Finally, there is a need for the development of evidence-based strategies to address maladaptive patterns of appearance- and performance-enhancing substance use in boys and men, particularly within adolescent and young adult populations.

Prevention and Treatment

There are several areas of future research needed in the area of eating disorder prevention and treatment among boys and men. Regarding prevention, most research has examined the impact of programs with regard to reducing risk factors for eating disorder and muscle dysmorphia psychopathology. Few research studies have included adequate assessments and the required duration of follow-up necessary for determining whether existing programs can actually *prevent* eating disorder onset. Future randomized controlled trials with at least 1 year of follow-up are necessary to help move this area of the literature forward. Regarding treatment, there remain no empirically supported treatments developed specifically to address unique issues for boys and men with eating disorders. While initial data suggests that outcomes using existing treatments for men tend to be comparable to women, this research has been plagued by low sample sizes (e.g., $n < 40$ men in most studies). Future research aggregating larger samples of boys and men with eating disorders will be critical to help determine what differences, if any, exist in treatment and longer-term outcomes. This information can then be used to adapt or develop new treatments to increase efficacy and effectiveness for boys and men.

Specific Populations and Sociocultural Considerations

Eating disorders can affect cisgender and transgender boys and men of all race/ethnicities, cultures, nationalities, sexual orientations, and body sizes. Given the limited state of the general literature on boys and men with eating disorders, there is a crucial need for more research on unique sociocultural factors related to eating disorders in boys and men, as well as studies on how eating disorder psychopathology may differ (e.g., prevalence, symptom presentation, treatment) among boys and men with diverse identities. Specifically, further research is needed in racial/ethnic minorities and in populations from around the globe where eating disorders may be particularly under-recognized. Ongoing investigations focusing on samples of sexual minority men and individuals identifying as transgender and gender non-binary are also needed, particularly in the realm of intervention research. Further understanding the intersection between athleticism and eating disorders in boys and men is also an important area of future empirical work. Additionally, given the ubiquity of social media use, particularly in adolescent boys who may be particularly vulnerable to eating disorder psychopathology, continued research examining how engagement with social media may impact eating disorder and muscle dysmorphia symptoms in boys and men is warranted. Finally, developmental considerations for men will be critical to better understand how eating disorder psychopathology may differ in boys and men across the lifespan so that interventions can be appropriately tailored.

Final Thoughts

The field of eating disorders is constantly evolving, and a major element of that evolution is a much-needed growth in an understanding of diversity in *how* eating disorder symptoms can present and *who* is affected by these serious conditions. Boys and men have historically been under-recognized in the field, and there are ongoing consequences of the predominantly female-centric origins of the theoretical and empirical literature on eating disorders. Although there has been progress in recognition, there is much work that still needs to be done at multiple levels to combat the perception that eating disorders are solely a "female issue," reduce under-recognition of symptoms by both patients and providers, overcome barriers to treatment-seeking and access, understand how varying identities and their intersectionality may relate to eating disorder risk, and establish appropriate treatment guidelines and standards for the medical, nutritional, behavioral, and psychosocial symptoms and complications of eating disorders in boys and men.

Disclaimer The opinions and assertions expressed herein are those of the authors and do not necessarily reflect the official policy or position of the Uniformed Services University or the Department of Defense.

Reference

1. Academy for Eating Disorders. Nine more truths about eating disorders: boys and men. 2020. https://www.aedweb.org/resources/online-library/publications. Accessed 8 Feb 2021.

Index

A
AAS-withdrawal hypogonadism, 154
Adolescence, 322, 324
Anabolic-androgenic steroids (AASs), 150–152, 154, 155, 161
clinical considerations, 158, 159
eating disorders, 156
muscle dysmorphia, 156, 157
Anorexia nervosa (AN), 39, 58, 105, 120, 123, 142, 199
Antiretroviral therapy (ART), 184
Appearance and performance enhancing drugs (APEDs), 23, 25, 178
Appearance and performance enhancing substances (APESs), 150
Asian American, 218, 220
Athletes, 285, 286
Athletes Training and Learning to Avoid Steroids (ATLAS), 178
Atypical anorexia nervosa, 143
Avoidant and restrictive food intake disorder (ARFID), 56, 68
assessment, 73–76
course and outcomes
course of illness, 72, 73
medical sequelae and comorbidity, 71, 72
psychiatric comorbidity, 72
epidemiology, 68–69
symptoms and presentation, 69–71
treatment, 76–79

B
Binge eating disorder, 39, 40, 59, 62, 63
Binge Eating Scale, 90, 91
Body Appreciation Scale-2 (BAS-2), 246
Body Avoidance and Checking Scale (BBACS), 246
Body dissatisfaction, 240–244, 322, 323
Body Dysmorphic Disorder Modification of the Yale Brown Obsessive-Compulsive Scale (BDD-YBOCS), 106, 107
Body fat dissatisfaction, 10, 12, 14, 15
Body image, 7
gender role endorsement, 13, 14
integrated model and future research, 14–16
mediating variables, social influences, 12
meta-analysis, 8
objectification theory, 12, 13
research on, 8
tripartite influence model, 9
gay community, 11
media influence, 9, 10
mediating variables, social influences, 12
parent influence, 11
partner influence, 11
peer influence, 10, 11
social influences, 9
Body image across, 318, 323–326, 328, 329

J. M. Nagata et al. (eds.), *Eating Disorders in Boys and Men*,
https://doi.org/10.1007/978-3-030-67127-3

Body Image Assessment Questionnaires
binge eating scale, 90, 91
boys/men
assessment burden, 95
options, 95–97
well-established clinical norms/ cut-offs, 94
Compulsive Exercise Test, 93
developed specifically for or conceptually inclusive of boys, 88
Drive for Leanness Scale, 93
Drive for Muscularity Scale, 93
Eating Disorder Examination-Questionnaire, 90
Eating Disorder Inventory, 90
Eating for Muscularity Scale, 92
Eating Pathology Symptoms Inventory, 91
Exercise Dependence Scale, 94
Loss of Control Over Eating Scale, 91
Male Body Attitudes Scale, 92
Male Body Checking Questionnaire, 93
measurement properties and psychometrics, 85
implications for, 86, 87
measurement invariance, 86
reliability, 85
validity, 86
muscularity-oriented eating test, 92
Obligatory Exercise Questionnaire, 94
traditional eating disorder symptoms, 88–89
Body Mass Index (BMI), 130, 131
Bodybuilding, 13
Bone density, 123
Bone health, 130
Bone mineral density (BMD), 130
Bulimia nervosa
diagnoses, 58
nutritional management, 144

C
Calcium, 142
Cardiovascular consequences, 120, 122
Cardiovascular toxicity, 153
Cheat meals, 26, 63
Children's Eating Attitudes Test (ChEAT), 239
Clenbuterol, 151
Cognitive behavioral therapy, 78, 206
Cognitive behavioral therapy for body image and self-care (CBT-BISC), 261
Cognitive-Behavior Therapy for Avoidant/ Restrictive Food Intake Disorder (CBT-AR), 78
Cognitive restructuring techniques, 30
Co-morbidity, 46
Compensatory behaviors, 62
Compulsive Exercise Test, 93, 284, 286, 288, 293, 294
Conceptual model, 15
Confirmatory factor analysis (CFA), 239
Countertransference, 208
Creatine, 25

D
Diagnostic and Statistical Manual of Mental Disorders, Fifth Edition (DSM-5), 56
Dialectical behavior therapy (DBT), 206, 260
Diet, 106
Disordered eating, 92, 93, 285, 286, 289
Drive for Leanness Scale (DLS), 93
Drive for Muscularity Scale (DMS), 28, 93, 107, 108
Dual-energy X-ray absorptiometry (DXA) scans, 130, 142

E
Eating disorder, 68
anorexia nervosa, 58
binge-eating disorder, 59, 62, 63
body image concerns and fear of weight gain, 61, 62
bulimia nervosa, 58
compensatory behaviors, 62
diagnostic considerations, 60, 61
other specified feeding or eating disorder, 59, 60
shame and psychosocial impairment, 63, 64
Eating Disorder Examination-Questionnaire (EDE-Q), 27, 90
Eating Disorder Inventory (EDI), 90
Eating Disorder in Youth Questionnaire (EDY-Q), 75
Eating disorder not otherwise specified (EDNOS), 39, 235
Eating disorders, 335
american boys and men
body image assessment, 239, 245
cross-cultural studies, 237
features, 237, 238
prevalence, 230–236
risk factors, 236
sociocultural influences, 246
assessment, 337
boys, preadolescence, 322–324
diagnosis, 336, 337

anorexia nervosa, 58
binge-eating disorder, 59, 62, 63
body image concerns and fear of weight gain, 61, 62
bulimia nervosa, 58
compensatory behaviors, 62
diagnostic considerations, 60, 61
other specified feeding or eating disorder, 59, 60
shame and psychosocial impairment, 63, 64
diagnostic assessment, 274
epidemiology, 269, 270
gender affirming healthcare, 272, 273
gender diversity, social context, 268, 269
health inqueities, 270
implications, 276, 277
intersectionality, 269
medical, 337
men, midlife, 326–328
nine truths, 336
perspectives, 336
protective factors, 271, 272
risk, 270, 271
screening, 273
sociocultural considerations, 338
specific populations, 338
treatment, 274–276, 337
Eating disorders (EDs), 3
accounts and findings, 5
bisexual men, 184
boys, 170, 171
cognitive dissonance-based program, 178, 183
dissonance-based content prevention, 183, 184
epidemiological data, 5
epidemiological surveillance, 5
history of, 4
in-person cognitive-behavioral programs, 179–182
internet-based programs targeting both weight, 190
presentations, 4
programs targeting weight, 190
school-based prevention programs
boys, 172–176
elementary and middle school, 171, 177
high school, 177, 178
school-based programs targeting weight, 186–189
screening programs, 185, 186
Eating for Muscularity Scale (EMS), 28, 92, 107, 108
Eating Pathology Symptoms Inventory (EPSI), 28, 91
Electrolyte abnormalities, 122
Electrolyte derangements, 142
Energy, for eating disorders, 138–140
Epidemiology, 38
co-morbidity, 46
impairment/burden
disordered eating symptoms, 45
disorders, 45
prevalence, 38
anorexia nervosa, 39
binge eating disorder, 39, 40
bulimia nervosa, 39
disordered eating symptoms, 41, 42
muscle dysmorphia, 40, 41
otherwise specified feeding/eating disorders and unspecified feeding/eating disorder, 40
socio-demographic distribution, 42
age, 42
ethnicity, 43
gender identity, 44
SES, 43
sexual orientation, 44
treatment-seeking, 46, 47
Equivalence, 86
Ethnicity, 43, 218–224
Exercise, 104, 106
assessing exercise, 292, 293
athletes, 285, 286
athlete-specific eating disorder prevention, 295, 296
biopsychosocial model, 290
body image, boys and men, 294, 295
clinical samples, 285
conceptualizations, 287
eating disorder treatment, 298
eating disorders, 284
implications, boys and men, 299
maintenance model, 288
non-treatment seeking samples, 284
objectification theory, 289, 290
relative energy deficiency in sports, 291
sociocultural model, 290
treatment recommendations, boys and men, 297
Exercise Addiction Inventory (EAI), 293
Exercise Dependence Scale (EDS-21), 94

F

Fitspiration, 312–314
Food Avoidance Emotional Disorder (FAED), 75

G

Gastrointestinal medical complications, 124
Gay communities, 11
Gender affirmation, 271, 272
Gender identity, socio-demographic distribution, 44
Gender role endorsement, 13–15
Growth and body composition, 123
Gull, Sir William, 5

H

Hematological medical complications, 124
Hypophosphatemia, 140, 142
Hypothalamic suppression, 133

I

Impairment/burden
  disordered eating symptoms, 45
  disorders, 45
Inappropriate compensatory behaviors, 58
Indexing muscularity, 27–29
Integrated model body image, 14–16
Internalization of muscular ideal, 9, 10

L

Landmark Minnesota Starvation Experiment, 138
Lasegue, Ernest-Charles, 5
Latin America, 230
Latino, 218, 221, 223, 224
Liver medical complications, 124
Loss of Control Over Eating Scale (LOCES), 91

M

Macronutrients, 141, 142
Male Body Attitudes Scale (MBAS), 92, 245
Male Body Checking Questionnaire (MBCQ), 93
Masculinity, 13, 14
Measurement invariance, 86
Media influence, body image, 9, 10
Medical complications of eating disorders
  bone density, 123
  boys and men, 121
  cardiovascular consequences, 120, 122
  electrolyte abnormalities, 122
  gastrointestinal and liver, 124
  growth and body composition, 123
  hematological, 124
  mortality, 120
  neurological, 124
  Refeeding syndrome, 122
Medical management of eating disorders, 128, 129
  Body Mass Index, 130, 131
  determining treatment goal weight, 131
  monitoring bone health, 130
  muscle dysmorphia and performance-enhancing substances, 133, 134
  refeeding protocols, 132
  testosterone testing, 132, 133
Micronutrients, 142, 143
Minority stress theory, 256
Mortality, 120
Morton, Richard, 5
Muscle Appearance Satisfaction Scale (MASS), 106, 107, 239
Muscle dysmorphia (MD), 30, 40, 41, 104, 150, 156, 240–244
  assessment of, 106–108
  classification, 105, 106
  comorbidity of, 105
  medical management, 133, 134
  prevalence of, 104
  prevention/treatment, 110
  proposed etiology of, 108–110
  research, 107, 112
  risk factors and etiology, 111
Muscle Dysmorphia Inventory (MDI), 106, 107
Muscle Dysmorphic Disorder Inventory (MDDI), 107
Muscle-seeking behaviors, 25
Muscular body ideal, 23
Muscularity dissatisfaction, 10, 12, 14
Muscularity-oriented disordered eating, 14, 22, 24–27, 133
  complicating issue, 31
  crucial qualitative differences, 22
  empirically assessing and indexing muscularity concerns and related eating pathology, 27–29
  medical considerations, 22, 23
  muscular body ideal, 23, 24
  research, 29, 30
Muscularity-Oriented Eating Test (MOET), 28, 92, 107, 108

N

Native American, 218, 221
Neurological medical complications, 124
Nine Item ARFID Scale (NIAS), 75

Nutritional and dietary supplements, 152
Nutritional management
  atypical anorexia nervosa, 143
  bulimia nervosa, 144
  diagnoses, considerations for, 143
  energy considerations, 138–140
  guideline, absence of, 138
  macronutrients, 141, 142
  micronutrients, 142, 143
  refeeding syndrome, 140, 141

O
Objectification theory, 12, 13, 15, 256
Obligatory Exercise Questionnaire (OEQ), 94, 292
Osteopenia, 123
Osteoporosis, 123, 142
Other specified feeding or eating disorders (OSFED), 40, 56, 59, 60

P
Parent influence, 11
Partner influence, 11
Peer influence, 11
Performance-enhancing substances (PES), 133, 134
Personality variables, 15
Physical activity, 285, 289
Picky eating, 74
Poor appetite, 69
Preadolescence
  boys
    disordered eating, 323, 324
    dissatisfaction, 322, 324, 325
    eating disorders, 325
  midlife
    body dissatisfaction, 326
    disordered eating, 327
    eating disorders, 328
Prevalence, 38
  anorexia nervosa, 39
  binge eating disorder, 39, 40
  bulimia nervosa, 39
  disordered eating symptoms, 41, 42
  men, 258
  minority stress theory, 256
  muscle dysmorphia, 40, 41
  objectification theory, 256
  otherwise specified feeding/eating disorders and unspecified feeding/eating disorder, 40
  in sexual minority men, 254, 257
  treatments, 259–261
  tripartite influence model, 255
Prohormones, 151, 161
Protein consumption, 141
Protein supplements, 161
Psychiatric effects, 153
Psychodynamic psychotherapy, 206–207
Psychopathology, 42
Psychosocial impairment, 74
Psychotherapy
  age of onset, 200
  cognitive behavioral therapy, 206
  co-morbidity, 200
  dialectical behavior therapy, 206
  eating behaviors, 199
  exercise, 199
  gender socialization, 202
  identity and personal meaning, 201, 202
  implications, 209
  interpersonal psychotherapy, 206
  men, 198, 204, 205
  motivation, 201
  psychodynamic, 207
  seeking help, 201
  sexual orientation, 200
  stigma and barriers to treatment, 201
  techniques, 207, 208
  traits and temperament, 200
  treatment, 203, 204

R
Race
  culture-specific variables, 222, 223
  eating disorder symptoms
    asian american men, 220
    black men, 219, 220
    latino men, 221
    native american, 221, 222
  implicit bias, 218
  prevalence rates, 219
  prevention, 223, 224
  treatment, 223, 224
Refeeding syndrome, 139
  medical complications, 122
  nutritional management, 140, 141
Relative Energy Deficiency in Sport (RED-S), 23, 291
Reliability, 85
Resilience, 272

S
Selective eating, 70, 72
Self-construction, 309
Selfies, 308, 311–313
Self-objectification, 12
Sexual orientation, 44
Shame and psychosocial impairment, 63, 64
Social comparison, 14
Social influences, 9
Social media, 26, 308–313
Social networking sites (SNS), 308–312
Sociocultural model, 271
Socio-demographic distribution, 42
  age, 42
  ethnicity, 43
  gender identity, 44
  SES, 43
  sexual orientation, 44
Socio-economic status (SES), 43
Sodium diet, 142
Sports supplement, 23
Stigmatization, 268, 276

T
Testosterone boosters, 152
Testosterone testing, 132, 133
Traditional ED behaviors, 24
Transgender and gender non-binary (T/GNB), 266, 268–277
Tripartite influence model, 9, 15, 255
  gay community, 11
  media influence, 9, 10
  mediating variables, social influences, 12
  parent influence, 11
  partner influence, 11
  peer influence, 10, 11
  social influences, 9

U
Unspecified feeding/eating disorder (UFED), 40

V
Validity
  Body Image Assessment Questionnaires, 86

Z
Z-score, 123

MIX
Papier aus verantwortungsvollen Quellen
Paper from responsible sources
FSC® C105338
FSC
www.fsc.org

If you have any concerns about our products,
you can contact us on
ProductSafety@springernature.com

In case Publisher is established outside the EU,
the EU authorized representative is:
Springer Nature Customer Service Center GmbH
Europaplatz 3, 69115 Heidelberg, Germany

Printed by Libri Plureos GmbH
in Hamburg, Germany